ASTROCYTE - PHYSIOLOGY AND PATHOLOGY

Edited by **Maria Teresa Gentile**
and **Luca Colucci D'Amato**

Astrocyte - Physiology and Pathology
http://dx.doi.org/10.5772/intechopen.69076
Edited by Maria Teresa Gentile and Luca Colucci D'Amato

Contributors
Hiroaki Miyajima, Katja Kanninen, Riikka Lampinen, Irina Belaya, Isabella Boccuni, Tarja Malm, Carlos Pérez-Monter, Aldo Torre-Delgadillo, Ramani Ramchandran, Emily Gronseth, Ling Wang, David Harder, Ilaria P Dal Pra, Anna Chiarini, Ubaldo Armato, Michael Lattke, Thomas Wirth, Pavel Montes De Oca Balderas, José Roberto González-Hernández, Michal Izrael, Michel Revel, Joseph Itskovitz-Eldor, Shalom Guy Slutsky, Ginger Withers, Christopher Wallace, Maria Teresa Gentile

Published by InTech
Janeza Trdine 9, 51000 Rijeka, Croatia

Publishing Process Manager Maja Bozicevic
Technical Editor SPi Global
Cover InTech Design team

First published March, 2018
Printed in Croatia
Legal deposit, Croatia: National and University Library in Zagreb

Additional hard copies can be obtained from orders@intechopen.com

Astrocyte - Physiology and Pathology, Edited by Maria Teresa Gentile and Luca Colucci D'Amato
p. cm.
Print ISBN 978-953-51-3885-3
Online ISBN 978-953-51-3886-0

For EU product safety concerns:
IN TECH d.o.o., Prolaz Marije Krucifikse Kozulić 3, 51000 Rijeka, Croatia,
info@intechopen.com or visit our website at intechopen.com.

Meet the editors

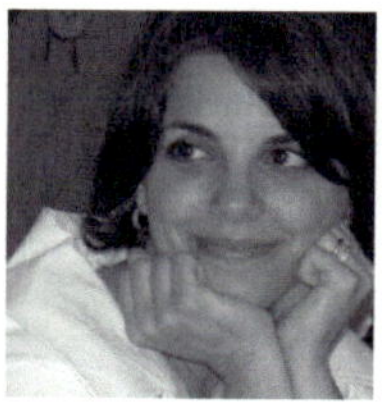

Dr. Maria Teresa Gentile obtained her master's degree in Molecular Biology from the University of Naples "Federico II" and PhD degree in Pharmacology from the Second University of Naples. She has worked on projects on cardiovascular risk factors of neurodegenerative disorders such as Alzheimer's disease and in particular on the molecular mechanisms underlying beta amyloid–induced endothelial dysfunction and its deposition in brain tissues in animal models of essential hypertension. At the moment, her interest is on the mechanisms that control cell proliferation in glioblastoma and melanoma, and possible new therapies obtained from natural compounds. She is performing her research program at the Laboratory of Molecular and Cellular Pathology of the University of Campania "Luigi Vanvitelli." She is the author of numerous scientific manuscripts and book chapters.

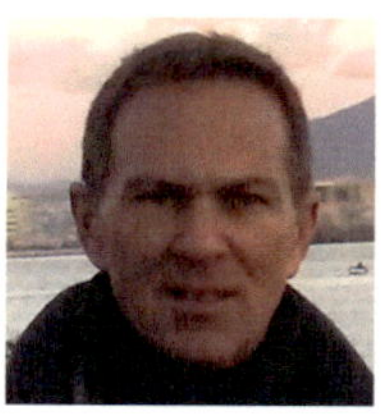

Luca Colucci D'Amato is an associate professor of General Pathology at the University of Campania "Luigi Vanvitelli," where he runs the Laboratory of Cellular and Molecular Pathology, after being a researcher at the National Research Council (CNR). He received his medical degree from the University of Naples "Federico II," where he, then,obtained a PhD degree in Molecular and Cellular Pathology. He also completed his residency in neurology at the same university. Soon after that, he devoted his efforts to biomedical molecular and cellular research, spending some research periods at the National Institutes of Health, Bethesda, MD, USA, the Bristol-Myers-Squibb Pharmaceutical Research Institute, Princeton, NJ, USA, and the Centre National de la Recherche Scientifique, Gif-sur-Yvette, France. His scientific interests focus on the molecular mechanisms underlying neural cell proliferation, differentiation, and survival under physiological and pathological conditions.

Contents

Preface

This book entitled "Astrocyte - Physiology and Pathology" is a review of the most updated studies about astrocytes. For decades, since their discovery in the late 1800s, astrocytes, together with the other glial cells, have been considered as a purely unfunctional glue for neurons. However, recent studies have demonstrated that astrocytes are active dynamic signaling players of the central nervous system (CNS). A team of authors from prestigious academic schools contributed to draw up a project, which is divided into three sections. The first section is introductory and describes the importance of astrocytes in the research of CNS diseases. The second section gives a detailed account of astrocyte's morphology and physiology, examining thoroughly all the astrocyte's types; giving an accurate description of their morphology, location, and function in the brain; and illustrating their physiology in terms of dealing with neurons through "gliotransmitters," ionic channels, and membrane "receptors expression. The third section of the book focuses on the role of astrocytes in neurodegenerative disorders such as Alzheimer's disease (AD) and amyotrophic lateral sclerosis (ALS), in particular on the molecular mechanisms behind the degeneration of motor neurons typical of ALS with attention to the intracellular signaling pathways activated and/or inhibited, and on the molecular events behind AD onset such as the role of astrocyte in Abeta toxicity and Tau phosphorylation or the role of astrocyte's mitochondria function and quality control with a look at the potential future therapeutic approach to modulate these events. Moreover, a deep insight into the molecular mechanisms and intracellular signaling pathways that are behind the role of astrocytes in tumor growth and progression has been reported with a look at brain tumors of both astrocytic and metastatic origins. Studies about astrocyte's interaction with the cells of the brain tissue, such as endothelial cells of blood-brain barrier, pericytes, and other cells of the perivascular niche, neurons, and all the intracellular signaling pathways stimulated or inhibited in order to facilitate tumor growth and progression, are thoroughly described. Furthermore, the most recent literature about therapeutic challenges that scientists are dealing with in order to prevent and/or curb brain tumor growth and progression is posted. Last but not least, two chapters focus on the important role of astrocytes in brain damage due to peripheral pathologic conditions such as liver disease or the genetic disease aceruloplasminemia. Altogether, these essays give an overview of the crucial role of astrocytes in the physiology of the CNS and in the pathogenesis of several CNS disorders suggesting that the shift from a neurocentric view to one that incorporates astrocytes in disease models for drug discovery is a critical step in renewing drug development strategies to treat neurodegenerative diseases.

Maria Teresa Gentile, PhD and Luca Colucci D'Amato, MD, PhD
Laboratory of Molecular and Cellular Pathology
Department of Environmental, Biological and Pharmaceutical Sciences and Technologies
University of Campania "Luigi Vanvitelli," Caserta, Italy

Section 1

Introduction

Chapter 1

Introductory Chapter: The Importance of Astrocytes in the Research of CNS Diseases

Maria Teresa Gentile and Luca Colucci D'Amato

Additional information is available at the end of the chapter

http://dx.doi.org/10.5772/intechopen.74710

1. Introduction

Glial cells were identified for the first time in the nineteenth century when the French physician René Dutrochet described for the first time, in 1824, small globules among the large ones within the mollusk nervous system. However, we have to wait until 1856 when the German pathologist Rudolph Virchow coined the term "nervekitt," nerve glue, to describe that sort of connective tissue of the central nervous system. Subsequently, Santiago Ramon y Cajal, Pio del Rio Hortega, and Otto Deiters pioneered this field with their experiments and gave them the name "glia" derived from the ancient Greek word that means glue. At that time, glia was considered as purely unfunctional glue for neurons [1]. However, research since the mid-1990 has shown that glia might play a particularly important role in the cognitive function as indicated by the correlation between the glia/neuron ratio in brain tissue and the state of evolution of species [2]. In fact, *C. elegans* possesses only 52 glial cells versus 302 neurons with a glia-to-neuron ratio of 0.18 [3], whereas the whole human-adult brain has a one-to-one ratio [4] and with a ratio of 1.4 in the cerebral cortex [5]. Moreover, comparison of glia-to-neuron ratio in different human cortical areas with that of macaques displayed a significant augmentation of the ratio in humans [6]. In the CNS, glia includes astrocytes, oligodendrocytes, microglia, and their progenitors NG2 glia and decades of studies demonstrated that they have a specific role in brain tissue homeostasis. In particular, astrocytes, whose name derived from Greek and means "star-like cell," are active dynamic signaling players of the central nervous system. They are key regulators of synaptic activity and plasticity, neural network, and cognitive functions controlling extracellular ion balance and neurotransmitter homeostasis. They perform many functions, including biochemical support of endothelial cells that form the blood-brain barrier, provision of nutrients to the nervous tissue, and regulation of neurogenesis and brain wiring [7]. Dysfunction of astrocytes can thereby induce major alterations in neuronal functions, contributing to the pathogenesis of several brain disorders. Astrocytes participate to a variety of essential physiological processes in the healthy brain such as the formation and maturation of the synapses, receptor trafficking, control of the homeostasis of ions and energy metabolites, and clearance of neurotransmitters. Astrocytes also regulate the extracellular space volume and modulate the synaptic plasticity [8, 9]. Dynamic bidirectional signaling between neurons and astrocytes has been extensively demonstrated in experimental animal models. However, recently Navarrete et al. [10] demonstrated that astrocyte from human brain tissue exhibit Ca^{2+}-induced excitability and can respond to neurotransmitters released by synapses. Moreover, morphological, genomic, and functional studies revealed that human astrocytes display specific characteristics compared to the rodent counterparts. In particular, human astrocytes express more proteins involved in calcium signaling and propagate calcium waves at a higher speed compared to murine astrocytes [11]. These observations lead to the idea that human astrocytes play an important role in the molding of the higher cognitive functions and that they give a significant contribution to cerebral pathology. As a matter of fact, transplantation of human astrocytes into mouse brain leads to an improvement of higher cognitive functions, such as long-term potentiation (LTP) and learning, pointing toward the importance of human astrocytes in the cognitive abilities of human brains [2].

Indeed, even if several neuropathologists, such as Alzheimer, Nissl, and Fromman, speculate a glial role in neurodegenerative disorders, until the mid-1990s, the neurocentric paradigm dominated. Nevertheless, growing evidences indicate that astroglial dysfunction contributes to the pathogenesis of several neurological and psychiatric disorders [12]. A common feature of several neurological diseases is reactive astrogliosis.

2. Reactive astrogliosis

Reactive astrogliosis is a spectrum of changes in astrocytes that occur in response of all forms of CNS injury and disease. In summary, injured tissues display upregulation of structural proteins, such as glial fibrillary acidic protein (GFAP) and vimentin, and hypertrophy of astrocytes' cell body and processes that elongate around the lesion core and release a cascade of inflammatory signals that can strongly affect the pathological outcome [13]. Moreover, some quiescent astrocytes re-enter the cell cycle [14]. However, these hallmarks can vary according to the severity of the disease and are regulated by inter- and intracellular signaling molecules in a context-specific manner [15]. In particular, in mild or moderate astrogliosis, which generally occurs far from CNS focal lesions, astrocytic proliferation is almost absent and the increased GFAP expression together with cell body and process hypertrophy, which is not altering astrocyte organization into individual distinct domains, are variable [16]. Moreover, moderate astrogliosis also results in the expression of copper-zinc superoxide dismutase, glutathione peroxidase or metallothionein, inducible nitric oxide synthase, and release of trophic factors and cytokines, including tumor necrosis factor and interleukins and interferons [17]. Furthermore, in mild or moderate forms, if the initial triggering insult is removed, reactive astrogliosis can revert and cells return to a condition similar to that observed in healthy tissue [15]. On the other hand, near focal lesions, severe diffuse astrogliosis is characterized by significantly increased astrocytic proliferation. The molecular factors that induce astrocytes' proliferation are not completely characterized, but several studies ascribe an important role to epidermal growth factor, fibroblast growth factor, endothelin 1, ATP, lipopolysaccharide, and nitric oxide [18–21]. Astrocytic proliferation causes overlapping of neighboring astrocytic processes with the disruption of the individual astrocyte domains and the consequent formation of a compact glial scar. Such scar, which represents the hallmark of reactive astrogliosis, is due to astrocyte interaction with different cell types of the brain tissue and is characterized by phenomena of necrosis, tumors, chronic neurodegeneration, infection, or inflammatory infiltration [15, 21]. These structural changes are not reversible and persist also after the resolution of the triggering insult [15]. More important, mature glial scars act as barriers to inflammatory cells to protect surrounding healthy tissue from nearby areas of intense inflammation. Reactive astrocytes can also protect CNS cells and tissue by up-taking excitotoxic glutamate, producing glutathione against oxidative stress, degrading amyloid-beta peptides, regulating extracellular space volume and ion balance, facilitating blood-brain barrier repair, and regulating CNS inflammation. Nevertheless, growing evidence also shows that reactive astrocytes can contribute to or be the primary source of CNS physiopathology. Reactive astrocytes from glial scars can indeed synthesize collagen and sulfate proteoglycans, which prevent axon regeneration [17].

3. Astrocytes: new tools for neurological disease research

Traditionally, astrocytes have been studied as a homogeneous group of cells, even if the peculiar morphology of mature mammalian astrocytes was observed since 1865 thanks to the studies on mouse brain by Otto Deiters [22]. A detailed morphological study of glial cells came from Camillo Golgi and Ramon y Cajal in 1872 who, independently, by means of the black staining reaction, observed two different types of astrocytes: the protoplasmic and the fibrous astrocytes. However, for a long time, astrocytes received little or no consideration as target for neurological studies because the neurocentric paradigm dominated. New and recent findings demonstrated that astrocytes are positioned to promote both the regeneration of the damaged neurons and to protect existing neurons from degeneration. For this reason, astrocytes represent an important focus in the development of new therapeutic tools for neurodegenerative disorder that have been historically viewed as purely neuronal in their pathology. Within the past 5 years, important progress has been made deriving astrocytes from induced pluripotent stem cells (IPSC). Researchers are now able to generate patients-specific astrocytes that recapitulate the patients' genetic background. Once healthy astrocytes have been obtained and characterized, they can be used to replace dying astrocytes or to promote the survival of existing neurons. This kind of application has not yet been tested in humans; however, there is a growing body of *in vitro* and *in vivo* evidence that indicates that these therapies would be beneficial for many neuronal diseases [23]. Indeed, in an amyotrophic lateral sclerosis (ALS) mouse model, researchers have shown that the direct transplantation of human (h)iPSC-derived neural progenitor cells prolonged the lifespan of the animal [24]. In these experiments, NPCs differentiated into astrocytes and exhibited an upregulation of vascular endothelial growth factor (VEGF), which induces the activation of the AKT-dependent intracellular signaling, which has previously been shown to be important for cell survival and proliferation in ALS [25]. The authors also hypothesized that the introduction of progenitor-derived astrocytes with normal expression of glucose transporters could restore glucose homeostasis in this model [26]. Moreover, these versatile human astrocytes could be used alone or in co-culture with neurons in both target-based and phenotypic high-throughput drug-screening research studies, promoting the discovery of novel therapeutics tools useful in the treatment of neurodegenerative disorders. For decades, therapeutic development for neurodegenerative disorders has focused only on diseased neurons. Due to the crucial role of astrocytes in physiology of the central nervous system and in the pathogenesis of several neurodegenerative diseases, it is not surprising that the traditional drug development strategy which follows the neurocentric paradigm has not produced effective therapies. Developing new drugs that complement and combine therapies which target both neuronal and astrocytic degeneration could provide a new direction to increase the success of therapeutic development for neurodegenerative diseases in the future. The shift from a neurocentric view to one that incorporates astrocytes in disease models for drug discovery is a critical step in renewing drug development strategies to treat neurodegenerative diseases.

Author details

Maria Teresa Gentile* and Luca Colucci D'Amato

*Address all correspondence to: matergen@yahoo.it

Department of Environmental, Biological and Pharmaceutical Sciences and Technologies, University of Campania "Luigi Vanvitelli", Caserta, Italy

References

[1] Kettenmann H, Ransom BR. The Concept of Neuroglia: A Historical Perspective. In *Neuroglia*. Oxford University Press; 2013. DOI: http://dx.doi.org/10.1093/acprof:oso/9780195152227.003.0001

[2] Han X, Chen M, Wang F, Windrem M, Wang S, Shanz S, Xu Q, Oberheim NA, Bekar L, Betstadt S, Silva AJ, Takano T, Goldman SA, Nedergaard M. Forebrain engraftment by human glial progenitor cells enhances synaptic plasticity and learning in adult mice. Cell Stem Cell. 2013;**12**(3):342-353

[3] Oikonomou G, Shaham S. The glia of *Caenorhabditis elegans*. Glia. 2011;**59**(9):1253-1263

[4] Azevedo FA, Carvalho LR, Grinberg LT, Farfel JM, Ferretti RE, Leite RE, Jacob Filho W, Lent R, Herculano-Houzel S. Equal numbers of neuronal and nonneuronal cells make the human brain an isometrically scaled-up primate brain. The Journal of Comparative Neurology. 2009;**513**(5):532-541

[5] Pelvig DP, Pakkenberg H, Stark AK, Pakkenberg B. Neocortical glial cell numbers in human brains. Neurobiology of Aging. 2008;**29**(11):1754-1762

[6] Sherwood CC, Stimpson CD, Raghanti MA, Wildman DE, Uddin M, Grossman LI, Goodman M, Redmond JC, Bonar CJ, Erwin JM, Hof PR. Evolution of increased glia-neuron ratios in the human frontal cortex. Proceedings of the National Academy of Sciences of the United States of America. 2006;**103**(37):13606-13611

[7] Vasile F, Dossi E, Rouach N. Human astrocytes: Structure and functions in the healthy brain. Brain Structure & Function. 2017;**222**(5):2017-2029

[8] Araque A, Carmignoto G, Haydon PG, Oliet SH, Robitaille R, Volterra A. Gliotransmitters travel in time and space. Neuron. 2014;**81**(4):728-739

[9] Dallérac G, Rouach N. Astrocytes as new targets to improve cognitive functions. Progress in Neurobiology. 2016;**144**:48-67

[10] Navarrete M, Perea G, Maglio L, Pastor J, García de Sola R, Araque A. Astrocyte calcium signal and gliotransmission in human brain tissue. Cerebral Cortex. 2013;**23**(5):1240-1246

[11] Bazargani N, Attwell D. Astrocyte calcium signaling: The third wave. Nature Neuroscience. 2016;**19**(2):182-189

[12] Dossi E, Vasile F, Rouach N. Human astrocytes in the diseased brain. Brain Research Bulletin. 2018;**136**:139-156

[13] Sofroniew MV. Astrocyte barriers to neurotoxic inflammation. Nature Reviews. Neuroscience. 2015;**16**(5):249-263

[14] Buffo A, Vosko MR, Ertürk D, Hamann GF, Jucker M, Rowitch D, Götz M. Expression pattern of the transcription factor Olig2 in response to brain injuries: Implications for neuronal repair. Proceedings of the National Academy of Sciences of the United States of America. 2005;**102**(50):18183-18188

[15] Sofroniew MV. Molecular dissection of reactive astrogliosis and glial scar formation. Trends in Neurosciences. 2009;**32**(12):638-647

[16] Wilhelmsson U, Bushong EA, Price DL, Smarr BL, Phung V, Terada M, Ellisman MH, Pekny M. Redefining the concept of reactive astrocytes as cells that remain within their unique domains upon reaction to injury. Proceedings of the National Academy of Sciences of the United States of America. 2006;**103**(46):17513-17518

[17] Chen Y, Swanson RA. The glutamate transporters EAAT2 and EAAT3 mediate cysteine uptake in cortical neuron cultures. Journal of Neurochemistry. 2003;**84**(6):1332-1339

[18] Gadea A, Schinelli S, Gallo V. Endothelin-1 regulates astrocyte proliferation and reactive gliosis via a JNK/c-Jun signaling pathway. The Journal of Neuroscience. 2008;**28**(10): 2394-2408

[19] Levison SW, Jiang FJ, Stoltzfus OK, Ducceschi MH. IL-6-type cytokines enhance epidermal growth factor-stimulated astrocyte proliferation. Glia. 2000;**32**(3):328-337

[20] Neary JT, Zimmermann H. Trophic functions of nucleotides in the central nervous system. Trends in Neurosciences. 2009;**32**(4):189-198

[21] Sofroniew MV, Vinters HV. Astrocytes: Biology and pathology. Acta Neuropathologica. 2010;**119**(1):7-35

[22] Deiters VS, Guillery RW. Otto Friedrich Karl Deiters (1834-1863). The Journal of Comparative Neurology. 2013;**521**(9):1929-1953

[23] Gorshkov K, Aguisanda F, Thorne N, Zheng W. Astrocytes as targets for drug discovery. Drug Discovery Today. 2018. pii: S1359-6446(17)30472-5

[24] Kondo T, Funayama M, Tsukita K, Hotta A, Yasuda A, Nori S, Kaneko S, Nakamura M, Takahashi R, Okano H, Yamanaka S, Inoue H. Focal transplantation of human iPSC-derived glial-rich neural progenitors improves lifespan of ALS mice. Stem Cell Reports. 2014;**3**(2):242-249

[25] Lunn JS, Sakowski SA, Kim B, Rosenberg AA, Feldman EL. Vascular endothelial growth factor prevents G93A-SOD1-induced motor neuron degeneration. Developmental Neurobiology. 2009;**69**(13):871-884

[26] Hall CE, Yao Z, Choi M, Tyzack GE, Serio A, Luisier R, Harley J, Preza E, Arber C, Crisp SJ, Watson PMD, Kullmann DM, Abramov AY, Wray S, Burley R, Loh SHY, Martins LM, Stevens MM, Luscombe NM, Sibley CR, Lakatos A, Ule J, Gandhi S, Patani R. Progressive motor neuron pathology and the role of astrocytes in a human stem cell model of VCP-related ALS. Cell Reports. 2017;**19**(9):1739-1749

Section 2

Astrocytes: A Molecular Point of View

Chapter 2

Signaling Pathways Regulating the Pathophysiological Responses of Astrocytes: A Focus on the IKK/NF-κB System

Michael Lattke and Thomas Wirth

Additional information is available at the end of the chapter

http://dx.doi.org/10.5772/intechopen.72283

Abstract

Astrocytes are highly responsive to changes in their microenvironment, and undergo prominent functional alterations in pathological conditions, a process called astrogliosis. In such conditions, astrocytes can gain immune cell-like functions, form glial scars and promote brain repair and regeneration. However, astrogliosis can also contribute to disease pathogenesis by exacerbating inflammation and perturbing the normal physiological functions of astrocytes. The IKK/NF-κB signaling system is a master regulator of inflammation, cell survival and differentiation, which also controls astrocyte functions, in particular their responses to pathological conditions. Activation of IKK/NF-κB signaling in astrocytes is a key driver of neuroinflammation and astrogliosis, which can interfere with normal brain development and homeostasis and can aggravate various central nervous system (CNS) pathologies. Besides IKK/NF-κB signaling, several other signaling pathways regulate pathophysiological responses of astrocytes, in particular hypertrophy, proliferation and the reactivation of neural stem cell-like properties of astrocytes. Further dissection of the role of these signaling pathways in the control of physiological functions and pathophysiological plasticity of astrocytes will reveal new insights into the pathogenesis of neurological diseases and might indicate new neuroprotective and regenerative therapeutic approaches.

Keywords: NF-kappa B, astrocytes, neuroinflammation, astrogliosis, neurodegeneration, brain development, brain homeostasis, signal transduction

1. Introduction

Astroglial cells, which comprise one of the major cell populations in the central nervous system (CNS), show a remarkable morphological and functional diversity and they are highly important for brain development and homeostasis. For example, prototypical parenchymal astrocytes regulate the local cerebral blood flow and the transport of metabolites through the blood-brain-barrier (BBB) according to local demand [1]. These metabolites are then converted by astrocytes to metabolites required by neurons and other cells in the brain parenchyma [1]. Astrocyte also directly contact synapses with their cell processes and they are actively and specifically involved in synaptic signaling. They take up potassium ions and neurotransmitters like glutamate released by neurons and release gliotransmitters to modulate synaptic transmission [1]. These active functions in synaptic signaling led to the concept of the tripartite synapse, that is, the view that astrocytes processes are a third integral component of synapses beside the pre- and postsynaptic neuronal compartments [1]. Astrocytes also have important functions in development, as structural scaffold and in neuronal maturation [1]. Furthermore, neural stem cells (NSCs) in development (radial glia) and the adult brain show extraordinarily high similarity to astrocytes, and recent studies indicate that classical parenchymal astrocytes can regain NSC-like properties [2]. Therefore, NSCs might even be considered to be a part of a broad continuous spectrum of astrocyte-like cells [2].

For many of their diverse functions in normal brain development and homeostasis, astrocytes need to closely monitor and respond to changes in their environment. Therefore, it is not surprising that astrocytes also strongly respond to pathological conditions. This can result in the gain of novel functions, like immune cell-like functions, but also in the disruption of their normal homeostatic functions, adding an additional layer of complexity to astrocyte biology. Due to the important functions of astrocytes and their prominent alterations in pathologies, astrocytes are known or suspected to be involved in the pathogenesis of a large number of neurological conditions, from acute injury and inflammatory diseases to neurodegenerative and even psychiatric disorders [3, 4].

Astrocytes express a large set of receptors allowing them to detect a wide spectrum of changes in their environment, which activate various signaling pathways. Many of these receptors detect molecules occurring in pathological conditions, for example, pathogen-derived molecules, molecules derived from damaged cells (pathogen-associated molecular patterns/Danger associated molecular patterns (PAMPs/DAMPs)), and cytokines [5, 6]. Signaling of most of these receptors converges on one major signaling pathway, the IKK/NF-κB signaling pathway. This pathway is a master regulator of inflammation, and one of the main pathways controlling the pathophysiological responses of astrocytes, as will be discussed in detail in this chapter.

2. Astrogliosis: responses of astrocytes to pathological conditions

Most CNS pathologies, ranging from acute damage in traumatic brain injury (TBI) or CNS infections to inflammatory disorders like multiple sclerosis (MS), epilepsy and classical chronic neurodegenerative diseases like Alzheimer's disease (AD) are associated with similar characteristic histopathological alterations of astrocytes, which are generally referred to as astrogliosis [1]. Astrogliosis is usually associated with local inflammatory processes elicited by these pathological conditions. Similarly, microglia, the resident macrophages of the CNS, show characteristic alterations in these conditions, called microgliosis, which usually occur together with astrogliosis. [3, 7, 8].

A common feature of astrogliosis is astrocyte hypertrophy, along with an upregulation of proinflammatory mediators and intermediate filaments like the classical astrocyte and astrogliosis marker GFAP [1, 5, 6, 9]. Depending on the severity and type of insult, this hypertrophic response can also be accompanied by astrocyte proliferation and can result in the formation of dense glial scars [10].

The production of inflammatory mediators like cytokines (e.g. TNF, IL-1β) and chemokines (e.g. MCP1 (CCL2), RANTES (CCL5) and IP-10 (CXCL10)) by reactive astrocytes is crucial for the recruitment of peripheral immune cells into the CNS and their subsequent activation [3, 5]. This astrocyte-mediated immune cell recruitment is essential to fight infections and repair tissue damage, but exacerbated or chronic immune cell infiltration also drives autoimmune pathologies like MS, and can aggravate other pathologies associated with neuroinflammation, like neurodegenerative disorders [3, 11].

In response to pathological conditions, beside recruiting professional immune cells, astrocytes themselves contribute to inflammation and immune responses by producing a variety of acute phase response factors, like complement proteins (e.g. C1q, C3) or Lcn2 [12, 13]. While these factors can have important protective functions, for example, by inhibiting bacterial growth in case of an infection, they can also promote synapse elimination and neuronal cell death [12, 13]. Interestingly, reactive astrocytes also upregulate MHC class II genes and have phagocytic capabilities [14, 15]. Therefore reactive astrocytes might act as professional antigen-presenting cells, similar to macrophages and dendritic cells [14, 15].

Overall, these inflammation-related and immune cell-like properties gained by reactive astrocytes suggest that astrocytes, beside microglia, are a second major component of the innate immune system of the brain.

The inflammatory functions of astrocytes are important for a fast and strong early response of the CNS to pathological conditions, which can be crucial to limit damage, for example, in infections or acute injury. This local response is particularly important in the CNS, because as an immune-privileged organ it has limited surveillance by peripheral immune cells. But inflammation increases cellular stress by various mechanisms, therefore chronic or exaggerated inflammatory astrocyte activation can have severe adverse effects resulting in neurotoxicity [16]. These early inflammatory responses of astrocytes are similar to the early responses of microglia and macrophages to pathological conditions, often described as proinflammatory M1 polarization [17]. Therefore, this type of astrocyte responses was recently described as A1 activation [16].

In addition to increased inflammatory stress, this type of astrocyte activation can also disrupt their normal homeostatic functions, like BBB maintenance, or the clearance of extracellular neurotransmitters (e.g. glutamate) and potassium ions released during synaptic activity [1, 18, 19]. Disruption of these astrocyte functions can cause edema formation and alters neuronal excitation and network activity, which can result in behavioral changes, epileptic seizures and excitotoxic neurodegeneration [3, 18, 19].

Beside the described prominent proinflammatory phenotype, which in some conditions can have adverse consequences, reactive astrocytes also seem to occur in more "benign" states, which has been described as A2 activation, in analogy to a similar anti-inflammatory, pro-regenerative state of microglia and macrophages (M2 polarization) [16, 17].

In chronic neurodegenerative or neuroinflammatory pathologies, A1 astrocyte activation seems to dominate, whereas after acute injury or ischemia, this A2 activation seems to determine the overall functional consequences of astrogliosis [16]. In these acute insults, reactive A2 astrocytes upregulate neurotrophic factors and can gain overall neuroprotective functions [16].

After acute brain injury, for example, in models of cortical stab wound injury or spinal cord injury (SCI), but not in chronic neurodegenerative or neuroinflammatory pathologies, astrocytes also respond by proliferation and the formation of dense astroglial scars [10, 20, 21]. It is often assumed that this glial scar is required to restrict the spreading of tissue damage in the acute stage of the injury, but interferes with CNS regeneration on the long term, for example, by preventing axonal regrowth through the scar tissue. However, several studies indicate that also on the long term, the astrocytes of the glial scar rather promote repair and regeneration [10, 20]. Specifically, ablation of proliferating astrocytes has been shown to interfere with the repair of the BBB in cortical stab wound injury and SCI models, and prevented axonal regrowth after SCI stimulated by a conditioning lesion and neurotrophin application [20, 22, 23]. In addition, recent studies suggest that astrocytes not only protect the surviving of neurons in the damaged tissue, but might also reactivate a NSC-like potential, and might thereby contribute to the (very limited) generation of new neurons after injury [21, 24–26].

3. The IKK/NF-κB signaling pathway: a central signaling hub in inflammation, cell survival, proliferation and differentiation

The IKK/NF-κB pathway is a master regulator of inflammation, which is also implicated in a wide range of other biological processes, including cell death/survival, proliferation and differentiation [27–29]. This signaling pathway integrates signals from a large number of different receptors, converging in the activation of the IκB kinase (IKK) complex, the key activator of the NF-κB family of transcription factors in canonical NF-κB signaling [28]. In mammals, the NF-κB family includes the five members—RelA, RelB, c-Rel, p105/p50 and p100/p52, which form homo- and heterodimers [28]. In the basal state, these dimers are kept inactive in the cytoplasm by binding to proteins of the inhibitor of NF-κB (IκB) family [28].

The IKK complex, consisting of the kinase subunits IKK1 and IKK2 (also called IKKα and IKKβ) and the regulatory subunit NEMO (IKKγ), can activate NF-κB dimers by phosphorylating IκB proteins through IKK2 as active kinase subunit [28]. This induces the poly-ubiquitination and subsequent proteasomal degradation of the IκB proteins, resulting in the release of the NF-κB dimers [28]. These dimers then can translocate to the nucleus, where they can activate or repress a large number of target genes [28].

Various inflammation-mediating receptors activate NF-κB through this canonical signaling pathway, including the TNF receptor TNFR1 and the IL-1β receptor as prototypical examples [28]. Upon activation, these receptors recruit K63-ubiquitin ligases like the cIAP proteins, and the linear ubiquitin assembly complex (LUBAC) [30, 31]. These ubiquitin ligases build K63- and linear (M1-) poly-ubiquitin chains on receptor-associated scaffolding proteins, which form the backbone for the assembly of large signaling complexes [30, 31]. The TAK1/TAB2/3 and IKK kinase complexes then bind to these poly-ubiquitin chains, allowing the phosphorylation of IKK2 at two conserved serine residues by TAK1 and IKK2 itself [30, 31]. This dual phosphorylation of IKK2 is the key step in the activation of the IKK complex, which is then capable of phosphorylating IκB proteins [30, 31].

Beside TNFR1 and the IL-1β receptor, among the receptors activating this canonical NF-κB signaling pathway there are also many pattern recognition receptors (PRRs), like Toll-like receptors (TLRs) and NOD-like receptors (NLRs) [6, 28, 32]. These receptors are sensors of molecular danger signals, like conserved pathogen-derived molecules (pathogen-associated molecular patterns, PAMPs) and molecules released by damaged cells (danger-associated molecular patterns, DAMPs), which are driving the initiation of inflammatory responses [6, 28, 32].

Some other extracellular signals, like CD40L, LTβ, BAFF or RANKL, can activate an alternative NF-κB signaling pathway, by activation of IKK1 via the NF-κB inducing kinase (NIK). This induces the proteasomal processing of the NF-κB precursor subunit p100, resulting in the degradation of an inhibitory IκB domain of p100 [27]. This processing leaves the active subunit p52, which can translocate to the nucleus as a p52/p52 or RelB/p52 dimer [27].

In addition, several other stimuli, including neurotrophins and general cellular stress, like DNA damage and high levels of reactive oxygen species, can activate NF-κB signaling. In these cases, NF-κB activity is often regulated via atypical NF-κB signaling pathways, which involve various posttranslational modifications of IKK and NF-κB subunits [28, 33–35].

As diverse as the range of NF-κB activating stimuli are the target genes of the NF-κB transcription factors. NF-κB signaling controls the expression of a large number of inflammatory cytokines, chemokines, cell adhesion molecules, immunoreceptors and acute phase response genes [36]. As NF-κB signaling is activated by a wide range of inflammatory stimuli, and induces a large number of proinflammatory target genes, it can both initiate inflammatory responses and enhance them by positive feedback loops via NF-κB activating cytokines. These properties make the NF-κB signaling system a critical master regulator of inflammatory processes. In fact, IKK/NF-κB activation alone is sufficient to initiate and maintain inflammatory responses in many tissues, which often phenotypically closely resemble classical autoimmune/inflammatory diseases. This has been shown by us and others by conditional genetic activation of IKK/NF-κB in pancreatic acinar or β-cells, hepatocytes, cardiomyocytes and airway or intestinal epithelial cells [37–43]. Vice versa, genetic inactivation of IKK/NF-κB signaling strongly suppresses inflammation in many mouse models of pathological conditions. This often ameliorates pathology, for example, in a model of cerebral ischemia with inactivated neuronal IKK/NF-κB signaling [44], or in an MS model with inactivated IKK/NF-κB signaling in all neuroectodermal cells [45].

Among the large spectrum of NF-κB targets are also many genes controlling cell proliferation, differentiation and survival, like growth factors, cyclins and apoptosis regulators of the Bcl-2 and IAP families [29, 36]. Therefore NF-κB signaling represents a crucial link between inflammation and cancer [29, 36]. In addition, in the CNS, NF-κB signaling regulates neuronal differentiation and function, for example, dendrite formation and synaptogenesis, via various target genes like neurotrophins or IGF2 [34, 46–48].

In conclusion, the NF-κB signaling pathway is a central signaling hub integrating a large spectrum of signals to regulate a similar broad range of biological processes. One important function is the transduction of pathophysiological alarm signals, which is crucial for the cellular responses to these signals, in particular for inflammatory responses. Due to its diverse other biological functions, the NF-κB signaling pathway is a critical molecular link between inflammation and various physiological processes known to be dysregulated in inflammatory conditions.

4. Activation of the IKK/NF-κB pathway in astrocytes

Considering the responsiveness of astrocytes to pathological conditions and the central role of NF-κB in the transduction of such responses, it is not surprising that NF-κB signaling in astrocytes is activated in many pathological conditions and regulates many of these pathophysiological responses.

Astrocytes express a large number of cytokine receptors including TNFR1 and IL-1RI; PRRs including TLRs (TLR2,3,5,9); NLRs including NOD2 and NLRP3 and RIG-1 like receptors (RLRs), which can activate NF-κB signaling in pathological conditions [5, 49, 50].

Accordingly, astrocytes activate NF-κB signaling in vitro after stimulation with ligands of these receptors, and in vivo in various neuropathological conditions associated with neuroinflammation.

For example, in vitro, stimulation of primary mouse astrocytes with TNFα or IL-1β induces nuclear accumulation of RelA indicating NF-κB activation (e.g. [45]). In vivo, astroglial NF-κB activation was described, for example, in MS [51], traumatic brain injury (TBI) [52], in chronic neurodegenerative pathologies such as ALS [53] and Huntington's disease (HD) [54], but remarkably also in a post-mortem study in autism spectrum disorders [55].

5. Functions of astroglial IKK/NF-κB signaling: a central regulator of the pathophysiological responses of astrocytes

To investigate the specific functions of NF-κB signaling in astrocytes in vivo, we and other groups have developed conditional transgenic mouse models allowing the genetic activation or inactivation of NF-κB signaling specifically in astrocytes and closely related cell types.

One much-studied mouse model was developed by the group of John R. Bethea, the GFAP-IκBα-dn transgenic mouse line [56]. In this mouse model, astroglial NF-κB signaling is strongly inhibited by overexpression of a dominant-negative, non-degradable mutant of the NF-κB inhibitor IκBα [56]. The transgene expression is driven by the GFAP promoter, which restricts its expression to astrocytes and closely related cell types [56].

Vice versa, to genetically activate IKK/NF-κB signaling, we generated a mouse model allowing the inducible overexpression of a constitutively active mutant of IKK2 specifically in astrocytes (GFAP.tTA/tetO.IKK2-CA) [57]. Using a so-called Tet-off conditional expression system, the expression of this transgene is driven by the GFAP promoter and can be reversibly repressed by the administration of doxycycline, allowing both constitutive and time-controlled transient activation of astroglial IKK/NF-κB signaling [57, 58].

Other strategies to manipulate astroglial IKK/NF-κB signaling include the Cre-mediated deletion of components of the IKK complex to block NF-κB activation [45], or deletion of IκBα to enhance astroglial NF-κB signaling [59].

A number of studies using these or similar approaches have revealed important functions of astroglial NF-κB signaling in normal CNS development and homeostasis, as well as critical roles in the regulation of astroglial responses to pathological conditions.

5.1. Astroglial IKK/NF-κB signaling is a central regulator of neuroinflammation

In line with the key role of IKK/NF-κB signaling in the regulation of inflammation in other cell types, and the important role of astrocytes in neuroinflammation, a number of studies have established that astroglial IKK/NF-κB activation is a critical step in the initiation and propagation of neuroinflammatory processes.

In the initial description of the GFAP-IκBα-dn model, it was shown that IKK/NF-κB inhibition in astrocytes in SCI reduced the expression of the proinflammatory chemokines CCL2 (MCP-1) and CXCL10 (IP-10), which are important regulators of immune cell recruitment [56]. This study also showed that the upregulation of the astrogliosis-promoting cytokine TGFβ2 after SCI is mediated by astroglial NF-κB signaling [56].

A subsequent study on the role of NF-κB signaling in experimental autoimmune encephalitis (EAE), a model of MS, showed that inhibition of NF-κB signaling in all neuroectodermal cells (Nes-Cre/NEMO fl/fl and Nes-Cre/IKK2 fl/fl) prominently reduced the expression of a large spectrum of inflammatory mediators in this pathology [45]. This study indicated that inhibition of astroglial NF-κB signaling was predominantly responsible for this amelioration of neuroinflammation, which was confirmed later by astrocyte-specific NF-κB inhibition using the GFAP-IκBα-dn model [60]. GFAP-IκBα-dn transgenic mice in this study showed a similar reduction of the expression of inflammatory mediators after EAE [60]. These mediators included various chemokines and cell adhesion molecules involved in the recruitment of peripheral immune cells, and the major proinflammatory cytokines TNF, IL-1β and IFN-γ, as well as inflammatory effector genes like complement factors [45, 60].

These findings suggest that astroglial IKK/NF-κB signaling is important for the recruitment and activation of immune cells in neuroinflammatory conditions. Indeed, in both mentioned models, a reduced infiltration of immune cells after EAE induction was found in mice with inhibited astroglial IKK/NF-κB signaling [45, 61], although originally also an increase of (regulatory) T cell infiltration was described for the GFAP-IκBα-dn model [60].

Similar to the situation in EAE and SCI, inhibition of astroglial NF-κB signaling by GFAP-IκBα-dn also resulted in a reduced induction of multiple proinflammatory factors in models of retinal ischemia-reperfusion injury [62] and optic neuritis [63]. While this reduced microgliosis and astrogliosis in ischemic injury [62], infiltration of peripheral immune cells in optic neuritis was not obviously altered, although this was not quantified in this study [63].

Overall, these studies demonstrate that astroglial NF-κB signaling mediates the coordinated induction of various inflammatory mediators in various neuropathologies. However, the consequences of this proinflammatory signaling for local glial reactivity and the infiltration of peripheral immune cells depend on the specific pathological context. Whether these context-dependent effects in different pathologies are due to different levels of NF-κB activation, or whether additional signaling pathways are required for astrocytes to modulate neuroinflammation, was not investigated by these studies. Also, they could not address the question, whether astroglial NF-κB activation can only modulate neuroinflammation induced by other processes in these specific pathologies, or whether it is actually a driving force of neuroinflammation, which is sufficient to initiate neuroinflammation.

To address these questions, we generated the GFAP.tTA/tetO.IKK2-CA model, which allows astroglial NF-κB activation in normal physiological conditions, that is, in the absence of an external pathogenic trigger that could induce neuroinflammation [57]. Remarkably, both in the developing, early postnatal brain and in the adult brain, the selective activation of astroglial NF-κB in this model was sufficient to initiate and maintain a prominent global neuroinflammatory response [57, 58, 64]. This inflammatory response was characterized by strong astrogliosis and microgliosis, as well as a prominent infiltration of innate immune cells, and, in adult animals, also T cells [57, 58, 64]. On a molecular level, in particular the chemokines CCL2(MCP-1), CCL5(Rantes) and CXCL10(IP-10), the cell adhesion molecule Madcam1, the MHC class II protein CD74 and some acute phase effector genes (Lcn2, C3) were highly upregulated by astroglial IKK/NF-κB activation [57, 58]. These inflammatory mediators and effectors were upregulated both in brain tissue and in primary astrocytes, suggesting that they are direct targets of IKK/NF-κB signaling in astrocytes [57, 58]. In contrast, TNF and IL-1β were induced in adult cerebellar tissue of these animals [58], but not in primary astrocytes [57]. This indicates that these major proinflammatory cytokines are not direct NF-κB targets in astrocytes, but that they are produced by other cell types as an indirect consequence of astroglial IKK/NF-κB activation.

In conclusion, these studies show that astroglial IKK/NF-κB signaling is a key regulator of inflammatory responses in the CNS, whose activation is required and can be sufficient to initiate and maintain neuroinflammation. Specifically, astroglial IKK/NF-κB activation alone is sufficient to induce the infiltration of peripheral immune cells into the brain, probably via the strong induction of chemokines. However, in specific disease contexts this can also occur independently of astroglial IKK/NF-κB signaling, and other cell types or signaling pathways are likely required for the production of major cytokines to activate these immune cells. Furthermore, astroglial IKK/NF-κB activation can trigger astrogliosis and induce a number of acute phase response factors, which might be important for the rapid response of the CNS to acute pathological insults, to limit potential further damage, for example, in an infection or injury.

5.2. Astroglial IKK/NF-κB activation can interfere with postnatal brain development

Astrocytes and related cell types, like radial glia, have important functions in CNS development [1], and neuroinflammatory conditions like brain infections, which are associated with NF-κB activation in astrocytes, are known to be major risk factors for neurodevelopmental disorders [65, 66]. This suggests that NF-κB-mediated astroglial responses during CNS development might contribute to the pathogenesis of such inflammation-associated neurodevelopmental disorders.

Indeed, in line with this hypothesis, we found that constitutive activation of astroglial IKK/NF-κB signaling during early postnatal brain development in the GFAP.tTA/tetO.IKK2-CA model resulted in lethality due to neuroinflammation-associated hydrocephalus formation [57]. Hydrocephalus is a known complication of neuroinflammatory insults, in particular during brain development [57]. In the GFAP.tTA/tetO.IKK2-CA model, hydrocephalus formation was caused by impaired differentiation of the ependymal cells lining the cerebral ventricles, which failed to develop motile cilia [57]. These cilia are required to facilitate the flow of the cerebrospinal fluid through the cerebroventricular system, and defects of these cilia can cause hydrocephalus also in other mouse models [57]. Ependymal cells are closely related to astrocytes and develop postnatally from radial glia, which are common progenitors of both astrocytes and ependymal cells [2]. Thus, at least some ependymal cells expressed the IKK2-CA transgene [57]. Therefore, it is not clear whether this defect is cell-intrinsic, or whether non-cell-autonomous effects of astrocyte-mediated neuroinflammation contribute to this defect [57]. Beyond hydrocephalus formation, astroglial IKK/NF-κB activation in the GFAP.tTA/tetO.IKK2-CA model resulted in additional defects in late developing brain regions, specifically in a disorganization of the hippocampus, most prominently in the dentate gyrus, and a delayed maturation of the cerebellum [57]. These defects might be caused by an impaired migration of neural progenitors, as this migration is guided by chemokine gradients, which are likely disturbed by the massive NF-κB-mediated upregulation of chemokines by astrocytes, and the overall inflammatory environment [57].

These findings demonstrate that astroglial IKK/NF-κB activation can interfere with normal brain development, providing a potential molecular link between neuroinflammation and neurodevelopmental disorders. On the other hand, inhibition of IKK/NF-κB signaling in astrocytes does not cause obvious defects of brain development and homeostasis [45, 56]. Therefore, it will be interesting to study to what extent inhibition of astroglial IKK/NF-κB signaling can ameliorate inflammation-associated neurodevelopmental defects.

5.3. Roles of astroglial IKK/NF-κB signaling in normal adult brain homeostasis and function

Mice with IKK/NF-κB inhibition in astrocytes do not show obvious phenotypes in normal physiological conditions [45, 56], demonstrating that astroglial NF-κB signaling is not broadly required for normal brain development, homeostasis and function. However, two studies reported subtle behavioral phenotypes of mice with reduced basal astroglial IKK/NF-κB signaling, specifically a sex-specific impairment in learning and memory in female GFAP-IκBα-dn mice [67], and reduced food intake in mice with Cre-mediated astroglial IKK2 inactivation (GFAP-Cre/IKK2 fl/fl) [68].

On the other hand, as described in Section 5.1, activation of astroglial IKK/NF-κB signaling in normal physiological conditions in the adult brain in the GFAP.tTA/tetO.IKK2-CA model induces prominent global neuroinflammation [58, 64]. This indicates that activation of IKK/NF-κB signaling in astrocytes might have more severe consequences for brain homeostasis and function than its inhibition. Interestingly however, this prominent global neuroinflammatory phenotype had obvious consequences for brain homeostasis only in one specific brain region, the cerebellum [58]. In the cerebellum, with some delay massive neurodegeneration was observed, which predominantly affected Purkinje cells, the output neurons of the cerebellum and resulted in severe motor impairment [58]. This was found to be due to the dysfunction of the Bergmann glia, a specific population of astrocytes with radial glia-like morphology, which is essential for the function and survival of the Purkinje neurons [58]. IKK2 activation in Bergmann glia resulted in prominent astrogliosis-like alterations, including prominent upregulation of GFAP and morphological alterations disrupting their specialized morphology [58]. These alterations were shown to represent an irreversible "point of no return" resulting in inevitable Purkinje cell degeneration [58]. Of note, this phenotype resembles alterations found in inflammatory cerebellar neurodegenerative disorders, for example, in paraneoplastic cerebellar degeneration, which are also characterized by prominent selective Purkinje cell degeneration [58]. Therefore, these findings suggest a mechanism how cerebellar neuroinflammation caused by various insults might result in the common pathology of Purkinje cell degeneration: Inflammation-induced IKK/NF-κB activation in Bergmann glia would cause irreversible Bergmann glia dysfunction, which consequentially would drive Purkinje cell degeneration [58].

Interestingly, it was also found that astroglial IKK/NF-κB activation in the GFAP.tTA/tetO.IKK2-CA model resulted in the downregulation of the glutamate transporters EAAT1 (GLAST) and EAAT2 (GLT-1) in the cerebellum and the medulla oblongata [58]. Downregulation of these transporters is found in many neurological disorders, including cerebellar neurodegenerative disorders, and is believed to contribute to the pathogenesis of these disorders [18, 69]. By impairing the uptake of the excitatory neurotransmitter glutamate by astrocytes, downregulation of these transporters can result in neuronal hyperexcitation and excitotoxic neurodegeneration [18, 69].

Another recent study found that astroglial IKK/NF-κB activation also impairs the astroglial uptake of the neurotransmitter GABA, at least in the hypothalamus, which resulted in increased activity of specific neurons in hypothalamic nuclei [68]. In this model, a constitutively active IKK2 allele was activated by GFAP-Cre-mediated recombination (GFAP-Cre/Rosa26-LSL-IKK2CA) [68]. This resulted in more moderate astroglial IKK/NF-κB activation, which was not sufficient to induce neuroinflammation in heterozygous mice [68]. In this model, astroglial IKK/NF-κB activation led to mild astrogliosis-like changes, specifically increased astrocyte numbers and altered morphology (shortened processes) [68]. These alterations resulted in changes in the systemic metabolism, which is controlled by the hypothalamus, specifically in a metabolic syndrome-like phenotype with insulin resistance, increased blood pressure and increased fat deposition [68].

Given the important functions of astrocytes in neuronal metabolism and signaling, and their prominent alterations in pathological conditions, it is likely that astroglial IKK/NF-κB activation also causes additional more subtle alterations in neuronal communication in the CNS. Indeed, we have found a moderate reduction of striatal dopamine levels in the GFAP.tTA/tetO.IKK2-CA model [64]. However, more research is needed to examine the functions of astroglial IKK/NF-κB in the modulation of neurotransmitter signaling.

Another mechanism beside the uptake of neurotransmitters and release of gliotransmitters, by which astrocytes modulate neuronal communication, is the regulation of synapse formation, maturation and elimination. On a molecular level, complement proteins, including C3, which is highly induced by astrocytes upon NF-κB activation, contribute to the elimination of synapses [70]. Indeed, it has recently been demonstrated, that astroglial NF-κB activation by GFAP-Cre-mediated IκBα deletion promotes synapse elimination and alters neuronal signaling via C3 induction [70].

5.4. Roles of astroglial IKK/NF-κB signaling in models of specific pathological conditions

Astrogliosis and neuroinflammatory processes are occurring in most neurological disorders, most prominently in autoimmune/inflammatory disorders and acute injury. Often these processes contribute to the pathogenesis of these disorders, but depending on the conditions they can also have protective roles. Astroglial IKK/NF-κB signaling is a key regulator of these pathophysiological responses, therefore a number of studies have addressed the role of astroglial IKK/NF-κB signaling in specific CNS disease and injury models.

The first neuropathological condition, in which the role of astroglial NF-κB signaling was studied using the GFAP-IκBα-dn model, was SCI, a condition in which inflammatory processes are believed to prominently contribute to pathogenesis [56, 71]. In line with the idea that astroglial NF-κB signaling promotes neuroinflammation and that this aggravates pathogenesis of SCI, functional recovery was improved in mice with inhibited astroglial NF-κB signaling [56]. Histologically, microgliosis and astrogliosis were less pronounced in the absence of astroglial NF-κB signaling after SCI [71]. This was associated with improved white matter preservation, probably due to reduced secondary inflammatory white matter damage [56], which also improved axonal integrity [71]. Also, a reduced intra-lesional deposition of chondroitin sulfate proteoglycans (CSPGs) was observed [56]. CSPGs are important components of the glial scar, which interfere with regenerative axonal outgrowth [56]. In this model of contusive SCI, even some degree of axonal sprouting across the lesion was observed upon inhibition of astroglial NF-κB signaling, but not in wildtype animals [71]. This indicates that NF-κB-mediated scar formation contributes to the inability of the CNS to regenerate lost axons. However, this regenerative response was not able to bridge the lesion in a complete spinal cord transection, showing that astroglial NF-κB inhibition is not sufficient to allow axonal regeneration [71]. In conclusion, these studies show that astroglial NF-κB signaling might contribute to the pathogenesis of SCI by aggravating inflammatory secondary tissue damage and by interfering with regenerative processes.

Another well studied neurological disorder with an obviously strong inflammatory pathogenic component is MS, the most common autoimmune disease of the CNS. A number of studies have therefore investigated whether astroglial NF-κB signaling contributes to pathogenesis of demyelination in this disease [45, 60, 61, 63, 72, 73].

In an early study indicating that indeed astroglial NF-κB signaling might contribute to MS pathogenesis, the core components of the IKK complex were inactivated in neuroectodermal cells (neurons, astrocytes and oligodendrocytes) in a mouse model using nestin-promoter driven Cre expression (Nes-Cre x IKK1 fl/fl or IKK2 fl/fl or NEMO fl/fl) [45]. After induction of EAE, mice with conditional IKK2 and NEMO inactivation, but not with IKK1 inactivation, displayed prominently reduced neurological deficits [45]. This indicates that canonical, but not non-canonical NF-κB signaling in astrocytes, oligodendrocytes and neurons, contributes to EAE pathogenesis [45]. These reduced neurological deficits were accompanied by reduced demyelination and immune cell infiltration, and a reduced expression of proinflammatory genes in primary astrocytes [45]. Because microglia and astrocytes are the main cell types in the CNS parenchyma that regulate inflammatory processes, and microglia are not targeted by the Nes-Cre-driven ablation approach, the authors concluded that reduced proinflammatory signaling by NF-κB inhibition in astrocytes is likely responsible for the amelioration of the phenotype [45]. This hypothesis was confirmed by astrocyte-specific NF-κB inhibition in EAE in the GFAP-IκBα-dn model [60, 61]. Astrocyte-specific NF-κB inhibition in this model also reduced neurological deficits after EAE induction, along with a reduced expression of inflammatory mediators, and led to improved remyelination and neuronal survival at chronic stages [60, 61]. Vice versa, GFAP-Cre-mediated inactivation of A20, a negative feedback regulator of NF-κB signaling, in astrocytes, increased expression of proinflammatory NF-κB target genes and inflammatory infiltration after EAE, which resulted in aggravated neurological deficits and demyelination [72]. Interestingly, the observed myelin preservation after inhibition of astrocyte-specific NF-κB signaling is not restricted to EAE, which is driven by an autoimmune attack, that is, a very strong inflammatory insult. Increased myelin preservation was also observed in a model of cuprizone-induced toxic demyelination, where inflammatory events are not the primary cause but rather a co-pathogenic consequence of the myelin damage [73]. This indicates that NF-κB-mediated astroglial responses contribute to the pathogenesis of demyelination not only by inflammatory signaling, for example, by promoting the recruitment of peripheral immune cells, but that astrocytes gain additional pathogenic properties after NF-κB activation. In line with this idea, demyelination in the optic nerve, one of the earliest symptoms of MS, is reduced in EAE in the GFAP-IκBα-dn model even without any obvious differences in local immune cell infiltration [63]. It was proposed that astroglial NF-κB signaling in the latter paradigm contributes to myelin damage by increasing oxidative stress, as it induces the NAD(P)H oxidase subunits Cybb/NOX2 and Ncf1 [63].

Overall, these studies provide clear evidence that activation of NF-κB-mediated inflammatory responses of astrocytes aggravate demyelination and associated neurological defects in different animal models, indicating that these NF-κB-mediated astrocytic responses likely contribute to the pathogenesis of MS and other demyelinating disorders.

For other neurological disorders, the functions of astroglial NF-κB signaling are less well studied.

In a model of ischemic retinal injury, astroglial NF-κB inhibition in GFAP-IκBα-dn mice was shown to be neuroprotective, likely by suppressing the induction of Nos2 (iNos) and NADPH-oxidase genes after ischemia [62, 74]. This resulted in a reduction of oxidative stress, a crucial pathogenic factor in ischemia, at least in vitro [62, 74]. In contrast, an earlier study using a model with a different astrocyte-specific dominant-negative IκBα transgene did not find any consequences of astroglial NF-κB inhibition for the pathogenesis of cerebral ischemia [75].

A reduction of the expression of the oxidative stress promoting enzyme iNos by astroglial NF-κB inhibition in GFAP-IκBα-dn mice was also found in a model of hepatic encephalopathy [76]. In this model, astroglial NF-κB inhibition had a protective effect due to a prominent reduction of astrocyte swelling and edema formation [76].

These findings, as the described similar findings in EAE/optic neuritis [63], indicate that astroglial NF-κB signaling increases oxidative stress, which might contribute to the pathogenesis of a range of neuroinflammation-associated neuropathological conditions.

Classical chronic neurodegenerative disorders like AD, PD or ALS are also associated with neuroinflammatory processes, which are believed to contribute to the pathogenesis of these diseases. However, only few studies so far have addressed the role of astroglial NF-κB signaling in models of chronic neurodegeneration.

One study found that Aβ can activate NF-κB in astrocytes, resulting in C3 induction [70]. Further, this study showed that in AD C3 levels are elevated, and that inhibition of the C3 receptor C3aR can revert memory deficits in a mouse model of AD [70]. This suggests that astroglial NF-κB activation via C3 induction might contribute to AD pathogenesis. However, a direct link of astroglial NF-κB activation and disease pathogenesis in AD has yet to be demonstrated.

To study the role of astroglial NF-κB signaling in PD, we have analyzed the consequences of enhanced NF-κB activation in astrocytes in GFAP.tTA/tetO.IKK2-CA mice for neurodegeneration in the MPTP model of PD [64]. In this paradigm, astroglial NF-κB activation did not affect the degeneration of dopaminergic neurons in the substantia nigra, despite inducing prominent neuroinflammation in this brain region [64]. This argues against a prominent role of astroglial NF-κB signaling in PD pathogenesis. However, the mechanism of degeneration in this toxin-induced dopaminergic neurodegeneration model differs from the mechanism of degeneration in PD, therefore studies in other models of PD should be undertaken to further elucidate the role of astroglial NF-κB signaling in PD.

Finally, one study inhibited astroglial NF-κB signaling in a mouse model of ALS, using another independent GFAP-IκBα-dn transgenic mouse line [77]. Rather unexpectedly, despite the well documented contribution of astrocytes to ALS pathogenesis and a delayed onset of astrogliosis and microgliosis in this model, no alterations in disease onset or progression were found in this model [77]. This argues against a prominent contribution of astroglial NF-κB signaling to astrocyte dysfunction and neurodegeneration in ALS.

In conclusion, although astrocytes have crucial functions in neuroinflammation and neuronal homeostasis, and neuroinflammation and astrocyte dysfunction are widely accepted as pathogenic mechanisms in chronic neurodegeneration, direct evidence for the contribution of astroglial NF-κB signaling to the pathogenesis of these disorders is scarce. Given the huge socioeconomic impact of these disorders, and the prominent role of astroglial NF-κB signaling on the pathogenesis of other neurological disorders, further studies should address the role of astroglial NF-κB signaling in chronic neurodegeneration in more detail.

6. Other signaling pathways regulating pathophysiological responses of astrocytes: an overview

Although we have focused here on the role of NF-κB signaling in the regulation of pathophysiological responses of astrocytes, several other signaling pathways have been implicated in these responses. Interestingly, many pathways involved in astrocyte reactivity are also required for astrocyte differentiation in development. Activation of these pathways in pathological conditions seems to promote a partial de-differentiation of astrocytes, resembling more immature stages of astrocyte differentiation with increased proliferative and lineage potential.

One of these key developmental pathways contributing to astrocyte reactivity is the JAK/STAT3 pathway, which is activated by cytokines of the IL-6 family, like IL-6, LIF and CNTF [78, 79]. This pathway is closely interconnected with the NF-κB pathway, as, for example, IL-6 is induced in many inflammatory conditions, also by NF-κB activation in astrocytes [58]. Vice versa, JAK/STAT3 signaling induces target genes that are also induced by NF-κB signaling, like CXCL10 and LCN2 [78]. STAT3 activation in the context of pathological conditions was shown be a crucial driver of astrocyte hypertrophy and GFAP induction, two major hallmarks of astrogliosis [78]. Indeed, STAT3 directly regulates GFAP expression, in cooperation with SMAD transcription factors, which are activated by BMP and TGFβ signaling, another signaling system implicated in astrogliosis [80].

Interestingly, while both NF-κB and STAT3 signaling promote astroglial scar formation in SCI, STAT3 regulated aspects of astroglial scar formation seem to promote repair and regeneration [20], whereas NF-κB regulated aspects rather interfere with repair processes [56, 71]. This indicates that different types of astroglial scars exist, which are regulated by different molecular mechanisms and which can influence regeneration in different ways. Therefore, future studies should further investigate these mechanisms, as this might open up new strategies to promote regeneration after CNS damage, by converting astroglial scars to more pro-regenerative states.

STAT3 signaling also contributes to the proliferative response of astrocytes observed after acute injury [78], a response which is also regulated by Sonic hedgehog (SHH) signaling [21]. Interestingly, this proliferative response seems to be directly linked to the acquisition of NSC-like properties of astrocytes after injury, which similar to NSCs and immature astrocytes, can form multipotent neurospheres in vitro [21, 81]. This indicates that astrocytes after injury can partially de-differentiate, and can regain increased lineage plasticity, including the potential to generate new neurons. Indeed, recent studies have demonstrated that at least in the striatum, some astrocytes can generate neurons in vivo after cell cycle re-entry in response to ischemic or excitotoxic injury [25, 26]. In ischemic injury, this reactivation of proliferation and subsequent neurogenesis was associated with reduced Notch signaling [25], another pathway which is required for astrocyte differentiation and maturation, and which is also controlling NSC quiescence [82, 83].

This study further showed that genetic activation of Notch signaling can suppress this proliferative and neurogenic response in ischemia [25]. Vice versa, inhibition of Notch signaling in astrocytes by conditional RBPJ deletion is sufficient to elicit a neurogenic response in some striatal astrocytes [25]. These results indicate that Notch signaling is crucial to maintain the mature, quiescent state of astrocytes, and that downregulation Notch signaling promotes a de-differentiation response of astrocytes in pathological conditions.

It will be important to further dissect the mechanisms governing these neurogenic de-differentiation responses of astrocytes, which might open up new strategies for regenerative medicine. This could allow enhancing endogenous neuronal replacement in neurodegenerative conditions and improving the efficiency of neuronal reprogramming of astrocytes.

7. Conclusions and future directions

As we have described in this chapter, astrocytes are functionally diverse and plastic cells that are highly responsive to changes in the CNS microenvironment.

In most CNS pathologies, including acute injuries, autoimmune/inflammatory disorders like multiple sclerosis, and chronic neurodegenerative diseases like Alzheimer's disease, astrocytes show prominent pathophysiological responses, often rather superficially described with the unifying terms astrogliosis or astrocyte reactivity. These responses share common features, but include also many distinct aspects in different CNS pathologies, and can have important protective or pathogenic consequences in these pathologies.

Therefore, understanding the precise mechanisms as how these responses are controlled and how they influence CNS development, homeostasis and pathology, is highly relevant for translational and clinical neuroscience.

A large spectrum of extracellular signals activating several intracellular signaling pathways regulates the pathophysiological responses of astrocytes. One central signaling hub integrating many of these extracellular signals is the IKK/NF-κB signaling pathway. A number of studies summarized here have established that the IKK/NF-κB pathway in astrocytes is a key regulator of neuroinflammatory responses. These studies also demonstrated that astroglial IKK/NF-κB activation interferes with normal CNS development and homeostasis and contributes to the pathogenesis of various CNS disorders in mouse models.

These findings have important implications for the development of new strategies for the treatment of CNS disorders. Although pharmacological targeting of the IKK/NF-κB pathway has proven to be difficult due to its broad spectrum of functions, it might be an option for some very specific conditions, where a transient inhibition of a particularly strong inflammatory response might be beneficial, for example, in acute stages of autoimmune disorders or injury. In addition, the further investigation of the effector pathways of IKK/NF-κB signaling in astrocytes will hopefully identify specific aspects of this broad response that can be targeted with more selective approaches. Such approaches could include, for example, the inhibition of specific chemokines or the complement system, the prevention of the morphological changes of astrocytes that might cause disruption of the blood-brain-barrier or neuronal support functions, or the restoration of neurotransmitter uptake by astrocytes. Another important, unsolved question is, in which conditions astroglial NF-κB activation is actually beneficial. In most conditions investigated so far, astroglial NF-κB activation seems to have detrimental effects, but as this response is evolutionary conserved, it should have beneficial effects in some circumstances. One could speculate that acute CNS infections might require astroglial NF-κB activation to allow a rapid and strong response to stop spreading of the pathogens and to allow their efficient clearance. However, this has not been experimentally demonstrated yet.

As only shortly summarized here, also other signaling pathways have important functions in the regulation of astroglial responses to pathological insults, which, except for JAK/STAT signaling, have received only relatively limited attention so far. The functions of these pathways in astrocytes should be investigated in more detail in future studies, and the functional interaction of these pathways with each other has to be elucidated. Manipulation of the balance of these pathways might allow to improve regenerative responses of astrocytes, as indicated, for example, by the detrimental versus beneficial roles of NF-κB and STAT3 signaling in astroglial scars for regeneration in spinal cord injury models.

Finally, the investigation of the mechanisms which regulate the only recently recognized neurogenic responses of astrocytes, offers an exciting perspective for regenerative medicine. It might uncover approaches to stimulate endogenous replacement of lost neurons, which is an important mechanism of CNS repair in lower vertebrates, but has been largely lost in mammals.

Author details

Michael Lattke[1]* and Thomas Wirth[2]

*Address all correspondence to: michael.lattke@crick.ac.uk

1 Neural Stem Cell Biology Lab, The Francis Crick Institute, London, UK

2 Institute of Physiological Chemistry, University of Ulm, Ulm, Germany

References

[1] Sofroniew MV, Vinters HV. Astrocytes: Biology and pathology. Acta Neuropathologica. 2010;**119**(1):7-35

[2] Gotz M et al. Reactive astrocytes as neural stem or progenitor cells: In vivo lineage, in vitro potential, and genome-wide expression analysis. Glia. 2015;**63**(8):1452-1468

[3] Sofroniew MV. Astrocyte barriers to neurotoxic inflammation. Nature Reviews. Neuroscience. 2015;**16**(5):249-263

[4] Allaman I, Belanger M, Magistretti PJ. Astrocyte-neuron metabolic relationships: For better and for worse. Trends in Neurosciences. 2011;**34**(2):76-87

[5] Farina C, Aloisi F, Meinl E. Astrocytes are active players in cerebral innate immunity. Trends in Immunology. 2007;**28**(3):138-145

[6] Colombo E, Farina C. Astrocytes: Key regulators of neuroinflammation. Trends in Immunology. 2016;**37**(9):608-620

[7] Ransohoff RM, Perry VH. Microglial physiology: Unique stimuli, specialized responses. Annual Review of Immunology. 2009;**27**:119-145

[8] Ransohoff RM, Brown MA. Innate immunity in the central nervous system. The Journal of Clinical Investigation. 2012;**122**(4):1164-1171

[9] Liddelow SA, Barres BA. Reactive astrocytes: Production, function, and therapeutic potential. Immunity. 2017;**46**(6):957-967

[10] Pekny M, Pekna M. Astrocyte reactivity and reactive astrogliosis: Costs and benefits. Physiological Reviews. 2014;**94**(4):1077-1098

[11] Frank-Cannon TC et al. Does neuroinflammation fan the flame in neurodegenerative diseases? Molecular Neurodegeneration. 2009;**4**:47

[12] Jha MK et al. Diverse functional roles of lipocalin-2 in the central nervous system. Neuroscience and Biobehavioral Reviews. 2015;**49**:135-156

[13] Stephan AH, Barres BA, Stevens B. The complement system: An unexpected role in synaptic pruning during development and disease. Annual Review of Neuroscience. 2012;**35**:369-389

[14] Dong Y, Benveniste EN. Immune function of astrocytes. Glia. 2001;**36**(2):180-190

[15] Carpentier PA et al. Differential activation of astrocytes by innate and adaptive immune stimuli. Glia. 2005;**49**(3):360-374

[16] Liddelow SA et al. Neurotoxic reactive astrocytes are induced by activated microglia. Nature. 2017;**541**(7638):481-487

[17] Prinz M, Priller J. Microglia and brain macrophages in the molecular age: From origin to neuropsychiatric disease. Nature Reviews. Neuroscience. 2014;**15**(5):300-312

[18] Tilleux S, Hermans E. Neuroinflammation and regulation of glial glutamate uptake in neurological disorders. Journal of Neuroscience Research. 2007;**85**(10):2059-2070

[19] Jukkola P, Gu C. Regulation of neurovascular coupling in autoimmunity to water and ion channels. Autoimmunity Reviews. 2015;**14**(3):258-267

[20] Anderson MA et al. Astrocyte scar formation aids central nervous system axon regeneration. Nature. 2016;**532**(7598):195-200

[21] Sirko S et al. Reactive glia in the injured brain acquire stem cell properties in response to sonic hedgehog. [corrected]. Cell Stem Cell. 2013;**12**(4):426-439

[22] Bush TG et al. Leukocyte infiltration, neuronal degeneration, and neurite outgrowth after ablation of scar-forming, reactive astrocytes in adult transgenic mice. Neuron. 1999;**23**(2):297-308

[23] Faulkner JR et al. Reactive astrocytes protect tissue and preserve function after spinal cord injury. The Journal of Neuroscience. 2004;**24**(9):2143-2155

[24] Buffo A et al. Origin and progeny of reactive gliosis: A source of multipotent cells in the injured brain. Proceedings of the National Academy of Sciences of the United States of America. 2008;**105**(9):3581-3586

[25] Magnusson JP et al. A latent neurogenic program in astrocytes regulated by Notch signaling in the mouse. Science. 2014;**346**(6206):237-241

[26] Nato G et al. Striatal astrocytes produce neuroblasts in an excitotoxic model of Huntington's disease. Development. 2015;**142**(5):840-845

[27] Zhang Q, Lenardo MJ, Baltimore D. 30 Years of NF-kappaB: A blossoming of relevance to human pathobiology. Cell. 2017;**168**(1-2):37-57

[28] Hayden MS, Ghosh S. NF-kappaB, the first quarter-century: Remarkable progress and outstanding questions. Genes & Development. 2012;**26**(3):203-234

[29] Ben-Neriah Y, Karin M. Inflammation meets cancer, with NF-kappaB as the matchmaker. Nature Immunology. 2011;**12**(8):715-723

[30] Dondelinger Y et al. Poly-ubiquitination in TNFR1-mediated necroptosis. Cellular and Molecular Life Sciences. 2016;**73**(11-12):2165-2176

[31] Cohen P, Strickson S. The role of hybrid ubiquitin chains in the MyD88 and other innate immune signalling pathways. Cell Death and Differentiation. 2017;**24**(7):1153-1159

[32] Oviedo-Boyso J, Bravo-Patino A, Baizabal-Aguirre VM. Collaborative action of toll-like and NOD-like receptors as modulators of the inflammatory response to pathogenic bacteria. Mediators of Inflammation. 2014;**2014**:432785

[33] Morgan MJ, Liu ZG. Crosstalk of reactive oxygen species and NF-kappaB signaling. Cell Research. 2011;**21**(1):103-115

[34] Gutierrez H, Davies AM. Regulation of neural process growth, elaboration and structural plasticity by NF-kappaB. Trends in Neurosciences. 2011;**34**(6):316-325

[35] Miyamoto S. Nuclear initiated NF-kappaB signaling: NEMO and ATM take center stage. Cell Research. 2011;**21**(1):116-130

[36] Gupta SC et al. Inhibiting NF-kappaB activation by small molecules as a therapeutic strategy. Biochimica et Biophysica Acta. 2010;**1799**(10-12):775-787

[37] Sadikot RT et al. Selective I kappa B kinase expression in airway epithelium generates neutrophilic lung inflammation. Journal of Immunology. 2003;**170**(2):1091-1098

[38] Aleksic T et al. Cellular immune reaction in the pancreas is induced by constitutively active IkappaB kinase-2. Gut. 2007;**56**(2):227-236

[39] Baumann B et al. Constitutive IKK2 activation in acinar cells is sufficient to induce pancreatitis in vivo. The Journal of Clinical Investigation. 2007;**117**(6):1502-1513

[40] Maier HJ et al. Cardiomyocyte-specific IkappaB kinase (IKK)/NF-kappaB activation induces reversible inflammatory cardiomyopathy and heart failure. Proceedings of the National Academy of Sciences of the United States of America. 2012;**109**(29):11794-11799

[41] Vlantis K et al. Constitutive IKK2 activation in intestinal epithelial cells induces intestinal tumors in mice. The Journal of Clinical Investigation. 2011;**121**(7):2781-2793

[42] Salem HH et al. Long-term IKK2/NF-kappaB signaling in pancreatic beta-cells induces immune-mediated diabetes. Diabetes. 2014;**63**(3):960-975

[43] Sunami Y et al. Hepatic activation of IKK/NFkappaB signaling induces liver fibrosis via macrophage-mediated chronic inflammation. Hepatology. 2012;**56**(3):1117-1128

[44] Herrmann O et al. IKK mediates ischemia-induced neuronal death. Nature Medicine. 2005;**11**(12):1322-1329

[45] van Loo G et al. Inhibition of transcription factor NF-kappaB in the central nervous system ameliorates autoimmune encephalomyelitis in mice. Nature Immunology. 2006;**7**(9):954-961

[46] Kaltschmidt B, Kaltschmidt C. NF-KappaB in long-term memory and structural plasticity in the adult mammalian brain. Frontiers in Molecular Neuroscience. 2015;**8**:69

[47] Maqbool A et al. Sustained, neuron-specific IKK/NF-kappaB activation generates a selective neuroinflammatory response promoting local neurodegeneration with aging. Molecular Neurodegeneration. 2013;**8**:40

[48] Schmeisser MJ et al. IkappaB kinase/nuclear factor kappaB-dependent insulin-like growth factor 2 (Igf2) expression regulates synapse formation and spine maturation via Igf2 receptor signaling. The Journal of Neuroscience. 2012;**32**(16):5688-5703

[49] Lampron A, Elali A, Rivest S. Innate immunity in the CNS: Redefining the relationship between the CNS and its environment. Neuron. 2013;**78**(2):214-232

[50] Santello M, Volterra A. TNFalpha in synaptic function: Switching gears. Trends in Neurosciences. 2012;**35**(10):638-647

[51] Gveric D et al. Transcription factor NF-kappaB and inhibitor I kappaBalpha are localized in macrophages in active multiple sclerosis lesions. Journal of Neuropathology and Experimental Neurology. 1998;**57**(2):168-178

[52] Nonaka M et al. Prolonged activation of NF-kappaB following traumatic brain injury in rats. Journal of Neurotrauma. 1999;**16**(11):1023-1034

[53] Swarup V et al. Deregulation of TDP-43 in amyotrophic lateral sclerosis triggers nuclear factor kappaB-mediated pathogenic pathways. The Journal of Experimental Medicine. 2011;**208**(12):2429-2447

[54] Hsiao HY et al. A critical role of astrocyte-mediated nuclear factor-kappaB-dependent inflammation in Huntington's disease. Human Molecular Genetics. 2013;**22**(9):1826-1842

[55] Young AM et al. Aberrant NF-kappaB expression in autism spectrum condition: A mechanism for neuroinflammation. Frontiers in Psychiatry. 2011;**2**:27

[56] Brambilla R et al. Inhibition of astroglial nuclear factor kappaB reduces inflammation and improves functional recovery after spinal cord injury. The Journal of Experimental Medicine. 2005;**202**(1):145-156

[57] Lattke M et al. Nuclear factor kappaB activation impairs ependymal ciliogenesis and links neuroinflammation to hydrocephalus formation. The Journal of Neuroscience. 2012;**32**(34):11511-11523

[58] Lattke M et al. Transient IKK2 activation in astrocytes initiates selective non-cell-autonomous neurodegeneration. Molecular Neurodegeneration. 2017;**12**(1):16

[59] Lian H et al. IkappaBalpha deficiency in brain leads to elevated basal neuroinflammation and attenuated response following traumatic brain injury: Implications for functional recovery. Molecular Neurodegeneration. 2012;**7**:47

[60] Brambilla R et al. Transgenic inhibition of astroglial NF-kappa B improves functional outcome in experimental autoimmune encephalomyelitis by suppressing chronic central nervous system inflammation. Journal of Immunology. 2009;**182**(5):2628-2640

[61] Brambilla R et al. Astrocytes play a key role in EAE pathophysiology by orchestrating in the CNS the inflammatory response of resident and peripheral immune cells and by suppressing remyelination. Glia. 2014;**62**(3):452-467

[62] Dvoriantchikova G et al. Inactivation of astroglial NF-kappa B promotes survival of retinal neurons following ischemic injury. The European Journal of Neuroscience. 2009;**30**(2):175-185

[63] Brambilla R et al. Transgenic inhibition of astroglial NF-kappaB protects from optic nerve damage and retinal ganglion cell loss in experimental optic neuritis. Journal of Neuroinflammation. 2012;**9**:213

[64] Oeckl P et al. Astrocyte-specific IKK2 activation in mice is sufficient to induce neuroinflammation but does not increase susceptibility to MPTP. Neurobiology of Disease. 2012;**48**(3):481-487

[65] Stolp HB, Dziegielewska KM. Review: Role of developmental inflammation and blood-brain barrier dysfunction in neurodevelopmental and neurodegenerative diseases. Neuropathology and Applied Neurobiology. 2009;**35**(2):132-146

[66] Tsutsui Y, Kosugi I, Kawasaki H. Neuropathogenesis in cytomegalovirus infection: Indication of the mechanisms using mouse models. Reviews in Medical Virology. 2005;**15**(5):327-345

[67] Bracchi-Ricard V et al. Astroglial nuclear factor-kappaB regulates learning and memory and synaptic plasticity in female mice. Journal of Neurochemistry. 2008;**104**(3):611-623

[68] Zhang Y et al. Astrocytic process plasticity and IKKbeta/NF-kappaB in central control of blood glucose, blood pressure, and body weight. Cell Metabolism. 2017;**25**(5): 1091-1102 e4

[69] Custer SK et al. Bergmann glia expression of polyglutamine-expanded ataxin-7 produces neurodegeneration by impairing glutamate transport. Nature Neuroscience. 2006;**9**(10):1302-1311

[70] Lian H et al. NFkappaB-activated astroglial release of complement C3 compromises neuronal morphology and function associated with Alzheimer's disease. Neuron. 2015;**85**(1): 101-115

[71] Brambilla R et al. Transgenic inhibition of astroglial NF-kappa B leads to increased axonal sparing and sprouting following spinal cord injury. Journal of Neurochemistry. 2009;**110**(2):765-778

[72] Wang X et al. Astrocytic A20 ameliorates experimental autoimmune encephalomyelitis by inhibiting NF-kappaB- and STAT1-dependent chemokine production in astrocytes. Acta Neuropathologica. 2013;**126**(5):711-724

[73] Raasch J et al. IkappaB kinase 2 determines oligodendrocyte loss by non-cell-autonomous activation of NF-kappaB in the central nervous system. Brain. 2011;**134**(Pt 4):1184-1198

[74] Barakat DJ et al. Astroglial NF-kappaB mediates oxidative stress by regulation of NADPH oxidase in a model of retinal ischemia reperfusion injury. Journal of Neurochemistry. 2012;**120**(4):586-597

[75] Zhang W et al. Neuronal activation of NF-kappaB contributes to cell death in cerebral ischemia. Journal of Cerebral Blood Flow and Metabolism. 2005;**25**(1):30-40

[76] Jayakumar AR et al. NF-kappaB in the mechanism of brain edema in acute liver failure: Studies in transgenic mice. Neurobiology of Disease. 2011;**41**(2):498-507

[77] Crosio C et al. Astroglial inhibition of NF-kappaB does not ameliorate disease onset and progression in a mouse model for amyotrophic lateral sclerosis (ALS). PLoS One. 2011;**6**(3):e17187

[78] Ceyzeriat K et al. The complex STATes of astrocyte reactivity: How are they controlled by the JAK-STAT3 pathway? Neuroscience. 2016;**330**:205-218

[79] Namihira M, Nakashima K. Mechanisms of astrocytogenesis in the mammalian brain. Current Opinion in Neurobiology. 2013;**23**(6):921-927

[80] Koyama Y. Signaling molecules regulating phenotypic conversions of astrocytes and glial scar formation in damaged nerve tissues. Neurochemistry International. 2014;**78**:35-42

[81] Laywell ED et al. Identification of a multipotent astrocytic stem cell in the immature and adult mouse brain. Proceedings of the National Academy of Sciences of the United States of America. 2000;**97**(25):13883-13888

[82] Hasel P et al. Neurons and neuronal activity control gene expression in astrocytes to regulate their development and metabolism. Nature Communications. 2017;**8**:15132

[83] Ehm O et al. RBPJkappa-dependent signaling is essential for long-term maintenance of neural stem cells in the adult hippocampus. The Journal of Neuroscience. 2010;**30**(41): 13794-13807

Chapter 3

Evidence that Astroglia Influence Dendrite Morphogenesis and Synaptogenesis Independently in the Vertebrate Central Nervous System

Christopher S. Wallace and Ginger S. Withers

Additional information is available at the end of the chapter

http://dx.doi.org/10.5772/intechopen.73891

Abstract

In the absence of external spatial cues, dendritic arbors of neurons grown *in vitro* approximate those observed *in situ*. Absent, however, from these culture models is patterned orientation of dendritic trunks, and variation of branch geometry that provide identifiable characteristics of the cytoarchitecture of the intact brain. Although astroglia are present during key stages of dendritic development *in vivo*, little is known about whether local interactions with glia shape dendritic growth. Astroglial cells are good candidates for this kind of regulation because they can exert control over the formation of synapses, an event correlated with the maturational state of the dendrite. The present review highlights some key findings from vertebrate model systems offering evidence that astroglia can contribute to the shape, and growth, of the dendritic arbor. Drawing from our recent work using a co-culture system composed of neurons growing in differential contact with astroglia, we discuss findings that suggest: 1) growth of dendrites, and addition of synapses, can be independent; further, while astroglia promote synapse formation, they inhibit dendritic growth; 2) astroglia mediate dendrite growth through both paracrine, and contact-dependent mechanisms; and 3) astroglia appear to impose pattern by constraining the growth of dendrites within their zones of influence.

Keywords: dendrite morphogenesis, neuron-astroglia interactions, dendritic development, dendritic patterning, dendritic growth

1. Introduction

The size and shape of the dendritic arbor is a key factor in determining the connective potential of a neuron. While programs intrinsic to the neuron itself can instruct the general morphology of the dendritic arbor [1], it has long been recognized that the form dendrites take as they mature is under significant influence from extrinsic factors [2, 3]. The complexity of extrinsic influences, and the collective impact they have upon dendritic architecture, is evident when one compares the spatial patterning of dendritic arbors that have developed *in situ*, or within a tissue context, against those that form *in vitro*, largely deprived of patterned contact with other cells (e.g., see **Figure 1**). Although the importance of identifying and understanding how such extrinsic influences work has been recognized by neuroscientists for decades, relating specific influences to specific aspects of dendritic morphogenesis has proven challenging.

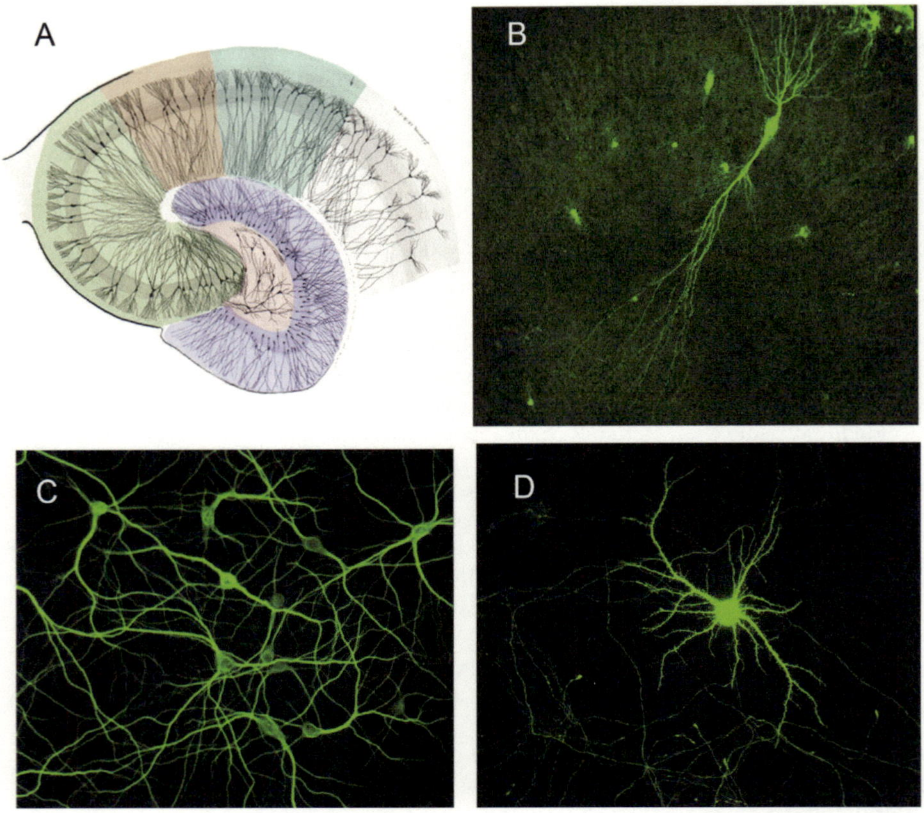

Figure 1. Comparing hippocampal pyramidal neurons grown under different conditions can help distinguish intrinsically determined features of the dendritic arbor from those under extracellular control. (A) Camera lucida drawing of the dendritic arbors of pyramidal neurons of the CA fields of the hippocampus and granule cells of the dentate gyrus, based on Golgi-Cox impregnation of an adult rat (modified from [4]). The dendritic arbor has pronounced apical and basilar domains that are physically segregated and oriented in opposite directions. (B) A hippocampal neuron labeled by biolistic transfection of eGFP in an organotypic slice culture from rat. (C) Dissociated hippocampal neurons growing in primary culture, immunostained with MAP2 to reveal the dendritic arbors of the neurons present in the field of view. (D) An individual cultured neuron, labeled by transfection with eGFP, from within a similarly dense field of neurons (unstained) as in (C). Based on the shape of the soma, and orientation of the primary dendrites, the major dendrite that points toward the upper left of the frame might be a candidate "apical" dendrite.

But while fundamental questions remain, new tools are being brought to bear in this area of active investigation, and a series of insights have unfolded over the last decade. For example, interactions within, and between, neurons are one important source of cues involved in ontogenesis of the dendritic arbor. The mechanism of "self-avoidance" between dendrites within a given arbor can help establish appropriate spacing of branches (for review, see [5]). Similarly, segregation of branch territories has also been recognized as important in understanding how the dendritic arbors of a single type, or class, of neuron within a brain region are arranged in a territorial configuration. Such an arrangement optimizes dendritic capture of incoming afferents and is now understood at a mechanistic level [6, 7]. It is hard to envision how these homotypic mechanisms contribute to the cases where branching pattern and density vary stereotypically along a single primary stalk of the arbor, however.

The hypothesis that astrocytes might also shape dendrites has received less attention. In 2010, Procko and Shaham proposed that glial cells might play such a role, although, at that time, direct evidence in vertebrate systems was lacking [8]. Mounting evidence, however, demonstrated that interactions between neurons and astroglia were crucial to other aspects of dendritic development [9–11]. Astroglia secrete factors that facilitate synapse formation, both in terms of the onset [12–16] and of rate [17, 18]. Because immature dendrites are not receptive to innervation [19], these synaptogenic effects could imply an astroglial contribution to dendrite maturation. In addition, astroglia produce factors that modulate synaptic efficacy [20] and regulate synapse pruning [21]. Moreover, a number of growth factors have been identified that selectively alter dendritic, but not axonal growth, of forebrain neurons, e.g., [22, 23] and these factors may be produced, or regulated by astroglia [24, 25]. Collectively, these findings point toward mechanisms whereby astroglia could influence the competence, or developmental state, of the dendrite. It is therefore becoming increasingly important to characterize these effects in more detail so as to determine the roles of astroglia as regulators of synapse formation versus sculptors of dendritic arbor size and shape.

In this regard, data from two human neurodevelopmental disorders, Rett Syndrome and Fragile X mental retardation, implicate astroglia as a regulatory influence on the growth of dendrites [26, 27]. In Rett Syndrome, single-gene mutations in the X-linked transcription factor methyl-CpG-binding protein 2 (*MeCP2*) are associated with infant death in males, while females begin to display signs of mental retardation, autism, and epilepsy between 6 and 18 months of age [28], coincident with the time when dendritic outgrowth is most robust. Mutations in the fragile X mental retardation 1 gene (*Fmr1*) cause similar cognitive and behavioral impairments, and individuals with Fragile X have abnormal dendrites [29]. Isolating how interactions between different cell types bearing the gene mutations could produce defects in dendritic development *in vivo* is difficult, such that *in vitro* models can be the best option for screening for effects of specific interaction between identified cell types. Accordingly, when wild-type neurons were co-cultured with astroglial cells bearing mutations in *MeCP2*, or *Fmr1*, they showed altered dendritic development. These are effects that would have been difficult to detect and attribute directly to astroglia, using *in situ* analyses of tissue from the transgenic animals. It is noteworthy that much of what we know about the development of dendrites has, in fact, been learned using *in vitro* models (for example, see [30–33]). The power of these models is that they permit direct microscopic observation and enable manipulation of the extent to which neurons can interact dynamically with astrocytes as they form dendrites.

2. Dendritic arbors of isolated neurons grown *in vitro* exhibit features that are intrinsically determined and lack those features patterned by extrinsic influences

The first microscopic views of the intact hippocampus, impregnated with Golgi stain, illustrated the extent to which dendritic arborization is patterned (**Figure 1A**). This distinctly polarized arbor, with zonal variation in branching pattern, also forms in organotypic slice cultures, a method that preserves some populations of afferents, astroglia, and microglia [34] as dendritic outgrowth and maturation takes place [35]. In contrast, dissociated cultures of hippocampal neurons isolated from embryonic rat brain remove spatial cues that come from organized inputs and contain predominantly neurons with an excitatory phenotype. These cells generate MAP2 positive dendritic arbors that proceed to form post-synaptic specializations expected of pyramidal cells *in vivo* [31]. Thus, an advantage of this *in vitro* model is that the developmental trajectory parallels development in the intact neuropil [23, 30]. And because they grow at low density while flat on a coverslip, benchmarks of morphological maturation can be readily observed and quantified. For example, processes become tapered and generate spines (see **Figure 1C** and **D**). Despite the physical isolation of these neurons, the dendritic arbors that form sometimes have a prominent dendrite that is somewhat thicker and distinct from the other dendrites that form off of the cell body, suggesting a rudimentary form of an apical dendrite. By comparing dendritic architecture of hippocampal pyramidal neurons from the intact brain, slice cultures, and dissociated neurons, we can separate basic features of the dendritic arbor that are expressed robustly across this range of extracellular contexts and therefore likely intrinsically determined from those features that require extracellular influences to be expressed.

3. Both the presence of astroglia and factors derived from astroglia alter the spatial patterning of dendritic arbors grown *in vitro*

3.1. Effects produced by secreted, soluble factors present in media conditioned by astroglia

In vitro approaches to studying neuron development were transformed when Gary Banker reported a new method that allowed dissociated embryonic hippocampal neurons from the rat to be grown on glass using defined serum-free medium [36]. There was one telling technical detail, however: long-term survival of neurons required astroglial cells to be present in the culture, although not in direct physical contact with neurons. In fact, these cultures were typically prepared with the astroglial cells grown as a separate monolayer culture on the bottom of the culture dish, while the neuronal cultures were grown on glass coverslips that were several millimeters away. These observations revealed that astroglia secreted trophic factors upon which the viability of neurons depended. Other data suggested that astroglia enabled more than just survival. Sympathetic ganglion cells, for example, formed axons readily *in vitro*, but dendrites could only be produced in the presence of glia [37]. The dendrite-specific factor necessary for this polarized outgrowth was later identified as BMP-7 [38].

Further evidence of the importance of developmental cross-talk between astroglia and dendritic morphogenesis emerged. Astroglia native to the cortex promoted dendrite formation of cortical neurons more effectively than astroglia from other regions of the brain [39–42]. These studies supported the hypothesis that astroglia could influence dendritic growth in a brain-region specific manner. Taken together, these findings suggest that the developmental interactions between astroglia and the forming dendritic arbor might be multiple and significant.

It was in this context that we sought to observe dendritogenesis *in vitro*, while controlling the extent to which developing neurons were exposed to astroglial cells. As a first step, cohorts of neurons were grown for several days under two conditions: in medium that had been conditioned by brief exposure to astroglia (24 h or less) versus in co-culture with a feeder layer of astroglia continuously present but with neurons isolated from physical contact. Neurons grown in conditioned medium formed dendritic arbors but did not form synaptic contacts. Conversely, sibling neurons grown with astroglia continuously present (yet not in direct contact) formed dendrites that displayed presynaptic contacts (**Figure 2**) [43]. Given previous reports that astroglia produced factors essential for synapse formation in retinal ganglion cells (reviewed in [44]) and in hippocampal neurons [17], the failure of synapses to form in glial-deprived cultures was not surprising.

What was unexpected, however, was that the dendritic arbors that formed in the glial-deprived neuron cultures were more extensive than those of neurons grown in an astroglial co-culture,

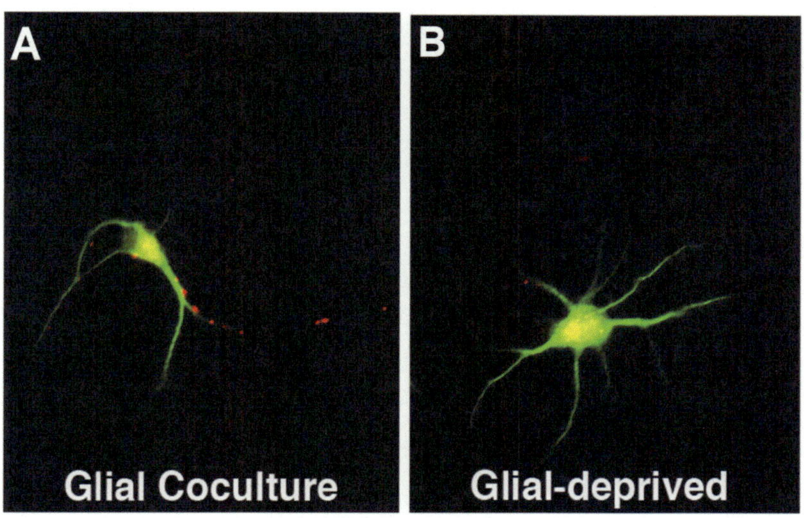

Figure 2. Dendritic arbors of neurons that are glial-deprived are more extensive but have few presynaptic contacts (B), compared to those co-cultured with astroglia (A). MAP2-stained dendrites are green, Synapsin1 puncta, representing presynaptic contacts, are red. Modified from Withers et al. [43].

with significantly more primary and higher-order branches [43]. These findings revealed that astroglia exert two effects on dendritic development that seem paradoxical. On the one hand, astroglia were permissive to synapse formation, and on the other hand, their presence limited dendritic outgrowth. A similar inhibitory effect by astroglia has been reported to occur in brain stem neurons *in vitro* [45] and the enabling effects of astroglia on synapses formation have been characterized in detail (see references above).

Thrombospondin (TSP) is the synaptogenic factor that is produced by astroglia and promotes the formation of presynaptic contacts onto dendrites both *in vitro* and *in vivo* [14]. Thus, in the glial-deprived paradigm, a straightforward prediction was that if TSP was added, the neurons growing under glial deprivation would form presynaptic contacts. They did. A second prediction could also be made: if TSP mediated the astroglial restriction of dendrite outgrowth as well, then those same neurons would be expected to have arbors that would be reduced in size compared with glial-deprived neurons not exposed to TSP. Instead, glial-deprived neurons + TSP still had dendritic arbors that were significantly larger than those growing in the presence of astroglia, and after 48 h of exposure, they were even greater than those growing under glial deprivation without TSP. A simple interpretation of these data is that the astroglia effects on dendritic growth are separate from the effects produced by TSP. The selective effects of TSP seem to suggest a mechanistic dissociation between the inhibition of dendritic growth and the formation of synapses.

3.2. Effects mediated by local contact between astroglia and neurons

Co-plating neurons and astroglia on the same coverslip offers opportunities for local interaction between the two cell types that could involve signals both soluble and contact-dependent. In our work, we have observed that neurons in full contact with astroglia had dendritic arbors with reduced size compared with neurons that did not contact astroglia at all. These effects could be mediated by the same mechanism as described earlier, but given that the neuron has

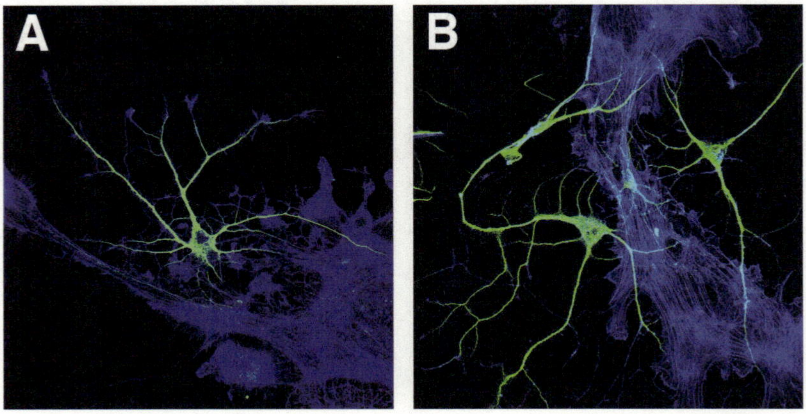

Figure 3. Asymmetry of dendritic arbors in partial contact with astroglia (A and B). The dendritic arbors are revealed by MAP2 immunostaining (green). Polymerized actin, stained with fluorescently conjugated phalloidin (blue), highlights astroglia, as well as growth cones at the tips of dendrites.

grown while adhering to an astroglial island, it seems very likely that the signal(s) originated from the astroglial cell on which it resided. The interesting case comes when physical contact is limited, when a neuron straddles an astroglial cell, such that part of the growing arbor touches and part does not (**Figure 3**). When in partial contact, the dendritic arbor forms asymmetrically, with the most extensive arborization not in direct contact. One interpretation of this biased growth is that it is the product of an interplay between the action of soluble factors produced by astroglia and a separate inhibition of growth when dendrites are in direct contact with the surface of astroglial cells.

4. If astrocytes sculpt dendrites *in vitro*, might they also influence dendrite arbor shape *in vivo*?

In vivo, the onset of astrogliogenesis occurs before robust dendritic outgrowth begins and immediately precedes peak synaptogenesis in the hippocampus [46–51]. For humans and nonhuman primates, the dendritic arbors of forebrain neurons take years to reach their full extent [52]. Dendritic development in rats is similarly protracted, with the elaboration of branches and the addition of synaptic contacts upon them occurring over weeks [53, 54]. This timing makes astroglia good candidates for secreting signals and providing physical cues to guide dendrite growth. Clues to the role astroglia might play *in vivo* could come from analyzing their spatial relationships with dendrites in mature tissue (see **Figures 4** and **5**) and the temporal sequence by which these relationships arise during development.

The effects of physical contact between a dendritic branch and astroglia *in vitro* provide an example of how functional domains within the dendritic field might be organized, at least in part, based on cross-talk between a specific dendritic branch and a neighboring glial cell. In support of this hypothesis, within intact neuropil, individual astroglia are arranged in non-overlapping territories that occupy a fraction of the dendritic arbor of an individual principal neuron [56]. Stains that identify dendrites and astroglia in tissue show their interwoven relationship (see **Figure 4A**, **C**, and **D**). Further, the spatial domain of a single astrocyte contacts synapses of multiple neurons [57], with fine processes extending dynamically to make physical contact at individual synapses [58]. There is an extensive literature documenting astroglial-synapse interactions that is well beyond the scope of this chapter, see [59]. These data fit well with the growing recognition that astroglia may contribute to the construction and function of cortical circuits and maps, physically defining and coordinating synaptic territories [60–62]. Further, dendrite-astroglia interactions during development could help to scale the growth of a synaptic network to match the available nutritional network [63], similar to the mechanisms involved in building the retina [64]. Control over dendrite arbor shape could be an important part of these mechanisms.

The arbors of pyramidal neurons in hippocampal subfield CA1 offer a useful model because this population of cells has elaborate arbors, yet the arrangement of arbor branches repeats with striking regularity (see **Figure 4B**). The story of how this pattern of arborization arises

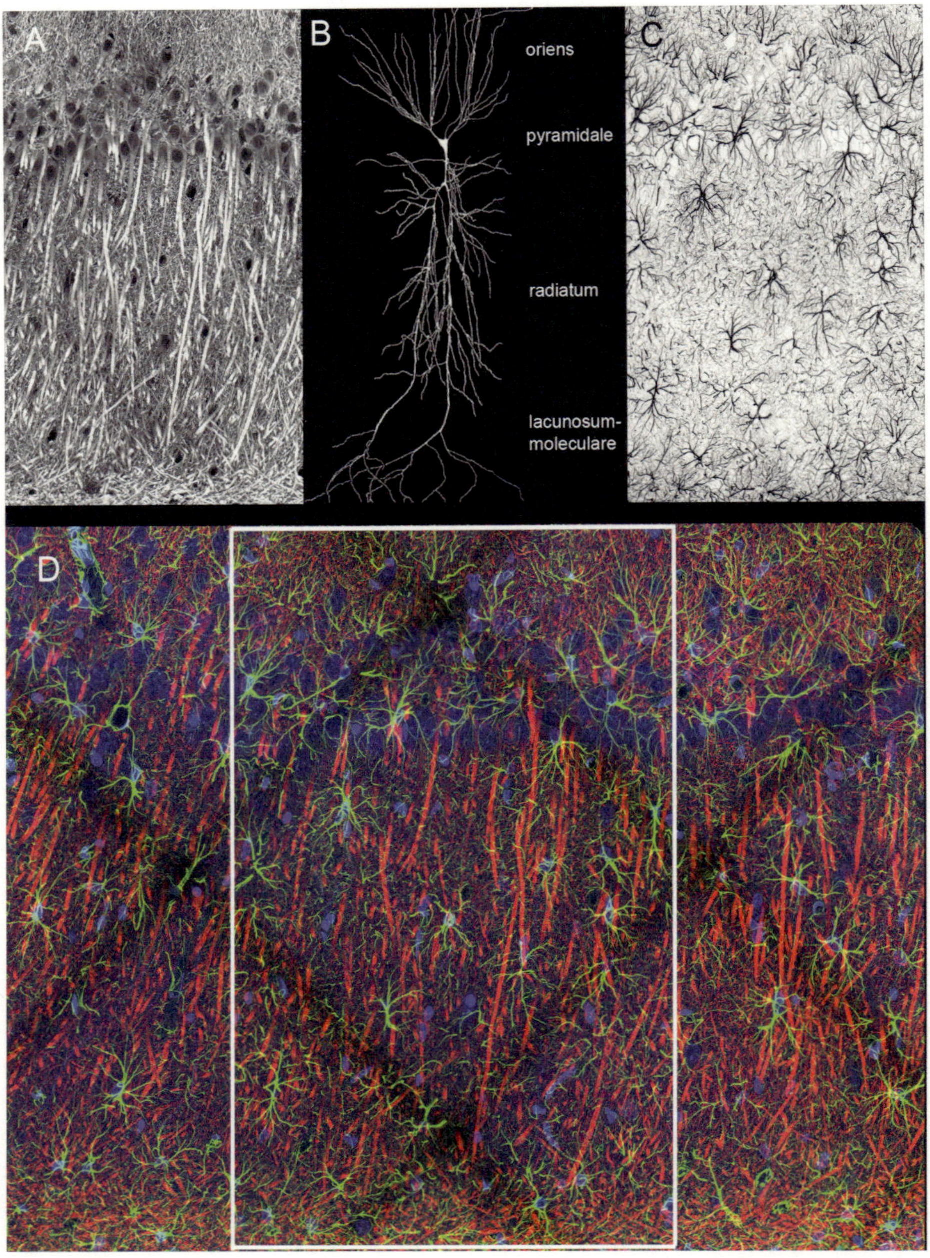

Figure 4. Cytoarchitecture of the CA1 field of the hippocampal formation from rat brain illustrates laminar variation in dendritic branching and astrocyte morphology. (A) Immunostaining for the dendritic marker MAP2. (B) The dendritic arbor of a typical CA1 (modified from [55]). (C) Immunostaining for the astrocytic marker GFAP from the same region as (A). (D) The colorized overlay, with dendrites in red, astroglia in green, and nuclei in blue. The white box surrounds the field shown in panels and (C). The field within which dendrites develop is tessellated with astroglia: the size of individual astrocytic territories is appropriate to exert local influences on a sub-laminar scale, and the astrocytes themselves appear to show cytoarchitectural variations across laminae.

in development is summarized nicely by Pokorny and Yamamoto [35]. In that report, dendrite branching and elongation, as measured in Golgi-impregnated pyramidal cells, was not synchronous but rather followed a distinct sequence. For example, the apical dendrite

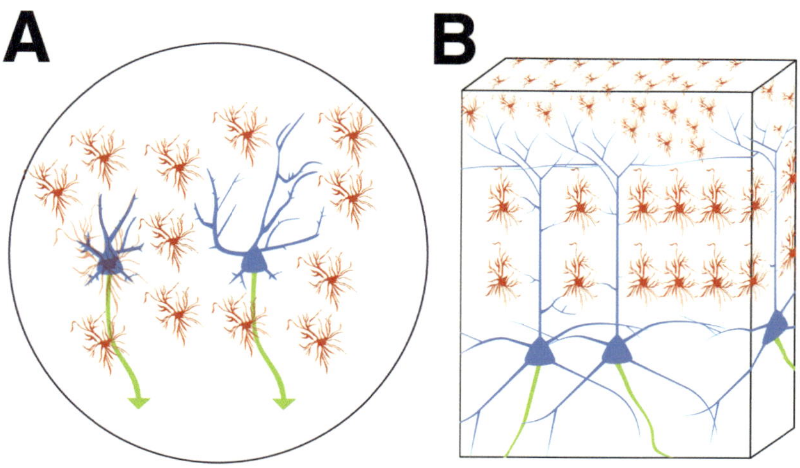

Figure 5. Illustration of how differential contact between astroglia and neurons can contribute to patterns of dendritic arborization. (A) Dendritic arbors of neurons grown *in vitro* are inhibited by contact with astroglia. (B) Dendritic arbors of CA1 hippocampal neurons show varied branching across laminae, coincident with changes in the distribution, and size, of astroglia. Astroglia, red; dendrites, blue; axons, green.

extended nearly to its mature length by postnatal day (P)10, but the lateral branches along the apical shaft had only extended a minor fraction of their mature length. There was also a temporal separation when these lateral branches formed. The number of lateral branches that arose from the apical shaft within the proximal stratum radiatum peaked at P15, whereas more distally, the number continued to be added out to P48. These zones within stratum radiatum correspond to afferent inputs from associative and commissural fibers (proximal stratum radiatum) and Schaffer collaterals (distal stratum radiatum). Branching within stratum lacunosum-moleculare, originating from the most distal portions of the apical dendrite, did not peak until after P48 and appeared to be more pronounced in the preterminal branches. The availability of afferents, which enter during embryonic development (for a review, see [65]), could be an important source of cues for dendritic development.

During the time frame when CA1 pyramidal cells are growing dendrites, astroglial cells in this region go through a number of transitions in number, and structure, that could be meaningful for establishing arbor pattern. Though relatively sparse before P10, astrocytes are present at the time when the apical dendrite is forming, and during the first 2 weeks of postnatal development, astroglia extend long filopodia-like processes [66]. An intriguing possibility is that during early stages of dendritic branch formation, the long filopodial extensions on glia serve a function related to branch formation or guidance, analogous to the guidance processes extended by radial glial cells. By the time astroglia begin to extend elaborate spongiform processes more characteristic of mature astroglia, the architecture of the arbor has been established, although branch growth continues beyond P30, when astrocytes have established nonoverlapping territories characteristic of mature neuropil [66].

Striking changes in the shape or spatial orientation of astroglia also accompany the most active periods of dendritic branch formation and growth. Astroglia are initially spherical but take on a polarized shape with development [66, 67]. In the stratum radiatum, this shape change is oriented perpendicularly to the cell body layer, stratum pyramidale. In the stratum lacunosum-moleculare, the astroglia are elongated parallel to the cell body layer [67]. Coincidentally, this is the zone of the apical dendritic arbor that shows the most prominent lateral spread.

In vitro, local encounters between growing dendrites and astroglial cells can exert significant biases in the spatial patterning of the arbor. We have observed long filopodial-like processes extending from astroglia that resemble those reported in developing tissue *in vivo* (see the earlier section). These extensions could provide a mechanism for spatial capture of dendrites [43]. Time-lapse recordings of living cells have shown that, although slow growing, dendritic branches are dynamic structures that extend and retract growth cones and various forms of filopodia [68–70] (Withers and Wallace, unpublished observations). Cycles of extension and retraction create the opportunity for multiple physical or molecular interactions between these two cell types, analogous to neuron-astroglia interactions that occur during neuron migration [71, 72]. Collectively, such interactions could determine the trajectory of dendritic branch growth in three-dimensional space.

Comparison of dendritic arbors of neurons and arrangement of astrocytic processes in neuropil suggests that the structures of these two cell types co-vary in a nonrandom manner (see **Figure 4**). Such a view, however, only begins to represent more nuanced phenotypic heterogeneity of astroglia based on patterns of gene expression that are of emerging importance in current research, for review, see [73]. Likewise, these kinds of analyses only begin to disclose the developmental shifts in phenotype of astrocytes across lamina that may accompany distinct stages of dendritic branch formation. Such shifts appear to occur. As early as P8, GFAP-positive astroglia are densely arranged in the stratum lacunosum-moleculare, while remaining comparatively sparse in the stratum radiatum [67]. Additionally, two different transporters for glutamate show a different time course of expression and distinctive localization in different populations of astroglia in the developing hippocampus [48]. While such complexities are far from resolved, there is enough data available, we argue, to make the case that (1) patterning of dendritic branches is subject to the influence of astroglia and that (2) this relatively neglected developmental effect is distinct from the actively studied influences on synapse formation. The purpose of this chapter was to build on the hypothesis proposed by Procko and Shaham [8] by adding supporting evidence based on direct analysis of dendritic arbor formation in principle neurons of the central nervous system. Both the documented impact of astrocytes on dendritic arbor formation *in vitro*, and the fact that astrocytes are present but distributed differentially, during the extended period of dendritic outgrowth *in vivo*, support the argument that astrocytes could be a key part of the network of extrinsic influences that locally refines dendritic arbor geometry during development.

Acknowledgements

This work was supported by funding from NIH 1R15HD061831 and NSF DBI-1039958 and a generous gift to Whitman College from the family of Dr. Robert F. Welty. We thank the many undergraduate students who have contributed to the research findings described here and NoahLani Litwinsella for the artwork in **Figure 5**.

Author details

Christopher S. Wallace and Ginger S. Withers*

*Address all correspondence to: wallaccs@whitman.edu

Department of Biology, Whitman College, Walla Walla, WA, USA

References

[1] Banker G, Waxman A. Hippocampal neurons generate natural shapes in cell culture. In: Lasek RJ, Black MM, editors. Intrinsic Determinants of Neuronal Form and Function. New York: Alan R Liss; 1988;61-82

[2] Hillman D. Parameters of dendritic shape and substructure: Intrinsic and extrinsic determination. In: Lasek RJ, Black MM, editors. Intrinsic Determinants of Neuronal Form and Function. New York: Alan R Liss; 1988;83-113

[3] Hillman D. Neuronal shape parameters and substructures as a basis of neuronal form. The Neurosciences, Fourth Study Program. 1979;477-498

[4] Larriva-Sahd JA. Some predictions of Rafael Lorente de No 80 years later. Frontiers in Neuroanatomy. 2014;**8**:147

[5] Lefebvre JL, Sanes JR, Kay JN. Development of dendritic form and function. Annual Review of Cell and Developmental Biology. 2015;**31**:741-777

[6] Grueber WB, Sagasti A. Self-avoidance and tiling: Mechanisms of dendrite and axon spacing. Cold Spring Harbor Perspectives in Biology. 2010;**2**(9):a001750

[7] Petrovic M, Schmucker D. Axonal wiring in neural development: Target-independent mechanisms help to establish precision and complexity. BioEssays. 2015;**37**(9):996-1004

[8] Procko C, Shaham S. Assisted morphogenesis: Glial control of dendrite shapes. Current Opinion in Cell Biology. 2010;**22**(5):560-565

[9] Corty MM, Cell FMR. Biology in neuroscience: Architects in neural circuit design: Glia control neuron numbers and connectivity. The Journal of Cell Biology. 2013;**203**(3): 395-405

[10] Shao Z, Watanabe S, Christensen R, Jorgensen EM, Colon-Ramos DA. Synapse location during growth depends on glia location. Cell. 2013;**154**(2):337-350

[11] Clarke LE, Barres BA. Emerging roles of astrocytes in neural circuit development. Nature Reviews. Neuroscience. 2013;**14**(5):311-321

[12] Mauch DH, Nagler K, Schumacher S, Goritz C, Muller EC, Otto A, et al. CNS synaptogenesis promoted by glia-derived cholesterol. Science. 2001;**294**(5545):1354-1357

[13] Ullian EM, Harris BT, Wu A, Chan JR, Barres BA. Schwann cells and astrocytes induce synapse formation by spinal motor neurons in culture. Molecular and Cellular Neurosciences. 2004;**25**(2):241-251

[14] Christopherson KS, Ullian EM, Stokes CCA, Mullowney CE, Hell JW, Agah A, et al. Thrombospondins are astrocyte-secreted proteins that promote CNS synaptogenesis. Cell. 2005;**120**(3):421-433

[15] Eroglu C, Barres BA. Regulation of synaptic connectivity by glia. Nature. 2010;**468**(7321): 223-231

[16] Hughes EG, Elmariah SB, Balice-Gordon RJ. Astrocyte secreted proteins selectively increase hippocampal GABAergic axon length, branching, and synaptogenesis. Molecular and Cellular Neurosciences. 2010;**43**(1):136-145

[17] Barker AJ, Koch SM, Reed J, Barres BA, Ullian EM. Developmental control of synaptic receptivity. The Journal of Neuroscience. 2008;**28**(33):8150-8160

[18] Hama H, Hara C, Yamaguchi K, Miyawaki A. PKC signaling mediates global enhancement of excitatory synaptogenesis in neurons triggered by local contact with astrocytes. Neuron. 2004;**41**(3):405-415

[19] Fletcher T, DeCamilli P, Synaptogenesis BG. In hippocampal cultures: Evidence indicating the axons and dendrites become competent to form synapses at different stages of neuronal development. The Journal of Neuroscience. 1994;**14**(11):6695-6706

[20] Stellwagen D, Malenka RC. Synaptic scaling mediated by glial TNF-α. Nature. 2006; **440**(7087):1054-1059

[21] Stevens B, Allen NJ, Vazquez LE, Howell GR, Christopherson KS, Nouri N, et al. The classical complement cascade mediates CNS synapse elimination. Cell. 2007;**131**(6):1164-1178

[22] McAllister AK. Cellular and molecular mechanisms of dendrite growth. Cerebral Cortex. 2000;**10**(10):963-973

[23] Withers GS, Higgins D, Charette M, Banker G. Bone morphogenetic protein-7 enhances dendritic growth and receptivity to innervation in cultured hippocampal neurons. The European Journal of Neuroscience. 2000;**12**(1):106-116

[24] Corty MM, Freeman MR. Architects in neural circuit design: Glia control neuron numbers and connectivity. Journal of Cell Biology. 2013;**203**(3):395-405

[25] Yang Q, Feng B, Zhang K, Guo Y-Y, Liu S-B, Wu Y-M, et al. Excessive astrocyte-derived neurotrophin-3 contributes to the abnormal neuronal dendritic development in a mouse model of fragile X syndrome. PLOS Genetics. 2012;**8**(12):e1003172

[26] Ballas N, Lioy DT, Grunseich C, Mandel G. Non-cell autonomous influence of MeCP2-deficient glia on neuronal dendritic morphology. Nature Neuroscience. 2009;**12**(3):311-317

[27] Jacobs S, Nathwani M, Doering LC. Fragile X astrocytes induce developmental delays in dendrite maturation and synaptic protein expression. BMC Neuroscience. 2010;**11**:132

[28] Chahrour M, Zoghbi HY. The story of Rett syndrome: From clinic to neurobiology. Neuron. 2007;**56**(3):422-437

[29] Beckel-Mitchener A, Greenough WT. Correlates across the structural, functional, and molecular phenotypes of fragile X syndrome. Developmental Disabilities Research Reviews. 2004;**10**(1):53-59

[30] Craig AM, Banker G. Neuronal polarity. Annual Review of Neuroscience (Palo Alto, CA). 1994;**17**:267-310

[31] Kaech S, Banker G. Culturing hippocampal neurons. Nature Protocols. 2006;**1**(5): 2406-2415

[32] Maeder CI, Shen K, Hoogenraad CC. Axon and dendritic trafficking. Current Opinion in Neurobiology. 2014;**27**:165-170

[33] van Beuningen SF, Hoogenraad CC. Neuronal polarity: Remodeling microtubule organization. Current Opinion in Neurobiology. 2016;**39**:1-7

[34] Humpel C. Organotypic brain slice cultures: A review. Neuroscience. 2015;**305**:86-98

[35] Pokorny J, Yamamoto T. Postnatal ontogenesis of hippocampal CA1 area in rats. I. Development of dendritic arborisation in pyramidal neurons. Brain Research Bulletin. 1981;**7**(2):113-120

[36] Banker GA. Trophic interactions between astroglial cells and hippocampal neurons in culture. Science. 1980;**209**(4458):809-810

[37] Tropea M, Johnson MI, Higgins D. Glial cells promote dendritic development in rat sympathetic neurons *in vitro*. Glia. 1988;**1**(6):380-392

[38] Lein P, Johnson M, Guo X, Rueger D, Higgins D. Osteogenic protein-1 induces dendritic growth in rat sympathetic neurons. Neuron. 1995;**15**(3):597-605

[39] Le Roux PD, Reh TA. Regional differences in glial-derived factors that promote dendritic outgrowth from mouse cortical neurons *in vitro*. The Journal of Neuroscience. 1994;**14**(8):4639-4655

[40] Le Roux PD, Reh TA. Independent regulation of primary dendritic and axonal growth by maturing astrocytes *in vitro*. Neuroscience Letters. 1995;**198**(1):5-8

[41] Le Roux PD, Reh TA. Astroglia demonstrate regional differences in their ability to maintain primary dendritic outgrowth from mouse cortical neurons *in vitro*. Journal of Neurobiology. 1995;**27**(1):97-112

[42] Le Roux PD, Reh TA. Reactive astroglia support primary dendritic but not axonal outgrowth from mouse cortical neurons *in vitro*. Experimental Neurology. 1996;**137**(1):49-65

[43] Withers GS, Farley JR, Sterritt JR, Crane AB, Wallace CS. Interactions with astroglia influence the shape of the developing dendritic arbor and restrict dendrite growth independent of promoting synaptic contacts. PLoS One. 2017;**12**(1):e0169792

[44] Allen NJ. Astrocyte regulation of synaptic behavior. In: Schekman R, Lehmann R, editors. Annual Review of Cell and Developmental Biology, Annual Review of Cell and Developmental Biology. 2014;**30**:439-463

[45] Martin JL, Brown AL, Balkowiec A. Glia determine the course of brain-derived neurotrophic factor-mediated dendritogenesis and provide a soluble inhibitory cue to dendritic growth in the brainstem. Neuroscience. 2012;**207**(C):333-346

[46] Nedergaard M, Ransom B, Goldman S. New roles of astrocytes: Redefining the functional architecture of the brain. Trends in Neurosciences. 2003;**10**:523-530

[47] Fields RD, Araque A, Johansen-Berg H, Lim SS, Lynch G, Nave KA, et al. Glial biology in learning and cognition. The Neuroscientist. 2014;**20**(5):426-431

[48] Schreiner AE, Durry S, Aida T, Stock MC, Rüther U, Tanaka K, et al. Laminar and usbcellular heterogeneity of GLAST and GLT-1 immunoreactivity in the developing postnatal mouse hippocampus. The Journal of Comparative Neurology. 2014;**522**:204-224

[49] Fiala JC, Kirov SA, Feinberg MD, Petrak LJ, George P, Goddard CA, et al. Timing of neuronal and glial ultrastructure disruption during brain slice preparation and recovery *in vitro*. The Journal of Comparative Neurology. 2003;**465**(1):90-103

[50] Kirov SA, Goddard CA, Harris KM. Age-dependence in the homeostatic upregulation of hippocampal dendritic spine number during blocked synaptic transmission. Neuropharmacology. 2004;**47**(5):640-648

[51] Watson DJ, Ostroff L, Cao G, Parker PH, Smith H, Harris KM. LTP enhances synaptogenesis in the developing hippocampus. Hippocampus. 2016;**26**(5):560-576

[52] Huttenlocher PR. Morphometric study of human cerebral cortex development. Neuropsychologia. 1990;**28**(6):517-527

[53] Defelipe J, Alonso-Nanclares L, Arellano JI. Microstructure of the neocortex: Comparative aspects. Journal of Neurocytology. 2002;**31**:299-316

[54] Minkwitz HG, Holz L. The ontogenetic development of pyramidal neurons in the hippocampus (CA1) of the rat. Journal fur Hirnforschung. 1975;**16**(1):37-54

[55] Altemus KL, Lavenex P, Ishizuka N, Amaral DG. Morphological characteristics and electrophysiological properties of CA1 pyramidal neurons in macaque monkeys. Neuroscience. 2005;**136**(3):741-756

[56] Bushong EA, Martone ME, Jones YZ, Ellisman MH. Protoplasmic astrocytes in CA1 stratum radiatum occupy separate anatomical domains. The Journal of Neuroscience. 2002;**22**(1):183-192

[57] Halassa MM, Fellin T, Takano H, Dong JH, Haydon PG. Synaptic islands defined by the territory of a single astrocyte. The Journal of Neuroscience. 2007;**27**(24):6473-6477

[58] Haber M, Zhou L, Murai K. Cooperative astrocyte and dendritic spine dynamics at hippocampal excitatory synapses. The Journal of Neuroscience. 2006;**26**(35):8881-8891

[59] Benjamin Kacerovsky J, Murai KK. Stargazing: Monitoring subcellular dynamics of brain astrocytes. Neuroscience. 2016;**323**:84-95

[60] Lopez-Hidalgo M, Schummers J. Cortical maps: A role for astrocytes? Current Opinion in Neurobiology. 2014;**24**(1):176-189

[61] Giaume C, Koulakoff A, Roux L, Holcman D, Rouach N. Astroglial networks: A step further in neuroglial and gliovascular interactions. Nature Reviews. Neuroscience. 2010;**11**:1-13

[62] Eilam R, Aharoni R, Arnon R, Malach R. Astrocyte morphology is confined by cortical functional boundaries in mammals ranging from mice to human. eLife. 2016;**5**

[63] Mota B, Herculano-Houzel S. All brains are made of this: A fundamental building block of brain matter with matching neuronal and glial masses. Frontiers in Neuroanatomy. 2014;**8**:127

[64] Fruttiger M. Development of the retinal vasculature. Angiogenesis. 2007;**10**:77-88

[65] Frotscher M, Seress L. Morphological development of the hippocampus. In: The Hippocampus Book. Oxford, UK: Oxford University Press; 2007. pp. 115-131

[66] Bushong E, Martone M, Ellisman M. Maturation of astrocyte morphology and the establishment of astrocyte domains during postnatal hippocampal development. International Journal of Developmental Neuroscience. 2004;**22**(2):73-86

[67] Nixdorf-Bergweiler BE, Albrecht D, Heinemann U. Developmental changes in the number, size, and orientation of GFAP-positive cells in the CA1 region of rat hippocampus. Glia. 1994;**12**(3):180-195

[68] Cline HT. Dendritic arbor development and synaptogenesis. Current Opinion in Neurobiology. 2001;**11**(1):118-126

[69] Jontes JD, Buchanan J, Smith SJ. Growth cone and dendrite dynamics in zebrafish embryos: Early events in synaptogenesis imaged *in vivo*. Nature Neuroscience. 2000; **3**(3):231-237

[70] Wong WT, Wong ROL. Rapid dendritic movements during synapse formation and rearrangement. Current Opinion in Neurobiology. 2000;**10**(1):118-124

[71] Bolteus AJ, Bordey A. GABA release and uptake regulate neuronal precursor migration in the postnatal subventricular zone. The Journal of Neuroscience. 2004;**24**(35):7623-7631

[72] Kaneko N, Marin O, Koike M, Hirota Y, Uchiyama Y, Wu JY, et al. New neurons clear the path of astrocytic processes for their rapid migration in the adult brain. Neuron. 2010;**67**(2):213-223

[73] Ben Haim L, Rowitch DH. Functional diversity of astrocytes in neural circuit regulation. Nature Reviews. Neuroscience. 2017;**18**(1):31-41

Chapter 4

NMDA Receptors in Astroglia: Chronology, Controversies, and Contradictions from a Complex Molecule

Pavel Montes de Oca Balderas and
José Roberto González Hernández

Additional information is available at the end of the chapter

http://dx.doi.org/10.5772/intechopen.72975

Abstract

The neurocentric theory dismissed for decades the role of glia in information handling within the central nervous system (CNS). Nevertheless, almost 3 decades ago, this started to change and today astrocytes are considered relevant players for this function. Astrocytes "listen" to neuronal communication, regulate it, and respond at the cellular and synctitial level. Ionotropic glutamate NMDA receptor (NMDAR) is critical in CNS. It mediates synaptic neuronal communication and it is involved in different mechanisms. However, NMDAR is also expressed by astrocytes, but its functional role in these cells has not been deeply investigated and has been a matter of debate in the last decades. In this chapter, we briefly outline NMDAR intracellular transduction pathways initiated by Ca^{2+} flux. Then, we review chronologically NMDAR expression and function in astrocytes that have been a source of controversies and apparent contradictions. Finally, some insights are presented regarding NMDAR in astrocytes in the context of the tripartite synapse concept and the recently described Ca^{2+} flux–independent metabotropic-like NMDAR function in astrocytes. Given the complex molecular nature of NMDAR, its critical role, and the relevance of astrocytes, the study of astrocytic NMDAR promises to provide further understanding of CNS physiology and pathology.

Keywords: NMDAR, astrocyte, glutamate, flux-independent, signal transduction, tripartite synapse

1. Introduction

The glutamate (Glu) N-methyl D-aspartate receptor (NMDAR) plays a fundamental role in the central nervous system (CNS) mediating synaptic neuronal communication based on its ionotropic function. This Glu receptor is sensitive to different coagonist such as glycine (Gly) or D-serine (D-Ser), ions (Mg^{2+}, Zn^{2+}, H^{+}), or other molecules such as polyamines. It is involved in different functions that include memory, synaptic plasticity, and long-term potentiation and depression (LTP and LTD) among others [1, 2]. This central role in CNS is given mainly by its location in the postsynaptic membrane, where it mediates neuronal communication enabling extracellular (EC) Ca^{2+} and Na^{+} entry into the postsynaptic neuron. Functionally, at resting membrane potential, neuronal NMDAR is inactive because its pore is blocked by an Mg^{2+} ion. This scenario is modified when the presynaptic neuron depolarizes and releases vesicular Glu into the synaptic cleft. This in turn activates AMPA and Kainate ionotropic receptors that depolarize the postsynaptic membrane, thus allowing Mg^{2+} removal from the NMDAR pore and therefore its opening with the consequent cationic flux in response to Glu and coagonist binding. For this reason, neuronal NMDAR is considered a coincidence detector that requires both membrane depolarization and ligand binding [1, 2].

NMDAR is a tetramer of homodimers or a heterotrimer conformed by two obligate subunits GluN1 coupled to GluN2 and/or GluN3 subunits. There is only one gene (*Grin1*) for GluN1 subunit that is present in all NMDAR described so far, since it plays a central role in NMDAR assembly in the endoplasmic reticulum (ER). There, GluN1 regulates NMDAR exit from this organelle due to ER retention signals that are masked after its assembly. In addition, there are four GluN2(A-D) genes (*Grin2a-d*) and two genes for GluN3 (A and B; *Grin3a-b*). It is well known that the mRNA of some of these genes undergoes posttranscriptional modification by alternative splicing, generating molecular variants that confer specific functional properties to NMDAR. This diversity of subunits also allows the assembly of different NMDAR according to subunits expressed by the cell, resulting in receptors with different features in terms of modulation, traffic, location, and biophysical properties, given in part by their interaction with different molecular partners. In addition, there are some posttranslational modifications of these subunits that also generate functional variants of NMDAR, such as phosphorylation, myristoylation, and proteolytic cleavage, among others [1, 2]. In the CNS, the expression of NMDAR subunits is regionalized, and notably, NMDAR is expressed by nonneuronal cells but also is widely expressed in cells from different mammal tissues including skin, testis, and pancreas, among many others [1–3].

All NMDAR subunits share a common structure with an EC region of ≈500 amino acids (aa); three transmembrane domains and two loops, the first one intracellular (IC) and the second EC; and an IC C-terminal domain that ranges from ≈200 aa in GluN1 and GluN3 subunits to ≈500 aa in GluN2 subunits (**Figure 1**). The EC region is comprised of two functional domains: the N-terminal domain (NTD) involved in subunit-subunit molecular interactions and the ligand binding domain (LBD) that in close interaction with the EC loop shapes the ligand binding site, Glu for GluN2 subunits and Gly or D-Ser for GluN1 and GluN3 subunits. The IC C-terminal domain mediates NMDAR molecular interactions that regulate its functional properties, for instance in the synapse with the postsynaptic density proteins that mediate the assembly of molecular clusters [1, 2].

NMDAR is a cationic channel with partial selectivity for Ca^{2+} conduction, explained at least in part by the DRPEER motif that binds this ion and is present near the second transmembrane domain of GluN1 that directly contacts the pore wall [2]. The entry of Ca^{2+} through NMDAR

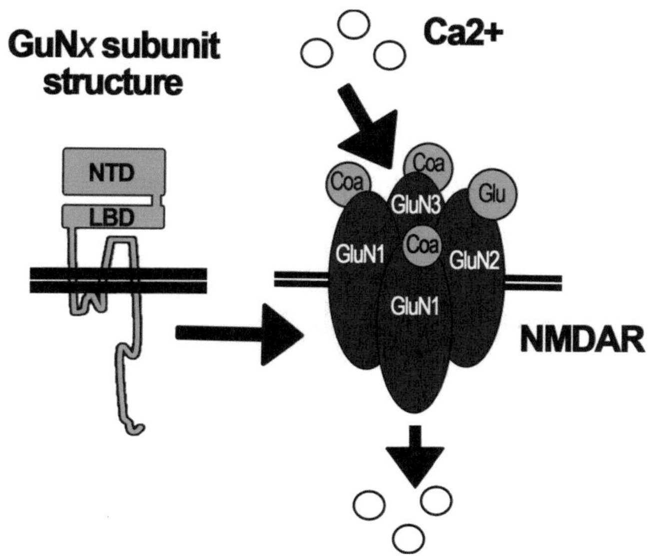

Figure 1. NMDAR subunit and channel structure (see text for details).

activates different IC signaling pathways that seem to depend upon its synaptic or extrasynaptic location (**Figure 2** and see below). It is well known that these pathways are involved in neuronal survival, growth, and differentiation, among other functions. On the other hand, it is also known that the excessive and persistent activation of NMDAR may result in the mechanism known as excitotoxicity, elicited by the excess of Ca^{2+} entry and the activation of IC pathways that lead to neuronal death (see below) [4, 5]. These Ca^{2+}-dependent IC pathways activated by NMDAR have also been referred to as Ca^{2+} flux–dependent metabotropic signaling [6].

Despite its wide expression and distribution in cells and tissues of mammals [3], NMDAR has been studied mainly in the neuronal context as a cationic channel [1, 2]. Nevertheless, now we know that NMDAR is expressed not only by other cells of the CNS such as astrocytes or oligodendroglia but also in non-CNS cells such as endothelium, platelets, and lymphocytes, among others [3, 7–9]. Moreover, there are some reports that have demonstrated NMDAR Ca^{2+} flux–independent functions and signaling [10–15], but only few of them have explored the molecular mechanisms that underpin this function.

Within the CNS, the role of astrocytes has transformed in almost a century from being considered supporting and metabolic cells to that of starring players in synaptic transmission among other functions. Indeed, since 1999, the concept of the tripartite synapse was coined by Araque et al. [16]. According to this idea, astrocytes play a relevant role beyond that of supporting cells, given their neurotransmitter receptor expression, neurotransmitter secretion, and IC Ca^{2+} waves elicited by neurotransmitters together with the early observed position of astrocytes that contact synapses and blood vessels. In this context, nowadays, a large amount of information supports the role of these cells in different CNS functions including synaptic transmission, synapse formation, development, LTP, and complex functions such as memory, sleep, and respiration, among many others [17] .

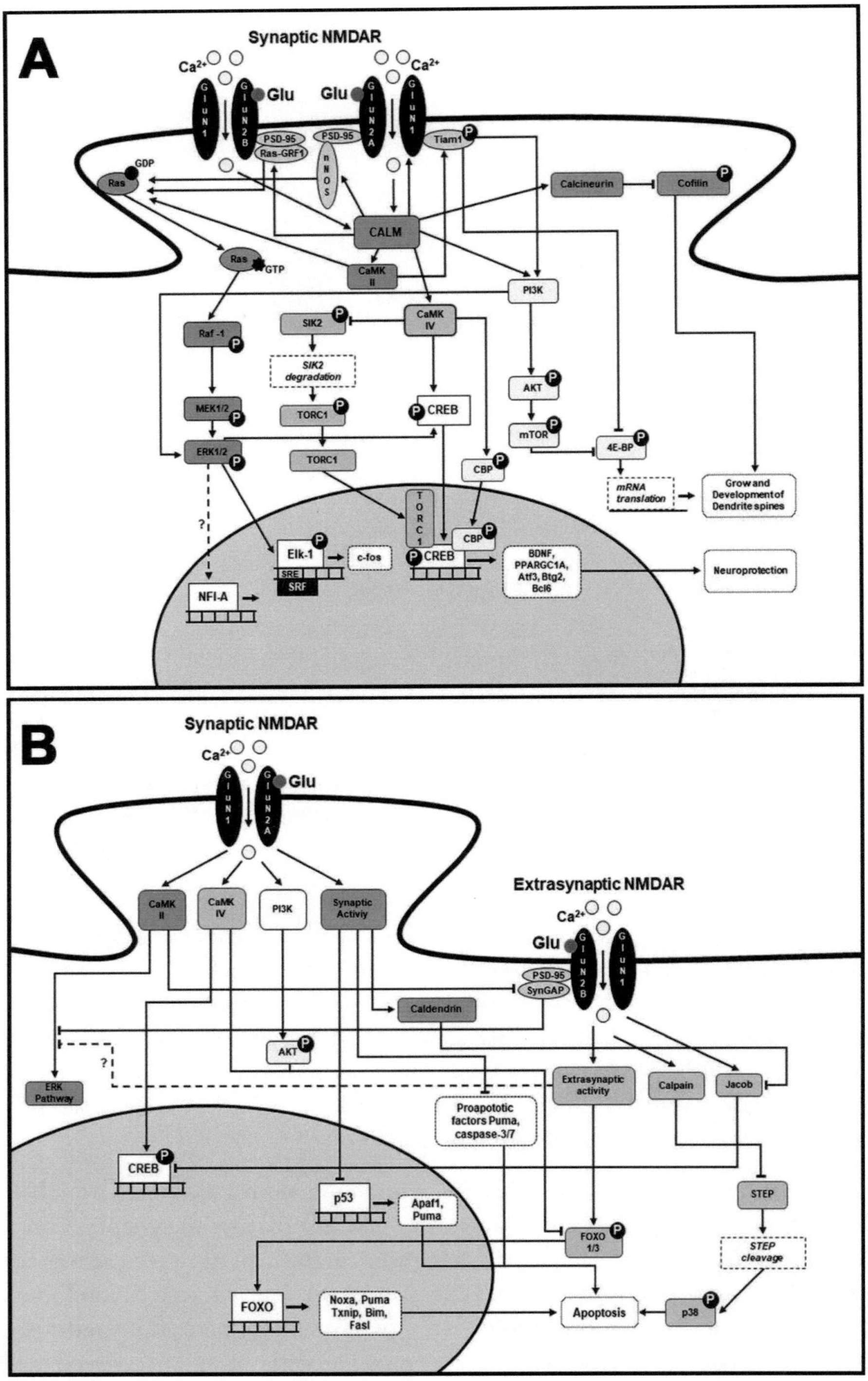

Figure 2. Ca^{2+} flux–dependent metabotropic signaling pathways in NMDAR. (A) Prosurvival, antiapoptotic pathways. (B) Prodeath, proapoptotic pathways (see text for details).

The aim of the present chapter is to review the expression and function of NMDAR in astrocytes, cells in which this topic has been a matter of debate and apparent contradictions. These have emerged mainly because astrocytes do not elicit action potentials as neurons do and thus NMDAR activation paradigm cannot be achieved, but also because NMDAR in astrocytes presents singularities not observed in neuronal NMDAR. Nevertheless, now there is a good amount of experimental evidence that has demonstrated NMDAR function in these cells.

In the first section of this chapter, we outline the Ca^{2+} flux–dependent metabotropic IC transduction pathways started by NMDAR activation, studied in the context of synaptic function, to substantiate the diversity of IC signals activated by this receptor. We then account chronologically the findings regarding the expression and function of NMDAR in astroglia that have been matter of some controversies and apparent contradictions. Finally, some insights are presented regarding NMDAR expression by astrocytes, with special attention to the tripartite synapse concept, and the Ca^{2+} flux–independent metabotropic-like NMDAR function recently reported. Given the complex molecular nature of NMDAR, its critical role in the CNS, both studied mainly in the neuronal context, and the relevance of astrocytes in the CNS evidenced in the last decades, the reexamination of NMDAR functions in astroglia may provide the basis to further gain insight into brain physiology and pathology.

2. NMDAR Ca^{2+} flux–dependent IC signaling

Until today, the canonical function of NMDAR is that of a cationic channel with partial selectivity for Ca^{2+}. This ion has been described in multiple signaling pathways ranging from bacteria to mammals and probably possesses the greatest universality and versatility as a second messenger [18]. Several IC signaling pathways are activated depending upon Ca^{2+} entry through NMDAR, and some mediate signaling to cell nucleus where gene expression is regulated (**Figure 2**) [5, 18, 19]. These Ca^{2+} dependent IC pathways triggered after NMDAR activation have been also referred as NMDAR metabotropic signaling [6]. The diversity of these IC pathways is influenced by NMDAR location and organism age among other variables [1, 20, 21]. Importantly, Ca^{2+}-dependent IC signaling mediates NMDAR function in LTP, memory, learning, neuronal plasticity, and survival, among other mechanisms but also mediates Glu excitotoxicity that leads to neuronal death [5].

Notably, there is a signaling dichotomy of NMDAR that has long been acknowledged [22]. A good amount of evidences supports divergent signaling between synaptic (prosurvival, antiapoptotic) and extrasynaptic (prodeath, proapoptotic) NMDAR [5], and even their genomic programs have been analyzed [23]. Interestingly, synaptic NMDAR is mainly assembled by GluN1/GluN2A subunits, whereas extrasynaptic NMDAR is mainly assembled by GluN1/GluN2B subunits [5, 24]. However, this dichotomy has presented inconsistencies in some tested models [25]. In the following subsections, we outline the IC signaling evoked by NMDAR that for convenience is separated into prosurvival, antiapoptotic signaling and prodeath, proapoptotic signaling. Since the review of these pathways is not the aim of this work, we invite the reader to please refer to the cited reviews and references therein for further information. Although some of these pathways have also been investigated in astrocytes, it must be considered that their involvement must be contextual since NMDAR in astrocytes contains different assembled subunits and these cells perform distinct functions.

On the other hand, as mentioned above, some reports have found that NMDAR also activates IC pathways independently of Ca^{2+} flux in neurons and astrocytes, also termed Ca^{2+} flux–independent metabotropic-like signaling, although its molecular mechanisms have been poorly studied. This kind of signaling is described in the section of NMDAR in astrocytes since recent work has demonstrated its occurrence in these cells, and then it is analyzed in the following section.

2.1. Prosurvival, antiapoptotic signaling

2.1.1. Calmodulin (CALM) pathway

One of the central pathways, if not the central one, associated with NMDAR Ca^{2+} flux is that of calmodulin (CALM). This small protein (148 aa) is a Ca^{2+} sensor that in turn activates the function of different enzymes, ion channels, aquaporins, and other proteins [26]. Consequently, CALM activation is a critical, necessary step for the activation of several downstream pathways associated with NMDAR. Malenka et al. demonstrated that CALM and CaMKII activation is necessary to induce LTP in rodent hippocampal slices. In their experiments, IC injection into CA1 pyramidal cells of calmidazolium (CALM antagonist) or a CALM-binding peptide blocked LTP [27]. Later, it was found that c-fos NMDAR-dependent activation required CALM activity in cultured rat hippocampal neurons, thus suggesting that CALM mediates signaling to cell nucleus [28]. In addition, CALM itself was found to modulate NMDAR function through its interaction with GluN1 subunit [29]. For a review of CALM functions in NMDAR signaling, please refer to the work by Xia and Storm [26].

2.1.2. Ca^{2+}/calmodulin-dependent protein kinase (CaMK) pathway

Consistent with the central role of CALM in NMDAR signaling, one of the most studied pathways is that of Ca^{2+}/calmodulin-dependent protein kinase (CaMK), of which two isoforms are active in NMDAR signaling. The role of these serine/threonine kinases was demonstrated by Bading et al. [28], who found in cultured rat hippocampal neurons that NMDAR triggered activation of CaMK (CaMKII, because of the inhibitors tested), since the addition of DL-2-Amino-5—phosphopentanoic acid (APV or AP-5), a competitive NMDAR antagonist, decreased CaMK activity. Furthermore, also in cultured rat hippocampal neurons, Ca^{2+}/CALM induced binding of CaMKII to the cytoplasmic domain of GluN2B, resulting in the translocation of the kinase to the synapse, allowing the persistent CaMKII activity and facilitated response to extracellular Ca^{2+}, mechanisms that regulate and potentiate synaptic strength [30]. CaMKII is involved in multiple neuronal functions such as LTP [31], dendritic spine density [32], and neuronal survival [20, 33], among others. These functions are achieved through activation of several downstream signaling pathways such as Ras/mitogen-activated protein kinase (MAPK) pathway and neuronal nitric oxide synthase (nNOS), among others (see below). For a review on the role of CaMKII in the synapse, please refer to the recent reviews [31, 34].

On the other hand, CaMKIV has also been involved in NMDAR-mediated functions. One of the earliest reports on NMDAR-dependent CaMKIV activation was that by Impey et al. [35]. Their results in cultured rat primary hippocampal neurons suggested that activation of CaMKIV is dependent upon NMDA, since APV treatment blocked its downstream signaling. In addition, NMDAR-mediated transcription was attenuated by treatment with CaMKIV inhibitors or in CaMKIV dominant-negative models [35]. CaMKIV has been extensively studied in downstream pathways, such as that of cAMP response element-binding protein (CREB; see below).

2.1.3. *Ras/mitogen-activated protein kinase (MAPK) pathway*

One of the most important and studied IC pathways activated by CaMKII is the Ras/MAPK pathway. Ras GTPase is a key molecule since when it is bound to GTP it activates different effectors. Raf-1 kinase is one of the effectors that in turn phosphorylates MEK1/2 (mitogen-activated protein kinase kinase) that phosphorylates and activates extracellular-regulated kinase (ERK1/2 or mitogen-activated protein kinase (MAPK)). ERK1/2 activation results in the regulation of different genes in the cell nucleus [36].

Bading and Greenberg [37] demonstrated that Glu treatment of cultured rat hippocampal cells resulted in the rapid and transient tyrosine phosphorylation of a 39-kilodalton protein suggested to be microtubule-associated protein kinase-2 (or ERK 2). NMDAR was responsible since APV blocked this effect that required Ca^{2+} influx. Later, Yun et al. [38] demonstrated that nitric oxide (NO), synthesized by nNOS, is a key player in NMDAR-mediated Ras activation. nNOS is a well-known target of CALM and it is activated after NMDAR mediated Ca^{2+} flux [39]. Moreover, NMDAR stimulation failed to activate Ras in $nNOS^{-/-}$ cultured cortical neurons, and ERK activation through NO and Ras is Ca^{2+} flux–dependent through NMDAR [38]. Later, it was found that Ca^{2+}/CALM-dependent Ras guanine nucleotide release factor (RasGRF1) directly interacts with GluN2B subunit, and this interaction mediates MAPK pathway activation [40]. For further details on this pathway, please refer to previous reviews [18, 41].

However, not always NMDAR activity leads to ERK activation. It has been shown that under certain circumstances ERK can be inhibited by NMDAR generating apoptotic signals (see below).

2.1.4. *Phosphoinositide 3-kinase (PI3K) pathway*

Phosphoinositide 3-kinase (PI3K) is a target of CALM [42]. Chandler et al. [43] demonstrated that PI3K-mediated NMDAR induced activation of ERK in cultured cortical neurons, since wortmannin (PI3K inhibitor) decreased phospho-ERK2 levels. This observation, together with PI3K catalytic subunit binding to phosphorylated GluN2 previously reported, let the authors suggest that NMDAR activation could directly mediate PI3K activation. This was later confirmed when it was found that exposure to NMDA significantly enhanced phospho-Akt levels in cultured rat cortical neurons [44]. This increase was blocked by MK-801, a pore blocker of NMDAR, or APV, but also by wortmannin and KN-93 (CaMKII inhibitor), indicating that PI3K and CaMKII play a role in NMDA activation of Akt/ERK signaling. The Akt pathway modulates actin dynamics and promotes the synthesis of proteins through the kinase mammalian target of rapamycin (mTOR) that in turn phosphorylates the factor 4E-binding protein (4E-BP) that controls mRNA translation [45].

2.1.5. cAMP response element-binding protein (CREB) pathway

One of the most studied pathways associated to NMDAR/CaMKIV is that of cAMP response element-binding protein (CREB), which plays a critical role in synaptic NMDAR-mediated neuroprotection. Impey et al. [35] showed that NMDAR activates transcription of CREB-responsive genes in cultured rat hippocampal neurons. CaMKIV was responsible for phosphorylating CREB-binding protein (CBP), a CREB coactivator. Moreover, mutation of CBP Ser301 impaired NMDAR and CaMKIV-stimulated transcription, whereas dominant-negative CaMKIV inhibited NMDAR-mediated activation of CREB-CBP. These authors showed that CaMKIV mediated a transient early phase of NMDAR-dependent CREB phosphorylation, while MAPK mediates a later persistent phase, suggesting the convergence between MAPK and CaMKIV pathways. In addition, the transducer of regulated CREB activity 1 (TORC1) modulates NMDAR-dependent CREB activation. Although the role of TORC1 in LTP had been previously demonstrated [46], Sasaki et al. [47] found NMDAR-dependent TORC1 transcription activation mediated by CaMKIV and salt-inducible kinase 2 (SIK2) degradation after oxygen-glucose deprivation (OGD).

Multiple genes related to cell survival are upregulated by NMDAR-dependent CREB activation. Nonetheless, it has been found that NMDAR activity-dependent shut off of genes is also an important process for neuronal survival. Zhang et al. [48] found in cultured mouse hippocampal neurons that NMDAR-mediated CREB regulation of Aft3 required nuclear Ca^{2+} transients and CaMKIV activity. Aft3 acts as a transcriptional repressor and protects neurons from apoptosis and extrasynaptic NMDAR-induced cell death triggered by NMDA or OGD. For a review, please refer to the work by Hardingham [5].

2.1.6. T-cell lymphoma invasion and metastasis 1 (Tiam1)

Tolias et al. [49] identified Rac-1 guanine nucleotide exchange factor (GEF) Tiam1 as a molecule involved in NMDAR downstream signaling. Tiam1 interacts and colocalizes with NMDAR that after activation allows Tiam1 phosphorylation, depending upon Ca^{2+} flux. It is suggested that such phosphorylation is mediated by CaMKII since it phosphorylates Tiam1 and increases Rac1 GTP exchange [50]. Using Tiam1 RNAi-infected neurons, this GEF was found to be necessary for NMDAR-dependent activation of Akt and phosphorylation of 4E-BP that mediates NMDAR-dependent mRNA translation [49].

2.1.7. Cofilin/calcineurin pathway

Calcineurin is a Ca^{2+}/CALM-dependent serine/threonine protein phosphatase that in neurons was found to downregulate NMDAR itself after its activation by Ca^{2+} entry through NMDAR [51]. In this work with acutely isolated adult rat neurons, the duration of NMDA channel openings is prolonged when calcineurin is inhibited by okadaic acid (phosphatase inhibitor) or its specific inhibitor FK506. On the other hand, it was found that NMDAR activation enhanced F-actin content in dendritic spines, associated to LTP, and such increase was mediated by cofilin deactivation that stimulates actin filament turnover and therefore growth and development of dendritic spines [52].

2.1.8. Serum response factor (SRF) and ETS domain containing protein (Elk-1)

The transcription factors serum response factor (SRF) and ETS domain containing protein (Elk-1) were found to mediate NMDAR Ca^{2+}-dependent transcriptional response in cultured rat hippocampal neurons [53]. In this work, it was determined that c-fos gene transcription through the serum response element (SRE) present in its promoter could be achieved by two different pathways: one by SRF independent of Elk-1 and the second dependent upon Elk-1 phosphorylation, mediated by ERK.

2.1.9. p53 and p53 upregulated mediator of apoptosis (PUMA) suppression

NMDAR has also been shown to inhibit proapoptotic factors. Lau and Bading [54] demonstrated in cultured mouse hippocampal neurons that synaptic NMDAR suppressed p53 expression. This effect was blocked by MK-801 and included the repression of proapoptotic p53 target genes apoptosis protease activating factor 1 (*apaf1*) and p53 upregulated modulator of apoptosis (PUMA). Léveillé et al. [55] demonstrated that in cultured mouse cortical neurons, blockage of NMDAR with MK-801 induced the activation of caspase-3/7 following an apoptotic insult. They also confirmed that synaptic NMDAR protected neurons by suppressing the expression of proapoptotic PUMA that through Bcl2 associated X protein (Bax) promotes mitochondrial release of apoptotic factors, such as cytochrome C, and facilitates the action of proapoptotic members of the Bax subfamily. Released cytochrome C binds to APAF-1, which oligomerizes and recruits procaspase-9 that then becomes activated, forming the apoptosome [56].

2.2. Prodeath, proapoptotic signaling

2.2.1. ERK pathway inhibition

Chandler et al. [43] found an ambivalent ERK regulation by NMDAR in rat neuronal cultures. High concentration of NMDA decreased phospho-ERK2 levels in 1 mM extracellular Ca^{2+}, but activated it in 100 μM extracellular Ca^{2+}. The inhibition was accompanied by a decrease of phospho-CREB. Later, Ivanov et al. [57] demonstrated in cultured rat hippocampal neurons that ERK activation or inhibition depended upon the pool of NMDAR activated. Synaptic NMDAR activated ERK, whereas extrasynaptic NMDAR inhibited it. However, more recently, it was reported that ERK pathway activation in cultured rat cortical neurons depended on the days *in vitro* (DIV) of the culture and NMDA concentration. However, effects were sensitive to ifenprodil (GluN2B receptor antagonists), thus suggesting that GluN2B containing NMDAR may activate or inhibit ERK pathway [21].

2.2.2. Synaptic Ras GTPase-activating protein (SynGAP)

Synaptic Ras GTPase-activating protein 1 (SynGAP1) has been shown to interact with PDZ domain containing proteins such as postsynaptic density protein 95 (PSD-95), in the PSD, where it exists as a macromolecular complex together with the NMDAR subunit GluN2B [58].

SynGAP is inhibited by its phosphorylation by CaMKII that in turn stops inactivation of Ras that leads to MAPK pathway activation [59]. In cultured rat hippocampal neurons, they used RNAi to specifically suppress SynGAP expression that resulted in sustained ERK activation following NMDAR stimulation instead of transient activity [58].

2.2.3. Forkhead box protein O (FOX O)

Forkhead box protein O (FOXO) class of transcription factors can promote neuronal death [60]. FOXO targets proapoptotic genes including Bcl2-interacting mediator of cell death (Bim), PUMA, and Fas ligand (FasL), among others. It has been demonstrated in cultured rat cortical neurons that synaptic NMDAR prevents FOXO nuclear export and suppression of FOXO1 gene through PI3K/Akt activation [61]. Similarly, Dick and Bading [62] found that in cultured rat hippocampal neurons, synaptic activity inhibits nuclear translocation of FOXO3 and that dominant negative CaMKIV(K75E) expression blocked protective activity. Contrarily, extrasynaptic NMDAR activity induced FOXO3 nuclear import resulting in apoptosis.

2.2.4. Juxtasynaptic attractor of caldendrin on dendritic boutons (Jacob)

A binding partner of the neuronal Ca^{2+}-binding protein caldendrin critical for extrasynaptic NMDAR signaling was identified named juxtasynaptic attractor of caldendrin on dendritic boutons protein (Jacob) [63]. These authors found that Jacob knockdown prevented CREB shut off after extrasynaptic NMDAR activation. When imported into the nucleus, Jacob causes CREB dephosphorylation and promotes apoptosis, effects prevented by Caldendrin, which binds Jacob in a Ca^{2+}-dependent manner elicited by synaptic NMDAR activity. Contrarily, extrasynaptic NMDAR activity promoted nuclear accumulation of Jacob and neuronal death [5, 63].

2.2.5. Calpain/p38 MAP pathway

The calpain pathway is another important pathway that is related to the extrasynaptic activity of NMDARs. Calpain is a Ca^{2+}-dependent protease that has been widely implicated in neurotoxicity [64]. Xu et al. [65] demonstrated that in cultured rat cortical neurons the activation of extrasynaptic NMDARs strongly activates calpains, whereas synaptic NMDAR fails to activate this protease. Striatal-enriched protein tyrosine phosphatase 61 (STEP61) is a substrate for calpain and is rapidly cleaved after strong glutamatergic stimulation such as during excitotoxic or ischemic insult [66, 67]. Extrasynaptic stimulation of NMDARs evoked calpain-mediated proteolysis of STEP61 and activation of p38 MAPK. p38 contributes to cell death induced by chronic NMDA or Glu exposure [65]. Previously, Kawasaki et al. [68] observed p38 activation after Glu treatment in mature cerebellar granule cells, mediated by NMDAR.

3. Chronological track of NMDAR expression and function in astroglia

When considering the role of NMDAR in astrocytes, it is convenient to first acknowledge the hypothesis made by nineteenth century scientists such as Fridtjof Nansen, William Lloyd

Adriezen, or Carl Ludwig Schleich who suggested that neuroglial cells could play a more relevant role than that of gluing the CNS, after the name neuroglia was coined by Virchow in 1856 [17]. After almost a century of studying CNS from the perspective of the neurocentric theory, this conception was found to be correct. Previous recent reviews have examined the expression of NMDAR in neuroglial cells [69, 70]. Here, we present a chronological comprehensive review about how the expression and function of NMDAR in astrocytes have been studied in the last 40 years. Throughout these decades, different controversies and apparent contradictions have been encountered, but today, NMDAR expression and function in astrocytes are well documented and accepted. Moreover, NMDAR in astrocytes could play a relevant role in CNS pathologies and therefore offer a window to develop new therapeutic strategies.

In this review, we focus in NMDAR expression and function of brain astrocytes, although we recapitulate some early approaches in other neuroglial cells. It must be noted however that different laboratories documented the expression and function of NMDAR in Muller, Bergman, and radial glial cells or spinal astrocytes mainly in the 1990s. Please refer to the reviews by Dzamba et al. [70] or Verkhratsky and Kirchhoff [69] who examined the work on these cells.

3.1. Is it there? The early years: 1960s, 1970s, and 1980s

In 1967, it was observed that cortical glial cells *in situ* did not respond to Glu [71]. Later, Hösli et al. [72] found that in spinal organotypic cultures, astrocytes depolarized after treatment with Glu (100 μM). However, it was postulated that such depolarization was due to K^+ released by neurons, since 4-aminopyridine (blocker of Kv1 receptors) inhibited such effect and it was observed only in astrocytes adjacent to neurons but not in isolated astrocytes. Remarkably, no change in membrane resistance was observed in these cells, but neither in astrocytes from the olfactory cortex that also responded to Glu [72, 73]. However, few years later, it was demonstrated that neuron-free cultured astrocytes from newborn rat hemispheres responded to Glu treatment (100 μM-1 mM) in a Na^+-dependent manner. These groups also demonstrated that NMDAR was not involved in Glu response of astrocytes, since NMDA treatment alone (100 μM-1 mM) did not generate membrane depolarization [74, 75]. Instead, Glu was found to open Na^+/K^+ channels in cultured rat astrocytes that shared many properties with neuronal kainate/quisqualate receptor [76]. This finding was confirmed by Pearce et al. [77] that measured Ca^{2+} efflux and breakdown of inositol phospholipids in cultured rat cortical astrocytes and found no response with 100 μM NMDA. Usowicz et al. [78] showed that type-2 cerebellar astrocytes also depolarized in response to Glu, and consistently with previous findings, these cells did not respond to NMDA application (30–100 μM). Consistently, Backus et al. [79] observed that cultured rat cerebral astrocytes had no change in membrane potential with NMDA, even with the coagonist Gly or in Mg^{2+}-free solution, conditions that would favor neuronal NMDAR response. These studies, most of them electrophysiological, the traditional approach to study neuronal NMDAR, set the basis to establish that astrocytes do not express NMDA-type Glu receptors.

3.2. Rethinking the idea: the 1990s

In the seminal study by Cornell-Bell et al. [80], who described for the first time Ca^{2+} waves in cultured rat astrocytes in response to Glu, establishing the possibility that this kind of signaling could be relevant for CNS function, small inconsistencies regarding the expression of

NMDAR in astrocytes were observed. Using the IC Ca^{2+} (iCa^{2+}) probe Fluo-3, they found that cultured astrocytes did not respond to NMDA (100 μM) and Gly, although a small decrease of iCa^{2+} is observable in their published recordings. Nevertheless, these authors noted that APV "attenuated" the Glu response, because peak frequency and the amount of iCa^{2+} between peak responses were reduced, although maximal amplitude was maintained. Indeed, APV depleted a Glu-dependent gradual increase of iCa^{2+} masked between peak responses. Despite these findings suggesting that NMDAR could somehow be functional in these cells, it was concluded that astrocytes did not express NMDAR, consistently with previous reports. Simultaneously, Jensen and Chiu [81] also reported a lack of iCa^{2+} response measured with fura-2 in cultured rat cortical astrocytes to NMDA with or without Mg^{2+}. The same year, the Cornell-Bell group reported in a different work that Glu induced the formation of filopodia in astrocytes of mixed hippocampal cultures; however, this effect was not achieved with NMDA alone (100 μM) [82].

After Ca^{2+} waves' discovery in cultured astrocytes, Dani et al. [83] demonstrated the existence of Ca^{2+} waves in fluo-3 labeled astrocytes from organotypically cultured slices of rat hippocampus. These waves were elicited by neuronal electrical stimulation or bath application of NMDA (20 μM). However, since these waves were secondary to Ca^{2+} rise in neurons, these authors inferred that they were indirectly elicited, resulting from neurotransmitter released from NMDA-stimulated neurons and not from a direct stimulation of NMDAR in astrocytes.

Later, Holzwarth et al. [84] also found no iCa^{2+} response measured with Fura-2 to NMDA in cultured rat cortical astrocytes, whereas Seifert and Steinhauser [85] did the same observation in acute isolated mice hippocampal astroglial cells by patch clamp. These results reinforced the notion that astrocytes lacked functional NMDAR. However, in parallel and contradiction with this conception, two different groups suggested astrocyte activity evoked by NMDAR. Steinhauser et al. [86] reported that in postnatal (9–12 days) mice hippocampal brain slices, in a small group of glial cells termed passive (34% of them glial fibrillary acidic protein + [GFAP+] and characterized by time-independent currents) NMDA (1 or 5 mM) elicited currents detected by patch clamp. However, these responses varied: 41% presented an inward current, 32% a small outward current, and 27% did not respond. Nevertheless, these authors did not unequivocally identify astrocytic NMDAR as the responsible receptor. The second work by Porter and McCarthy [87] was made in rat hippocampal slices from young animals (9–13 days) labeled with Fura Red AM or Calcium Green-1 and recorded with confocal microscopy. In this work, it was reported that 75% of recorded astrocytes, identified by GFAP, presented iCa^{2+} rise in response to NMDA (50 μM), blocked by APV, although only 45% of these responses persisted in the presence of tetrodotoxin (TTX) that blocks neuronal activity. These observations suggested that astrocytes have functional NMDAR, although authors considered that Glu release mediated by presynaptic NMDAR, even with TTX, offered an alternative explanation for their observations. On the other hand, the other 55% of cells confirmed that neuronal activity could also elicit astrocyte responses, as inferred by Dani et al. [83].

In the meanwhile, different groups looked for the expression of NMDAR with histological techniques. Conti et al. [88] initially suggested that in the cerebral cortex of adult rats, virtually all (95.7%) GFAP+ cells did not express the mRNA for GluN1 (NMDAR1 or NR1) as evidenced by *in situ* hybridization and electron microscopy (EM). Nevertheless, Gracy and Pickel [89] found by immunohistochemistry (IHC) combined with EM that in the basolateral amygdala 20% of staining with anti-GluN1 antibodies (Abs) corresponded to distal tips of astrocytic processes. Moreover, in a second work from Conti [90], it was found by IHC-EM, that in the cortex of adult rats, some distal processes and rare cell bodies of astrocytes were positive for GluN1 and GluN2A/B, although this was not evident by light microscopy. Similarly, Petralia et al. [91] found by IHC-EM and light microscopy in the dorsal cochlear nucleus some glial processes and wrappings of the synapses, and therefore possibly astrocytes, labeled with Abs against GluN1 and GluN2A/B. Likewise, Bockstaele and Colago [92] found in the nucleus coeruleus by IHC-EM the presence of GluN1 in astrocytic processes. Also, Farb et al. [93] reported that in the basal nuclei of the amygdala, glial processes were labeled by GluN1 Abs, detected by IHC-EM. Therefore, despite initial observations that supported the notion of astrocytes lacking NMDAR, several studies found evidences supporting its expression in tissue astrocytes of different brain regions.

Later, Pasti et al. [94] obtained further evidence with brain slices indicating that iCa^{2+} increase in cortical or hippocampal astrocytes in response to NMDA (100 μM) or neuronal electrical stimulation was a secondary effect of neuronal activity, not a direct action on putative astrocytic NMDAR. Consistently, Cai and Kimelberg [95] found no response to NMDA (100 μM) in GFAP+ acute isolated astrocytes from rat hippocampus. Notably, Gottlieb and Matute [96] in the same year found by IHC the expression of GluN2A and GluN2B subunits in rat hippocampus reactive astrocytes after transient ischemia. The expression of these subunits was maximal after 28 days of ischemia. This study constituted the first evidence suggesting that astrocytic NMDAR could play a role in the development of reactive astrocytes and therefore in pathology.

Two years after, Nishizaki et al. [97] detected currents by patch clamp elicited by NMDA (1 mM) in human cultured astrocytes obtained from the white matter surrounding a tumor. These currents were potentiated by Gly, sensitive to Mg^{2+}, independent of Glu transporters, but curiously were not sensitive to APV. Instead, they were partially sensitive to a G-protein inhibitor and increased when iCa^{2+} was depleted by inhibiting the sarcoendoplasmic reticulum Ca^{2+}/ATPase (SERCA), suggesting that currents were the result of store-operated Ca^{2+} entry (SOCE). In addition, it was observed with fura-2/AM that iCa^{2+} increased in response to NMDA, but this response was only partially inhibited by extracellular Ca^{2+} depletion and was also APV insensitive. With these findings, the authors suggested that NMDA elicited a response through a receptor distinct from NMDAR, perhaps through the activation of G-protein–coupled receptors (GPCR) that released Ca^{2+} from IC stores. However, Shelton and McCarthy [98] found no "clear" iCa^{2+} response to NMDA (100–400 μM) in rat astrocytes labeled with Calcium Green-1 AM from hippocampal slices obtained from 30 to 38 day animals, in Mg^{2+}-free solution with Gly and TTX. This contrasted with their previous observation in younger animals (9–13 days) [87] and led the authors to suggest that NMDAR expression could change during development. Simultaneously, Conti, et al. [99] reported that in human cortex, distal astrocyte projections had GluN1, GluN2A, and GluN2B labeling detected by IHC-EM, whereas astrocyte cell bodies were only occasionally labeled. Some of the labeled distal projections of astrocytes surrounded the axon terminal but others were present in areas not related with synapses.

3.3. It is there and it works: the 2000s

In 2001, Schipke et al. [100] identified functional NMDAR in cortical astrocytes of wild-type mice and transgenic mice with enhanced green fluorescent protein (EGFP) under control of GFAP promoter (EGFP-GFAP mouse). These authors isolated EGFP+ cells to obtain mRNA, perform RT-PCR, and test NMDAR subunit expression. In these experiments, GluN1, GluN2B, and GluN2C were expressed in astrocytes, whereas GluN2A, GluN2D, and GluN3 were not found. In addition, efforts were made to identify NMDAR subunits by western blot, but they were unsuccessful due to low cell yields. Patch clamp experiments in brain slices from 7 to 28 day animals showed that NMDA (100 μM) elicited currents in most (72%) of EGFP+ cells, but also in astrocytes from wild-type animals. Although the main component of these currents was found to be indirectly mediated by neuronal activity as previously identified, there was also a component related solely to direct NMDAR function in astrocytes. This response was blocked by MK-801 and Mg^{2+} suggesting that NMDAR was similar to neuronal NMDAR. Consistently, using Ca^{2+} indicators, it was found that NMDA increased iCa^{2+} observed mainly in distal projections, but also in the cell soma, consistently with previous ultrastructural observations that identified NMDAR mainly in distal projections.

This same year, Kondoh et al. [101] studied again NMDA (1 mM) responses by patch clamp in human astrocytes from the white matter surrounding a tumor. Essentially, the results reported were the same and consistent with their previous findings [97], but they also discarded that the cultured cells were from tumoral origin. Oddly, NMDA-elicited currents were potentiated by kynurenic acid (KYNA), a nonselective ionotropic Glu receptor antagonist. Also, the receptor mediating the response to NMDA was found to be less permeable to Ca^{2+}. With these observations, the authors suggested that astrocytes express a novel form of NMDAR, regulated by GPCR, as suggested by their sensitivity to a G-protein inhibitor, perhaps through the assembly of particular nondescribed subunits expressed in these cells.

Then, the group by Krebs et al. [102] reported that in rat hippocampus, NMDAR subunits GluN1 and GluN2B were observed in GFAP+ cells by IHC 3 days after transient ischemia, peaking at 28 days, and declining by 56 days, but were not detected in cells from intact animals. These observations were consistent with those made by Gottlieb and Matute [96]. In addition, GluN1 and GluN2B subunit expression was confirmed in astrocytes from postnatal (2–4 days) hippocampal neuron-glia cocultures subject to anoxia, where no neurons survived by day 3. In contrast, GluN2B was not found in pure cultured hippocampal astrocytes after anoxia. Functionally, NMDA (0.5–1 mM) elicited iCa^{2+} responses in astrocytes obtained from neuron-glia cocultures subject to anoxia or astrocytes acutely isolated from ischemic hippocampi. These responses were APV sensitive, and in acute isolated astrocytes, they were partially blocked by ifenprodil. These authors suggested that NMDAR function in astrocytes could provide the basis for new therapies to ameliorate the effects of stroke.

The same year, Zhang et al. [103] published a study reporting NMDAR participation in iCa^{2+} responses to Glu in cultured rat cortical astrocytes (87% of cells as described in their following publication) using APV. This is to our knowledge the first report that found response to NMDA in nonhypoxic cultured rat cortical astrocytes. A year after, the same group published these results but also found that NMDA (50–100 μM) elicited iCa^{2+} response that was sensitive to APV in a large proportion (72%) of cultured rat cortical astrocytes [104]. Interestingly, APV inhibition was reverted only after a 30-min incubation in APV-free solution.

Two years later, strong evidence was provided by the group of Verkhratsky indicating that NMDAR mediated currents in acute isolated and tissue mouse cortical astrocytes (17–22 days) [105]. Profiting the advantages of the EGFP-GFAP mouse model for the identification of astrocytes, these authors found three different components of currents elicited by Glu application in acute isolated astrocytes using AMPA/kainate receptor, NMDAR, and Glu transporter inhibitors (NBQX, APV, and L-TBOA, respectively). In particular, APV blocked the sustained component of the Glu-induced current. They also demonstrated that NMDA elicited robust currents potentiated by Gly in 87% of acute isolated astrocytes at −40 or −80 mV membrane potential, indicating their insensitivity to Mg^{2+}, in contrast with NMDAR-mediated currents in neurons and previous work with hippocampal astrocytes [100]. Robust currents required 10–100 μM NMDA but were observable with 30 nM NMDA, they were blocked by MK-801, and ifenprodil only partially reduced currents in 43% of cells. Importantly, electrical stimulation of neurons in brain slices from 17 to 22 day animals also evoked Mg^{2+}-insensitive cortical astrocyte currents of which the fast component was blocked by MK-801, suggesting NMDAR involvement. Glu transporters also mediated these currents, but in contrast with observations in isolated astrocytes, AMPA/kainate receptors were poorly involved, although preventing their desensitization increased current amplitude. Interestingly, miniature spontaneous currents were also observed in tissue astrocytes that were independent of TTX, partially blocked by APV (32%) but fully blocked by APV and NBQX combination. All in all, this work demonstrated that astrocytes express functional NMDAR that mediate neuron-astrocyte communication.

Contrary to these findings, the same year different groups reported that NMDAR is not involved in iCa^{2+} response of astrocytes. Wang et al. [106] investigated astrocyte Ca^{2+} activity in the barrel cortex of adult mouse (6–8 weeks) in response to whisker stimulation. In this work, it was found that iCa^{2+} activity in astrocytes was consistently triggered by whisker stimulation. However, iontophoretic application of APV did not modify astrocytic iCa^{2+} activity although postsynaptic currents were suppressed, suggesting that astrocytic NMDAR is not involved in their response. In addition, Serrano et al. [107] studied glial involvement in heterosynaptic depression in rat (14–21 days) hippocampal slices. Although these authors found that NMDA elicited iCa^{2+} responses in astrocytes that were blocked by APV, these responses were delayed minutes after NMDA application. Indeed, TTX revealed that these glial responses were indirect and mediated by neuronal activity, as previous works had reported. Likewise, Kato, et al. [108] found in cultured cortical astrocytes from newborn mouse that NMDAR antagonists MK-801, ifenprodil, or Ro25-6981 did not block iCa^{2+} rise in response to Glu, as it was observed in cultured neurons. Notably, Glu induced astrocytes' activation (measured by morphological changes and GFAP expression) in neuron/astrocyte cocultures or cultured astrocytes, but this effect was blocked by MK-801 or ifenprodil only in neuron/astrocyte cocultures. This supported that neuronal NMDAR mediated neuron-glia signaling mediated astrocyte activation, resembling previous observations made in tissue astrocytes. In addition, Edling et al. [109] found that c-fos induction by Glu in newborn rat cultured astrocytes was not blocked by MK-801.

In 2008, a transcriptome database for three cell types of the CNS (neuron, astrocyte, and oligodendrocyte) from mouse forebrain was published, describing developmental changes between postnatal days 1 and 30 [110]. In this work, astrocytes were isolated by fluorescence-activated cell sorter (FACS) from a transgenic mouse expressing EGFP under control of S100β promoter, an astrocyte marker. Results showed that *in vivo* but also cultured astrocytes express NMDAR subunits GluN1, GluN2C, and GluN3A, the subunits included in the arrays. In particular, GluN2C was enriched in mature astrocytes. Importantly, after expression profile analysis, the authors observed that cultured astrocytes expressed many of the genes expressed by *in vivo* astrocytes and did not express the enriched genes in neurons or oligodendrocytes. However, they concluded that cultured astrocytes do not represent the same cell type as *in vivo* astrocytes, but instead an immature stage of the astrocyte lineage or a reactive astrocyte phenotype.

Simultaneously, Serrano et al. [111] found evidence suggesting astrocytic NMDAR function in the hippocampus, in contrast to their previous findings. These authors first distinguished two populations of cells in hippocampal slices from the EGFAP-GFAP mouse (10–18 day). These cells had different current/voltage curves, GFP levels, and cell-coupling and therefore were designated linear and outward rectifying glial cells (probably NG^{2+} cells). NMDA (25 μM) depolarized both types of cells, but in linear glial cells, TTX blocked partially (43%) the depolarization, while in outward rectifying cells, TTX had no effect. These observations suggested the direct involvement of astrocytic NMDAR beyond an indirect role mediated by neuronal activity as suggested by their own work and other previous reports. These authors further suggested that diversity of glial cells in the hippocampus could underpin distinct observations regarding NMDAR function in hippocampal astrocytes.

3.4. NMDAR composition, peculiar function, and therapy window: the 2010s

Palygin et al. [112] reported again that acute isolated astrocytes from EGFP-GFAP mouse (3 months) elicited currents in response to NMDA (30 μM). These currents presented slow desensitization kinetics, were blocked by APV, and were insensitive to Mg^{2+} as previously reported by the same group [105]. In addition, NMDA (30 μM) also elicited iCa^{2+} responses in acute isolated astrocytes measured with Fura-2 that were 43% of that elicited with Glu. iCa^{2+} responses were also evoked in astrocytes from cortical slices by neuronal electrical stimulation and were proportional to stimulus intensity. The iCa^{2+} response was blocked by TTX (100%) or decreased by APV (34%) or UBP141 (29%; antagonist of GluN2C/D containing NMDAR). With these results, the authors confirmed that astrocytic NMDAR participated in neuron-glia signaling and suggested that they should be assembled with GluN2C/D subunits and GluN3 that could provide lack of Mg^{2+} block and low Ca^{2+} permeability.

The same year, Lee et al. [113] reported that human astrocytes also expressed functional NMDAR. In this work, all seven NMDAR subunits were detected by RT-PCR in cultured astrocytes from fetal brains or adult brains and by immunofluorescence in human cultured fetal astrocytes. They found iCa^{2+} responses measured with Fura-2 to Glu (20 μM- 2.5 mM) or quinolinic acid (QUIN; agonist of NMDAR; 40 nM- 5 μM) that were blocked by MK-801 or memantine (NMDAR antagonist). However, three aspects were atypical in these experiments:

(a) responses to Glu and QUIN were not transient but sustained even after 30 s of agonist removal; (b) disparate concentrations of Glu (500 μM) and QUIN (1 μM) were required to elicit a similar iCa^{2+} response; and (c) these experiments were made with a fluorometer despite employing live microscopy. On the other hand, cytotoxicity levels induced by Glu or QUIN were prevented by MK-801 or memantine, but again Glu and QUIN concentrations to achieve the same response were disparate (500 μM vs. 500 nM, respectively).

After, Jiang et al. [114] reported that in cultured rat cortical astrocytes the NO donor sodium nitroprusside (SNP) or NMDA (10 μM for 18 hrs) induced Carboxyl-terminal PDZ ligand of nNOS (CAPON) translocation form cytoplasm to cell nucleus. The authors assumed NMDAR function since SNP effect was prevented by MK-801. Extraordinarily, they observed that SNP induced GluN2B localization in the cell nucleus, supporting previous findings suggesting putative NMDAR nuclear translocation [115, 116]. On the other hand, Zhou et al. [117] characterized NMDAR subunit expression in mouse cultured astrocytes at different times and in a model of ischemia. They found GluN1, GluN2A, and GluN2B expression by RT-PCR and immunofluorescence (only GluN1 and GluN2B). The expression of GluN1 decreased with time (4 weeks), GluN2A was increased, and GluN2B was slightly increased. Ischemia, actually an incubation in medium without serum, glucose, and equilibrated with 85% N2 and 0% O2, caused a bell-shaped response in GluN1, GluN2A, and GluN2B gene expression.

The following year, a study by Palygin et al. [118] characterized pharmacologically the NMDAR in acute isolated cortical astrocytes from the EGFP-GFAP mouse (4–8 weeks). In these cells, NMDA (50 μM) evoked inward currents in all astrocytes tested that were inhibited by UBP141 (62%) and were Mg^{2+} independent, whereas in neurons, only a slight inhibition was observed (9%) and they were Mg^{2+} dependent. Ifenprodil did not block astrocyte responses (3%), whereas it had a marked effect on neurons (58%). Memantine at low concentration blocked mainly astrocyte responses (39%) but not neuronal responses (7%), whereas at high concentration, it blocked both responses by 72% in astrocytes and 46% in neurons. In addition, using cortical brain slices, astrocyte and neuronal synaptic responses to NMDA or afferent stimulation were recorded. Astrocyte currents were dependent (TTX blocked them) and proportional to neuronal activity, therefore termed glial synaptic currents (GSC), but had slower rise and decay times compared with neuronal responses. In these experiments, similar results were observed to those observed in acute isolated cells with UBP141, ifenprodil, and memantine. When MK-801 was applied to astrocytes intracellularly, their response was decreased and no further effect was achieved with UBP141 or APV, although Glu transporter inhibitors almost fully abolished astrocytic response. In addition, measuring simultaneously iCa^{2+} with Fluo-3 and currents in astrocytes, it was found that NMDAR contributes importantly (89%) to current response, whereas it mediated approximately half of iCa^{2+} response (50–55%). The Ca^{2+} permeability (Pa_{Ca}/P_{Na}) of astrocytic NMDAR was calculated and found lower than that of neurons (3.4 astrocytes vs. 7.5 neurons), as suggested previously. This value is similar to that of NMDAR containing GluN3 subunits and together with Mg^{2+} independence suggested that GluN3 subunits are assembled into NMDAR of astrocytes. These authors also obtained evidences suggesting that diheteromeric (GluN1/GluN3) NMDAR is present in astrocytes. Together, these findings indicated that NMDAR in cortical astrocytes is assembled with GluN1, GluN2C or D, and GluN3 subunits.

Later the same year, the same group reported the participation of NMDAR, AMPA, and P2X receptors and Glu transporters in astrocyte responses to synaptic activity using the same model [119]. Their results showed that the participation of these molecules change in time. In particular, NMDAR increases its participation in both evoked and spontaneous GSC from the young (1 month) to adult (6 months) animals, declining in old animals (18–21 months). The same behavior was observed for membrane current density and iCa^{2+}.

Also in 2011, Martins de Souza et al. [120] published a proteome analysis of cultured astrocytes (cell line 1321 N1) treated with MK-801 or clozapine, performed with 2D gel electrophoresis followed by MALDI-TOF/TOF mass spectrometry. MK-801 treatment (8–72 h) regulated the expression of different proteins that belong to the energy pathway, cell communication, or cell growth, among others.

One year later, Gerard and Hansson [121] published a paper in which they described that rat cortical astrocytes cocultured (9–11 days) with endothelial cells presented iCa^{2+} responses to NMDA (100 nM-100 μM) measured with Fura-2. These responses were fully blocked by APV or ifenprodil, indicating that NMDAR with GluN2B subunit mediated these responses, subunit that was detected by immunofluorescence. Interestingly, the amplitude of these responses was blocked only partially (50%) in Ca^{2+}-free solution or with Cd^{2+}. Moreover, Ca^{2+} depletion from IC stores with caffeine and thapsigargin almost fully blocked (90%) response amplitude, whereas a combination of IC Ca^{2+} depletion and extracellular Ca^{2+}-free solution fully blocked the response. These results indicated that the source of Ca^{2+} was mainly the IC pools. Consistently, xestospongin C (XesC; inhibitor of inositol tris-phosphate [IP3] receptors) importantly (80%) diminished iCa^{2+} response amplitude and in combination with Ca^{2+}-free extracellular solution reached more than 90% inhibition. These authors also found that lipopolysaccharide (LPS) treatment increased NMDA iCa^{2+} response or IL-1β secretion, effects blocked by APV or ifenprodil. These results constituted the first suggestion that in cultured astrocytes the NMDAR could elicit a metabotropic-like flux-independent response beyond its ionotropic function, although these authors did not rule out the possibility that this response was actually a Ca^{2+}-induced Ca^{2+} release (CICR). Few groups had previously reported that some neuronal functions were mediated by a metabotropic-like, Ca^{2+} flux–independent NMDAR [12].

In 2013, a new expression profile analysis for young (2.5 months) and old (15–18 months) mouse astrocytes and microglia was published [122]. In this work, astrocytes were isolated from mouse brain through FACS using Glu transporter-1 (GLT-1) labeling. The mRNA of these cells was obtained, and cDNA was synthesized and then hybridized in an expression array. Consistent with the work by Cahoy et al. [110], astrocytes were enriched with GluN2C subunit expression in young and old astrocytes. Similar to the previous transcriptome analysis, these authors also found glutamate ionotropic receptor NMDA-type subunit-associated protein 1 (Grina) high expression. In addition, young astrocytes expressed higher levels of GluN3A in comparison to old astrocytes. Unfortunately, when this review was written, the list of genes in the arrays used were not publicly available and therefore it could not be confirmed which other subunits of the NMDAR were included in this array. Certainly, the expression of GluN2 and GluN3 subunits without GluN1 would not result in NMDAR assembly in the ER and transport to the plasma membrane, given the current paradigm and therefore GluN1 subunit expression is inferred. Rusnakova et al. [123] also published a study in which expression of NMDAR subunits was confirmed by single cell quantitative RT-PCR in acute isolated astrocytes from postnatal EGFP-GFAP mouse brains at days 10, 20, 30, and 50. In this work, NMDAR subunits GluN1, GluN2A, GluN2B, GluN2C, GluN2D, and GluN3A were expressed with different levels by these cells. In addition, this study also confirmed the expression of these NMDAR subunits at 3, 7, and 14 days after ischemia.

A new transcriptome database was published later by the Barres group based on RNA library sequencing [124]. This database included several brain cell types: neurons, astrocytes, myelinating, new and precursor oligodendrocytes, microglia, endothelium, and pericytes. In particular, cortical astrocytes were isolated from a transgenic mouse expressing EGFP under control of aldehyde dehydrogenase (Aldh 1 l1) promoter. In the open database at the Stanford University site, astrocytes are reported to express all NMDAR subunits with different levels (https://web.stanford.edu/group/barres_lab/brain_rnaseq.html). These expression levels in astrocytes are paired with expression levels in neurons for comparison and were reported in fragments per kilobase of transcript sequence per million mapped fragments (FPKM) as follows: GluN1 (*Grin1*) astrocytes ≈3 vs. >60 neurons; GluN2A (*Grin2a*) ≈ 0.1 vs. ≈ 0.8; GluN2B (*Grin2b*) ≈ 0.6 vs. ≈ 3; GluN2C (*Grin2c*) >25 vs. <1; GluN2D (*Grin2d*) <0.5 vs. ≈ 1.4; GluN3A (*Grin3a*) ≈ 5 vs. ≈ 6; GluN3B (*Grin3b*) ≈ 0.2 vs. ≈ 0.3. Thus, this study confirmed previous findings in other expression databases [110, 122] indicating GluN1, GluN2C, and GluN3A expression in tissue astrocytes but also found low expression levels of the other NMDAR subunits.

Later, Haustein et al. [125] studied spontaneous Ca^{2+} transients in mouse hippocampal astrocytes infected with an adenovirus containing the genetically encoded Ca^{2+} indicator (GECI) GCaMP. In this work, APV application did not significantly modify soma or projection spontaneous Ca^{2+} transient peak responses, amplitude, or kinetics. However, if traces of these experiments in the work by Haustein et al. [125] are conscientiously analyzed, some subtle differences are observed that perhaps could not be detected due to the statistical analysis or the population of peaks analyzed. However, if this could be true, the effect of APV was contrary to that described by Lalo et al. [105], because in this case, it appears as if NMDAR blockade increased spontaneous iCa^{2+} transients.

The following year, one of us published a work in which serendipitously a metabotropic-like Ca^{2+} flux–independent NMDAR was found in cultured rat cortical astrocytes [15]. In these cells, the expression of the seven NMDAR subunits was found at the mRNA and protein level by immunofluorescence and of GluN1 by WB. Interestingly, it was found that acid-NMDA (1 mM; pH 6.0) elicited iCa^{2+} responses in Fluo-4 labeled astrocytes that were not blocked by MK-801 nor by Ca^{2+}-free extracellular solution, but they were blocked by APV, KYNA, XesC, ryanodine (inhibitor of ryanodine receptors), or GluN1 knockdown by siRNA. Later, we found that iCa^{2+} response was elicited by the NMDAR but in response to acid pH that regulates NMDAR canonic function [2], rather than to NMDA itself. Also, acid-NMDA treatment depleted mitochondrial membrane potential ($m\Delta\psi$). These results strongly suggested that cultured astrocytes express an NMDAR than generates Ca^{2+} release from IC pools, mediated by IP3R and ryanodine receptors as suggested earlier by Gerard and Hansson [121]. However, in contrast to their work, we ruled out that CICR was involved since MK-801 and extracellular Ca^{2+}-free solution did not block this response. These observations COULD help to explain the initial findings in cultured astrocytes that reported no electrophysiological response to NMDA or no iCa^{2+} response to low concentrations of NMDA. Nevertheless, the molecular mechanisms that enable this noncanonical function of the NMDAR still remain to be investigated.

The same year, Jimenez-Blasco et al. [126] reported that in cultured rat cortical astrocytes they observed iCa^{2+} rise measured with Fura-2 elicited by NMDA (1–100 μM). Curiously, NMDA effect was delayed by 500–1000 s after its application, presumably due to the low permeability of NMDAR in astrocytes. NMDA effect was partially sensitive to extracellular Ca^{2+}-free solution, suggesting NMDAR canonical ionotropic function, but it was fully blocked by Ca^{2+}-free solution in combination with SERCA inhibition by thapsigargin, evidencing also Ca^{2+} release from IC pools, although CICR was not ruled out. Moreover, iCa^{2+} rise was sensitive to U73122, inhibitor of phospholipase C (PLC), suggesting that IP3 synthesis could be involved in this effect, in agreement with our results. In addition, long-term NMDA treatment (20 μM, 8 h) promoted the activation of the PLC/protein kinase C (PKC)/p35/cyclin-dependent kinase (Cdk5) pathway that leads to nuclear factor erythroid 2-related factor 2 (Nrf2) activation and its nuclear accumulation, effect blocked by MK-801. Consistently, NMDA treatment activated the transcription of Nrf2-target genes.

Long-term effects of NMDA on astrocytes were reported also by Obara-Michlewska et al. [127], who tested the expression of inwardly rectifying K^+ channels (Kir4.1). In these experiments, the treatment of cultured rat astrocytes with NMDA (100 μM, 72 h) decreased the expression of Kir4.1 at the mRNA and protein level, effect reverted by MK-801 or APV. In addition, in a rat model of acute liver failure, memantine attenuated the decrease of Kir4.1 mRNA in the rat cortex.

On the other hand, Morquette et al. [128] described a role of astrocytes in the rat central pattern generator of the dorsal part of the trigeminal main sensory nucleus. In this study, it was found that astrocytes in this nucleus presented membrane currents or iCa^{2+} rise elicited by electric stimulation or NMDA treatment (1–2 mM), while neuronal activity turned from tonic to bursting and was also accompanied by iCa^{2+} rise. NMDA-elicited depolarizations in astrocytes were insensitive to TTX, whereas an inhibitory cocktail (CNQX, TTX, Cd^{2+}, and L-trans-pyrollidine-2,4-dicarboxylic acid [PCD] inhibitor of Glu uptake) blocked 53% of astrocyte response but almost fully blocked neuronal response, suggesting that astrocytic NMDAR was involved. Also, MK-801 diffused intracellularly in astrocytes blocked NMDA-elicited response in these cells. Together, these results strongly suggested that these astrocytes expressed functional NMDAR.

However, Otsu et al. [129] studied with the Ca^{2+} sensor Rhod-2 iCa^{2+} responses in glomerular astrocytes in the juvenile (14–21 day old) mouse olfactory bulb. In this work, it was found that electrical stimulation of odor sensory neurons elicited iCa^{2+} responses in glomerular astrocytes and neurons. Astrocyte responses were delayed and elicited only with high stimulus intensities in contrast to neuronal ones that were elicited even with single pulse stimulation. Astrocyte and neuronal responses were blocked by a combination of APV and CNQX, similar to the observations made by Lalo et al. [105] in cortical astrocytes. Nevertheless, considering the delay between both responses, these authors suggested that in astrocytes, responses were mediated by postsynaptic activity (dendrite Glu release), instead of a direct stimulation of astrocytic NMDAR or AMPAR. It must be noted that these observations were made measuring somatic Ca^{2+} dynamics, but the NMDAR role was not tested when a GECI mouse model was used. This could be relevant because it has been shown that somatic and projection iCa^{2+} responses have different molecular players [125, 130, 131].

In this year also, Dzamba et al. [132] analyzed the expression of NMDAR subunits in cortical astrocytes from the EGFP-GFAP mouse before and after ischemia by single cell quantitative RT-PCR. In these experiments, all NMDAR subunits were expressed by astrocytes of uninjured mouse with the exception of GluN3B that presented in very low levels, consistently with their previous work [123]. The expression of these genes was increased 7 and 14 days after ischemia, with the exception of GluN2C that was the highest expressed subunit in control conditions and GluN3B that did not increase nor was detected. In contrast, immunofluorescence experiments in brain slices showed only GluN3A expression in control animals, but after ischemia, NMDAR subunits GluN1 and GluN2B-D were also observed. iCa^{2+} responses were elicited in tissue astrocytes by NMDA (4–100 mM), were not blocked by TTX, but were sensitive to APV and memantine. In contrast to previous findings, ischemia reduced iCa^{2+} responses to NMDA. Also, cortical cultured astrocyte iCa^{2+} responses were elicited, but with higher NMDA concentration (500 μM), these responses were also reduced in astrocytes isolated from ischemic mice.

An additional study [133] tested the effect of MK-801 in GFAP expression in tissue hippocampal and cultured astrocytes from rat. In these experiments, MK-801 (6 days) increased GFAP expression in the hippocampus as measured by immunofluorescence and WB. Consistently, MK-801 (24 h) increased GFAP, BDNF, TrkB, and p75 expression at the mRNA and protein level in hippocampal cultured astrocytes. These results suggested that NMDAR activity mediates these effects in astrocytes. Moreover, with these results, the authors proposed that hippocampal astrocytes may participate in NMDAR hypofunction associated to the pathophysiology of schizophrenia.

In 2016, one study by Pinacho et al. [134] showed that MK-801 upregulated the expression of glycogen phosphorylase (PYGM) and RAC-1 when administered in mice but also in cultured rat cortical astrocytes (72 h).

Recently, Mehina et al. [135] studied astrocytes in mouse cortical slices and found that neuronal theta burst stimulation generated transient iCa^{2+} increase in astrocyte soma and projections, followed by a long-lasting decrease of cytoplasmic Ca^{2+} basal levels, perhaps related with observations made by Cornell-Bell et al. [80] with NMDA. Although the transient iCa^{2+} response in astrocytes was blunted by APV, this was not statistically significant; however, it did block the long-lasting decrease of cytoplasmic Ca^{2+} basal levels. Importantly, MK-801 applied intracellularly by the patch pipette also blocked the long-lasting decrease of basal Ca^{2+}, indicating that it was mediated by astrocytic NMDAR. Consistent with the role of NMDAR, it was also found that a NOS inhibitor mediated the decrease of basal Ca^{2+}, probably through its regulation of SERCA. These authors also showed that basal Ca^{2+} levels in astrocytes regulate long-lasting vascular tone, effect blocked by APV.

All in all, these studies have substantiated that astrocytes do express NMDAR at the mRNA, protein, and functional level. However, the reach of this conclusion has not been easy because apparent contradictory findings or controversies have been often reported. A critical issue through this achievement has been the distinction between neuronal and astrocytic NMDAR, considering their location at or near the synapse, but also presynaptic membranes, very close to the perisynaptic astrocyte projection (PAP), where the NMDAR may mediate astrocytic Ca^{2+} responses relevant for information handling in the brain. Nevertheless, other sites of NMDAR actions besides the PAP should not be discarded.

An additional source of controversy has been the selection of the experimental approach and model to test NMDAR in astrocytes. It seems clear now that canonical ionotropic NMDAR function is not conserved in cultured cells compared with tissue astrocytes. Classical electrophysiological experiments initially set the basis to conceive the lack of NMDAR in cultured astrocytes. However, the same approaches applied to tissue or acute isolated astrocytes suggested NMDAR function. In this regard, it is very interesting why and how the NMDAR becomes a different functional molecule when astrocytes are cultured and what may be the physiological relevance (if any) at the cellular and tissular level (see below).

An important source of controversy has been the *a priori* expectations that NMDAR in astrocytes should have similar biophysical and functional properties as its well-studied neuronal synaptic counterpart. Pharmacological studies have already demonstrated that NMDAR in astrocytes may be assembled by different subunits that confer particular functional properties. Its multisubunit nature, diversity of subunits, and multiple posttranslational and posttranscriptional modifications suggest that NMDAR function is more complex as it goes beyond synaptic function. Interestingly, in line with this conception, some reports have already documented a noncanonical metabotropic-like, flux-independent NMDAR function in astrocytes but also in neurons [10–12, 15]. Intriguingly, phosphatidylinositol metabolism was found associated with NMDAR-mediated Ca^{2+} flux in Muller and Bergman cells [136, 137]. As a matter of fact, metabotropic-like, flux-independent function is not necessarily new for ionotropic Glu receptors. It has been reviewed elsewhere that this kind of mechanisms occurs for kainate receptors, some of them described almost 2 decades ago [138]. However, the cellular and molecular mechanisms that make this possible are poorly studied and become very relevant considering NMDAR function in other cells and tissues and flux-independent function observed in neuronal-mediated mechanisms.

Some of the methodological and experimental sources of controversy that precluded the acknowledgment of NMDAR expression and function in astrocytes are shared with those that precluded the acceptance of astrocyte iCa^{2+} dynamic responses in CNS handling of information and function. Please refer to the review by Khakh and McCarthy [139] who deeply discussed these aspects.

4. Insights regarding astrocytic NMDAR

Given the relevance of NMDAR in CNS, the expression of NMDAR in astrocytes, and its role in information handling in CNS, the intuitive conclusion is that NMDAR in astrocytes is implicated in this function, as some electrophysiological works have already demonstrated, detecting iCa^{2+} signals in response to synaptic activity. However, electrical activity in astrocytes may have a secondary role in comparison to other cellular activities such as for instance synctitial communication, in contrast with their neuronal counterparts. Therefore, it is convenient to take into account the diversity of Ca^{2+}-dependent metabotropic IC signals elicited by NMDAR activation, outlined above, that could shape astrocyte activities. Since GluN2C is preferentially assembled into astrocytic NMDAR, then it is possible that IC pathways differ from GluN2A/B NMDAR, as some initial works have demonstrated. This is even more relevant when it is considered that astrocytes are involved not only in information handling, but also in energy administration, immune response to infection or tissue damage, development, or synaptogenesis, among other functions [17, 140]. In this regard, the IC pathways activated by Ca^{2+} entry through the NMDAR must be critical for the long-term effects that could occur not only to the astrocyte but also to its syncytium. Indeed, as described above, some groups have already started to study these long-term effects in astrocytes after chronic exposure to NMDA, and as history has demonstrated, cell culture is a useful tool to study these aspects. In addition, NMDAR has been shown to mediate IC signaling in astrocytes, function critically involved in neuronal survival. Furthermore, since astrocytes are also involved in the immune response and some evidences point to enhanced NMDAR activity in these cells after ischemia, thus it is possible to conceive that NMDAR in astrocytes is involved in immune function of these cells, as has been observed previously in lymphocytes [8]. Also, recent work has suggested that NMDAR of astrocytes could be involved in the hypofunction of NMDAR that has been proposed as an alternative hypothesis to understand schizophrenia [133]. More work is needed to investigate how NMDAR in astrocytes is related to other pathologies that have been related to astrocyte functions [141].

On the other hand, Ca^{2+} flux–independent metabotropic signaling by NMDAR in cultured astrocytes provides the grounds for a new framework of NMDAR activity, although more research is required to further confirm its occurrence in tissue astrocytes. Nevertheless, it must be noted that multifunctionality of cell membrane molecules is now well documented, and most of these mechanisms were initially described in cultured cells ([136]; and references therein). Indeed, it is possible that the effect observed by Nishizaki et al. [97] and Kondoh et al. [101] in cultured human astrocytes with a G-protein inhibitor could be related to NMDAR signaling inhibition itself instead of NMDA activation of an unknown receptor that elicited G-protein activation, or NMDAR regulation by a GPCR, as it was suggested. If true, this report could be the first hinting Ca^{2+} flux–independent metabotropic signaling by NMDAR. Therefore, this kind of signaling should not be discarded *a priori*, also considering that this Ca^{2+} flux–independent NMDAR function has also been observed in neuronal-mediated responses, and the number of works documenting this function is increasing [12, 142]. Moreover, flux-independent metabotropic signaling by other ionotropic Glu receptors have been known for almost 2 decades [138].

The experimental evidence indicates that in cultured astrocytes Ca^{2+} flux–independent metabotropic NMDAR signaling is dominant over its ionotropic function, that could be exacerbated by culture conditions, such as Glu concentration or the extracellular proteins present in fetal bovine serum. However, it is not possible to rule out that in tissue astrocytes some NMDAR, probably distributed at specific cellular locations, may elicit this kind of signaling. The currents observed in acute isolated astrocytes, the conservation of some classical ionotropic NMDAR function in astrocytes cocultured with endothelial cells, and its absence in pure cultured astrocytes support this notion [15, 105, 121], because cellular interactions may be involved in the conservation of canonical NMDAR function. Moreover, these observations may reflect a gradual conversion of NMDAR function due to some unknown mechanism that may be related to membrane dynamics. In addition, our observations suggest that there is some sort of segregation of Ca^{2+} flux–dependent and –independent functions of NMDAR in cultured astrocytes [143, 144]. Consistent with these putative Ca^{2+} flux–dependent and –independent functions of NMDAR, long-term effects in cultured astrocytes and even iCa^{2+} rise in human cultured astrocytes have been blocked by MK-801 or memantine, thus substantiating a canonical ionotropic function. This somehow contradicts the fact that most electrophysiological recordings in cultured astrocytes have never found NMDAR-mediated currents, with the exception of the work with human astrocytes from the white matter that intriguingly were not sensitive to APV. These apparent contradictions may have their source in the experimental settings employed, as described above. For instance, the cell model employed may cooperate in this variability given the diversity of astrocytes [145, 146]. Also, the intracellular crosstalk among Glu ionotropic and metabotropic receptors and their regulation in the experimental models employed may interplay and result in the apparent contradictions observed. In addition, it is of note that most experiments studying NMDAR in cultured astrocytes have used high agonist concentrations that are within the Glu concentration reached in the synaptic cleft after neurotransmission [147]. Also, it is interesting that different physiological solutions have been used with cultured astrocytes that could be related to the observations made. Notably, experiments with human astrocytes have shown unique behaviors of NMDAR suggesting perhaps that in human cells NMDAR may have specific molecular features that are still unknown.

However, the fact that cultured rat astrocytes present Ca^{2+} flux–independent metabotropic NMDAR signaling indicates at least the existence of a cellular and/or molecular mechanism that enables this function, although it could be overrepresented in cultured astrocytes due to culture conditions. This mechanism may be related to the expression of genes that let some authors conclude that cultured astrocytes represent an undifferentiated or activated phenotype of astrocytes. Nonetheless, since NMDAR is also expressed by endothelial cells, leukocytes, osteoblasts, platelets, or melanocytes, among other cells but also in a diversity of tissues including stomach, testis, thymus, ovaries, skin, pancreas, lung, kidney, or heart [3], it is likely that NMDAR function may encompass other mechanisms of action and regulation, beyond those described for synaptic or extrasynaptic NMDAR. For instance, leukocytes or endothelial cells are in contact with 40 times higher Glu (40 μM) in the blood than cells of CNS bathed by the cerebrospinal fluid (1 μM) [148]. Therefore, NMDAR in these cells must require particular cellular or molecular mechanisms to avoid its activation and the resulting entry of large quantities of Ca^2 that could activate them or even be cytotoxic. Also, Mg^{2+} blockade should not work in these cells since Glu concentrations are constant, unless it is regulated differently to neuronal NMDAR. One alternative for this Ca^{2+} flux–independent metabotropic-like function is that in cell culture, the NMDAR associates with molecular partners that enable this function. Interestingly, it has been reported that NMDAR has been found to associate with metabotropic dopamine receptors [149]. There is also a possibility that Ca^{2+} flux–independent metabotropic-like NMDAR function could be the result of proteolytic cleavage, as that already reported for NMDAR subunit GluN1 [150], that occurs to other membrane molecules [151]. In addition, GluN2C subunit–mediated IC signaling, found highly expressed in most transcriptome analysis of astrocytes, but that has been poorly studied, could be involved.

Of particular interest is the fact that, according to our results, higher H^+ concentration seems responsible to elicit NMDAR Ca^{2+} flux–independent metabotropic-like function. This is because three main points are relevant for CNS: (a) It is well known that presynaptic Glu release causes an increase of H^+ concentration in the synaptic cleft [152]. (b) Under certain processes such as inflammation, hypoxia/ischemia, or hypercapnia, among others, very low pH levels may be reached in the brain [153]. (c) The NMDAR is well known to be regulated negatively by acidic pH, and the amino acid sequences that mediate this effect have been identified [2]. Then, Ca^{2+} flux–independent metabotropic-like function of NMDAR in astrocytes presents singularities, or even antagonic features when compared with canonical NMDAR that could be relevant for astrocyte function and therefore for the maintenance of brain homeostasis. Thus, the study of the molecular mechanisms that make possible Ca^{2+} flux–independent function of the NMDAR may open new possibilities to modulate NMDAR function in certain pathologies.

On the other hand, which advantage presents the Ca^{2+} flux–independent metabotropic-like NMDAR in astrocytes? Perhaps the easiest answer is that some sort of NMDAR signaling could be initiated without extracellular Ca^{2+} entry that could pose a menace for cellular homeostasis. This could be more advantageous if it is considered that in our experiments we found that Ca^{2+} flux–independent metabotropic-like NMDAR is dependent on H^+ levels above physiological normal levels [15]. However, the nature of the IC pathways initiated by this Ca^{2+} flux–independent metabotropic-like NMDAR still remains to be investigated, because the PLC/PKC/p35/Cdk5/Nrf2 pathway activation was sensitive to MK-801 similar to CAPON nuclear translocation that may lead to MAPK activation through NOS. Thus, it seems that activation of these pathways by long-term treatment with NMDA requires Ca^{2+} flux. To further analyze this question, it is then necessary to define whether this metabotropic-like function is mediated by a channel NMDAR with posttranslational modifications that is also capable to initiate signal transduction as has been observed in neuronal NMDAR [12, 142] or by a nonchannel NMDAR. In the first case then, some specific mechanism of channel blockade must act to avoid fast measurable Ca^{2+} flux through NMDAR. In the second case, perhaps other molecular mechanisms could result in a nonchannel NMDAR, as described above. However, this question requires further research to fully understand the mechanism that enables Ca^{2+} flux–independent metabotropic-like NMDAR in astrocytes and perhaps in neurons or other cell types.

All the above-described effects mediated by NMDAR in astrocytes must occur when it is located in (a) the astrocyte synaptic membrane (AsSm) of the PAP that directly contacts the synapse, analog to the postsynaptic membrane, and/or in (b) PAP extrasynaptic sites that could even include the soma. However, IHC-EM experiments have indicated that NMDAR in astrocytes is preferentially located in their projections. In addition, Lalo et al. [105] have already described the GSC, suggesting that Glu sensing takes place at the PAP or near it, thus somatic NMDAR function seems unlikely, although this needs to be tested. The PAP is a dynamic structure that surrounds the synaptic bouton (**Figure 3**) extending and retracting as a function of synaptic activity. The more neuronal activity, the more neurotransmitter and the more PAP coverage [125, 154, 155]. But, is the NMDAR present in the AsSm of PAPs? Or is NMDAR located in extrasynaptic sites in the PAP where it would only be activated by some Glu spillover? If it is located in AsSm, then NMDAR could be sensing tiny amounts of Glu, whereas if it is in extrasynaptic sites, then only high synaptic activity would lead to its activation. This is in fact a common feature of iCa^{2+} signaling in astrocytes, and it is observed with high synaptic activity, as described by different groups [105, 125]. However, this observation could be the result of the integration of synaptic activity carried out by astrocytes and thus

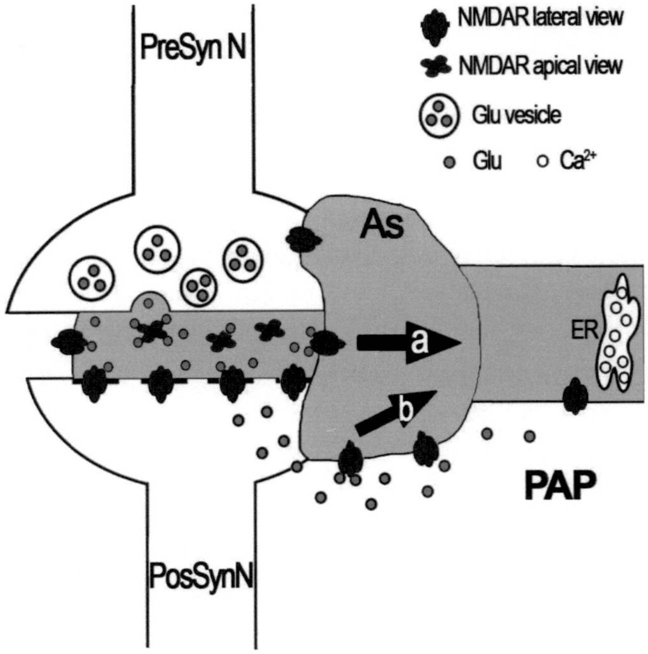

Figure 3. Astrocytic NMDAR putative locations. NMDAR may be located in the astrocyte synaptic membrane (AsSm) and/or astrocytic extrasynaptic membranes. IC signaling (a or b) in both places could be specific, b requiring Glu spillover. In a and/or b, the Ca^{2+} flux–independent metabotropic-like NMDAR could be involved, reaching IC Ca^{2+} pools such as the ER in the PAP. As, astrocyte; PreSynN, presynaptic neuron; PosSynN, postsynaptic neuron (see text for details).

does not necessarily rule out the presence of NMDAR in front of the synapse. Instead, it is possible that not enough receptors located at the AsSm are activated when low synaptic activity is elicited and thus the whole cell currents are not recorded. Therefore, at this point, it is not clear the exact location of astrocytic NMDAR; however, in this context, the density and organization of receptors at cell membrane in either location are relevant for the final result (**Figure 3**).

At this point, it is convenient to recall that Glu has been suggested to exert only metabotropic signaling (through mGluR, although the putative Ca^{2+} flux–independent function of NMDAR could participate) in extrasynaptic sites of the PAP, in view of the location of IC Ca^{2+} stores ≈1 μm far from the AsSm [156]. However, according to our biophysical modeling work, Ca^{2+} and IP3 diffusion coefficients (10X larger for IP3), together with mGluR location, support that synaptic astrocyte Glu metabotropic signaling may occur and reach IC Ca^{2+} stores within millisecond time scales depending upon PLC activity and number [157]. Moreover, PAP leaf-like morphology would optimize IP3 straightforward diffusion to IC Ca^{2+} stores. In contrast, although Glu has a ≈ 1.5 faster diffusion coefficient than IP3, the need to escape from the synaptic cleft and override the PAP enwrapping in the EC space and Glu multidirectional diffusion would perhaps make this alternative more difficult to occur, although not impossible when very high Glu secretion is reached (**Figure 3**).

Considering the ambivalent nature of NMDAR signaling described above (synaptic vs. extrasynaptic), an additional immediate question that comes up is which kind of signaling (prosurvival or prodeath) results from astrocytic NMDAR? Since astrocytes are resistant to different insults including high levels of Glu, then intuitively the answer should be prosurvival signaling. In fact, this has been confirmed by different works, but with some differences in comparison with synaptic NMDAR signaling described above. Activation of PLC/PKC/p35/Cdk5/Nrf2, a prosurvival pathway, and CAPON nuclear translocation were described in cultured astrocytes in response to NMDAR [114, 126]. On the other hand, MK-801 treatment of cultured astrocytes upregulated glycogen phosphorylase and regulated the expression of growth and metabolic genes [134]. Together, these observations indicate that NMDAR in cultured astrocytes provide signaling that help to maintain homeostasis. In line with this idea, ischemia increases NMDAR subunits, perhaps providing better tools for cell survival.

5. Conclusions

Research regarding NMDAR expression and function in astrocytes has been full of apparent contradictions and controversies and some of them still remain puzzling. Nevertheless, it now seems clear that tissue astrocytes do express NMDAR subunits that are assembled into functional receptors that mediate membrane currents, but are different from the well-studied neuronal NMDAR. On the other hand, cultured astrocytes also express NMDAR subunits, but it is well documented that NMDAR ligands do not elicit recordable membrane currents. However, few groups have found that NMDAR in cultured astrocytes evoke Ca^{2+} flux–independent metabotropic-like signaling, with the exception of human cultured astrocytes in which currents present certain singularities. Intriguingly, some reports have documented that long-term effects of NMDAR agonists in cultured astrocytes are prevented by the pore blocker MK-801. Thus, more research is needed to elucidate NMDAR function and its consequences in cultured astrocytes. Although NMDAR function in cultured astrocytes may represent a rare phenomena that result from culture conditions, it cannot be discarded *a priori* that it may occur in tissue astrocytes. This possibility is supported by NMDAR wide expression in non-CNS cells that could also be relevant for NMDAR Ca^{2+} flux–independent effects also observed in neurons.

Moreover, the apparent contradictions and controversies found in the last decades in the study of NMDAR in astrocytes together with its wide expression in cells and tissues let us realize that the biology of NMDAR is much more complex than that described for synaptic NMDAR. This seems to be true even within the synapse, where presynaptic NMDAR has casted new complexities in its synaptic function. Also, the NMDAR subunit phylogenetic conservation reinforces this idea. However, the understanding of NMDAR function in astrocytes and other cells and tissues may lead to envision new therapeutic strategies as has been suggested previously.

Acknowledgements

PMOB wishes to thank the invitation from Dr. Maria Teresa Gentile and Dr. Luca Colucci D'Amato to collaborate as an author in this book. PMOB also deeply thanks his family who has supported him despite the lack of funding and the difficulties to do science in his institution and our country. JRGH appreciates the unconditional support of his family and PMOB support and invitation to participate in this review.

Author details

Pavel Montes de Oca Balderas* and José Roberto González Hernández

*Address all correspondence to: pavel73@hotmail.com

Unit of Dynamic Neurobiology, Department of Neurochemistry, Instituto Nacional de Neurología y Neurocirugía, Mexico

References

[1] Paoletti P, Bellone C, Zhou Q. NMDA receptor subunit diversity: Impact on receptor properties, synaptic plasticity and disease. Nature Reviews. Neuroscience. 2013;**14**:383-400

[2] Traynelis SF, Wollmuth LP, McBain CJ, Menniti FS, Vance KM, Ogden KK, et al. Glutamate receptor ion channels: Structure, regulation, and function. Pharmacological Reviews. 2010;**62**:405-496

[3] Hogan-Cann AD, Anderson CM. Physiological roles of non-neuronal NMDA receptors. Trends in Pharmacological Sciences. 2016;**37**:750-767. DOI: 10.1016/j.tips.2016.05.012

[4] Aarts MM, Tymianski M. Novel treatment of excitotoxicity: Targeted disruption of intracellular signalling from glutamate receptors. Biochemical Pharmacology. 2003;**66**: 877-886

[5] Hardingham GE, Bading H. Synaptic versus extrasynaptic NMDA receptor signalling: Implications for neurodegenerative disorders. Nature Reviews. Neuroscience. 2010;**11**: 682-696

[6] Schwarzschild MA, Cole RL, Meyers MA, Hyman SE. Contrasting calcium dependencies of SAPK and ERK activations by glutamate in cultured striatal neurons. Journal of Neurochemistry. 1999;**72**:2248-2255. DOI: 10.1046/j.1471-4159.1999.0722248.x

[7] Kalev-Zylinska ML, Green TN, Morel-Kopp MC, Sun PP, Park YE, Lasham A, et al. N-methyl-D-aspartate receptors amplify activation and aggregation of human platelets. Thrombosis Research. 2014;**133**:837-847

[8] Lombardi G, Dianzani C, Miglio G, Canonico PL, Fantozzi R. Characterization of ionotropic glutamate receptors in human lymphocytes. British Journal of Pharmacology. 2001;**133**:936-944

[9] Spencer GJ, McGrath CJ, Genever PG. Current perspectives on NMDA-type glutamate signalling in bone. The International Journal of Biochemistry & Cell Biology. 2007;**39**: 1089-1104

[10] Kessels HW, Nabavi S, Malinow R. Metabotropic NMDA receptor function is required for beta-amyloid-induced synaptic depression. Proceedings of the National Academy of Sciences of the United States of America. 2013;**110**:4033-4038

[11] Nabavi S, Fox R, Alfonso S, Aow J, Malinow R. GluA1 trafficking and metabotropic NMDA: Addressing results from other laboratories inconsistent with ours. Philosophical Transactions of the Royal Society B: Biological Sciences. 2013;**369**:20130145

[12] Dore K, Aow J, Malinow R. The emergence of NMDA receptor metabotropic function: Insights from imaging. Frontiers in Synaptic Neuroscience. 2016;**8**:1-9. DOI: 10.3389/fnsyn.2016.00020

[13] Weilinger NL, Lohman AW, Rakai BD, Ma EMM, Bialecki J, Maslieieva V, et al. Metabotropic NMDA receptor signaling couples Src family kinases to pannexin-1 during excitotoxicity. Nature Neuroscience. 2016;**19**:432-442. DOI: 10.1038/nn.4236

[14] Vissel B, Krupp JJ, Heinemann SF, Westbrook GL. A use-dependent tyrosine dephosphorylation of NMDA receptors is independent of ion flux. Nature Neuroscience. 2001;**4**:587-596

[15] Montes de Oca Balderas P, Aguilera P. A metabotropic-like flux-independent NMDA receptor regulates Ca^{2+} exit from endoplasmic reticulum and mitochondrial membrane potential in cultured astrocytes. PLoS One. 2015;**10**:e0126314. DOI: 10.1371/journal.pone.0126314

[16] Araque A, Parpura V, Sanzgiri RP, Haydon PG. Tripartite synapses: Glia, the unacknowledged partner. Trends in Neurosciences. 1999;**22**:208-215

[17] Verkhratsky A, Butt AM, editors. Glial Physiology and Pathophysiology: A Handbook. 1st ed. Chichester: Wiley-Blackwell; 2013

[18] Haddad JJ. N-methyl-D-aspartate (NMDA) and the regulation of mitogen-activated protein kinase (MAPK) signaling pathways: A revolving neurochemical axis for therapeutic intervention? Progress in Neurobiology. 2005;**77**:252-282. DOI: 10.1016/j.pneurobio.2005.10.008

[19] Pláteník J, Kuramoto N, Yoneda Y. Molecular mechanisms associated with long-term consolidation of the NMDA signals. Life Sciences. 2000;**67**:335-364. DOI: 10.1016/S0024-3205(00)00632-9

[20] Hardingham GE, Fukunaga Y, Bading H. Extrasynaptic NMDARs oppose synaptic NMDARs by triggering CREB shut-off and cell death pathways. Nature Neuroscience. 2002. DOI: 10.1038/nn835

[21] Sava A, Formaggio E, Carignani C, Andreetta F, Bettini E, Griffante C. NMDA-induced ERK signalling is mediated by NR2B subunit in rat cortical neurons and switches from positive to negative depending on stage of development. Neuropharmacology. 2012;**62**:925-932. DOI: 10.1016/j.neuropharm.2011.09.025

[22] Waxman EA, Lynch DR. N-methyl-D-aspartate receptor subtypes: Multiple roles in excitotoxicity and neurological disease. The Neuroscientist. 2005;**11**:37-49. DOI: 10.1177/1073858404269012

[23] Zhang SJ, Steijaert MN, Lau D, Schütz G, Delucinge-Vivier C, Descombes P, et al. Decoding NMDA receptor signaling: Identification of genomic programs specifying neuronal survival and death. Neuron. 2007;**53**:549-562. DOI: 10.1016/j.neuron.2007.01.025

[24] Tovar KR, Westbrook GL. Mobile NMDA receptors at hippocampal synapses. Neuron. 2002;**34**:255-264. DOI: 10.1016/S0896-6273(02)00658-X

[25] Zhou X, Ding Q, Chen Z, Yun H, Wang H. Involvement of the GluN2A and GluN2B subunits in synaptic and extrasynaptic N-methyl-D-aspartate receptor function and neuronal excitotoxicity. The Journal of Biological Chemistry. 2013;**288**:24151-24159. DOI: 10.1074/jbc.M113.482000

[26] Xia Z, Storm DR. The role of Calmodulin as a signal integrator for synaptic plasticity. Nature Reviews. Neuroscience. 2005;**6**:267-276. DOI: 10.1038/nrn1647

[27] Malenka RC, Kauer JA, Perkel DJ, Mauk MD, Kelly PT, Nicoll RA, et al. And protein kinase activity an essential role for postsynaptic Calmodulin in long-term potentiation. Nature. 1989;**340**:554-557. DOI: 10.1038/340301a0

[28] Bading H, Ginty D, Greenberg M. Regulation of gene expression in hippocampal neurons by distinct calcium signaling pathways. Science (80-). 1993;**260**:181-187. DOI: 10.1017/CBO9781107415324.004

[29] Ehlers MD, Zhang S, Bernhardt JP, Huganir RL. Inactivation of NMDA receptors by direct interaction of Calmodulin with the NR1 subunit. Cell. 1996;**84**:745-755. DOI: 10.1016/S0092-8674(00)81052-1

[30] Bayer K-U, De Koninck P, Leonard AS, Hell JW, Schulman H. Interaction with the NMDA receptor locks CaMKII in an active conformation. Nature. 2001;**411**:801-805. DOI: 10.1038/35081080

[31] Lisman J, Yasuda R, Raghavachari S. Mechanisms of CaMKII action in log term potentiation. Nature Reviews. Neuroscience. 2012;**13**:169-182. DOI: 10.1002/ana.22528.Toll-like

[32] Engert F, Bonhoeffer T. Dendritic spine changes associated with hippocampal long-term synaptic plasticity. Nature. 1999;**399**:66-70

[33] Hardingham GE, Arnold FJ, Bading H. Nuclear calcium signaling controls CREB-mediated gene expression triggered by synaptic activity. Nature Neuroscience. 2001;**4**:261-267. DOI: 10.1038/85109

[34] Coultrap SJ, Bayer KU. CaMKII regulation in information processing and storage. Trends in Neurosciences. 2012;**35**:607-618. DOI: 10.1016/j.tins.2012.05.003

[35] Impey S, Fong AL, Wang Y, Cardinaux JR, Fass DM, Obrietan K, et al. Phosphorylation of CBP mediates transcriptional activation by neural activity and CaM kinase IV. Neuron. 2002;**34**:235-244. DOI: 10.1016/S0896-6273(02)00654-2

[36] Shi G-X, Andres DA, Cai W. Ras family small GTP-ase-mediated neuroprotective signaling in stroke. Central Nervous System Agents in Medicinal Chemistry. 2011;**11**:114-137. DOI: 10.1002/ana.22528.Toll-like

[37] Bading H, Greenberg ME. Stimulation of protein tyrosine phosphorylation by NMDA receptor activation. Science (New York, NY). 1991;**253**:912-914. DOI: 10.1126/science.1715095

[38] Yun HY, Gonzalez-Zulueta M, Dawson VL, Dawson TM. Nitric oxide mediates N-methyl-D-aspartate receptor-induced activation of p21 ras. Proceedings of the National Academy of Sciences of the United States of America. 1998;**95**:5773-5778

[39] Weissman BA, Jones CL, Liu Q, Gross SS. Activation and inactivation of neuronal nitric oxide synthase: Characterization of Ca^{2+}-dependent [125I] Calmodulin binding. European Journal of Pharmacology. 2002;**435**:9-18. DOI: 10.1016/S0014-2999(01)01560-6

[40] Krapivinsky G, Krapivinsky L, Manasian Y, Ivanov A, Tyzio R, Pellegrino C, et al. The NMDA receptor is coupled to the ERK pathway by a direct interaction between NR2B and RasGRF1. Neuron. 2003;**40**:775-784. DOI: 10.1016/S0896-6273(03)00645-7

[41] Fan X, Jin WY, Wang YT. The NMDA receptor complex: A multifunctional machine at the glutamatergic synapse. Frontiers in Cellular Neuroscience. 2014;**8**:160. DOI: 10.3389/fncel.2014.00160

[42] Joyal JL, Burks DJ, Pons S, Matter WF, Vlahos CJ, White MF, et al. Calmodulin activates phosphatidylinositol 3-kinase. The Journal of Biological Chemistry. 1997;**272**:28183-28186. DOI: 10.1074/jbc.272.45.28183

[43] Chandler LJ, Sutton G, Dorairaj NR, Norwood D. *N*-methyl-D-aspartate receptor-mediated bidirectional control of extracellular signal-regulated kinase activity in cortical neuronal cultures. The Journal of Biological Chemistry. 2001;**276**:2627-2636. DOI: 10.1074/jbc.M003390200

[44] Sutton G, Chandler LJ. Activity-dependent NMDA receptor-mediated activation of protein kinase B/Akt in cortical neuronal cultures. Journal of Neurochemistry. 2002;**82**:1097-1105. DOI: 10.1046/j.1471-4159.2002.01031.x

[45] Hay N, Sonenberg N. Upstream and downstream of ran GTPase. Genes & Development. 2004;**18**:1926-1945. DOI: 10.1515/BC.2000.052

[46] Kovacs KA, Steullet P, Steinmann M, Do KQ, Magistretti PJ, Halfon O, et al. TORC1 is a calcium- and cAMP-sensitive coincidence detector involved in hippocampal long-term synaptic plasticity. Proceedings of the National Academy of Sciences. 2007;**104**:4700-4705. DOI: 10.1073/pnas.0607524104

[47] Sasaki T, Takemori H, Yagita Y, Terasaki Y, Uebi T, Horike N, et al. SIK2 is a key regulator for neuronal survival after ischemia via TORC1-CREB. Neuron. 2011;**69**:106-119. DOI: 10.1016/j.neuron.2010.12.004

[48] Zhang S-J, Buchthal B, Lau D, Hayer S, Dick O, Schwaninger M, et al. A signaling Cascade of nuclear calcium-CREB-ATF3 activated by synaptic NMDA receptors defines a gene repression module that protects against extrasynaptic NMDA receptor-induced neuronal cell death and ischemic brain damage. The Journal of Neuroscience. 2011;**31**:4978-4990. DOI: 10.1523/JNEUROSCI.2672-10.2011

[49] Tolias KF, Bikoff JB, Burette A, Paradis S, Harrar D, Tavazoie S, et al. The Rac1-GEF Tiam1 couples the NMDA receptor to the activity-dependent development of dendritic arbors and spines. Neuron. 2005;**45**:525-538. DOI: 10.1016/j.neuron.2005.01.024

[50] Fleming IN, Elliott CM, Buchanan G, Downes CP, Exton H, Buchanan FG, et al. Ca^{2+}/Calmodulin-dependent protein kinase II regulates Tiam1 by reversible protein phosphorylation. The Journal of Biological Chemistry. 1999;**274**:12753-12758

[51] Lieberman DN, Mody I. Regulation of NMDA channel function by endogenous Ca^{2+}-dependent phosphatese. Nature. 1994;**369**:235-239

[52] Fukazawa Y, Saitoh Y, Ozawa F, Ohta Y, Mizuno K, Inokuchi K. Hippocampal LTP is accompanied by enhanced F-actin content within the dendritic spine that is essential for late LTP maintenance in vivo. Neuron. 2003;**38**:447-460. DOI: 10.1016/S0896-6273(03)00206-X

[53] Xia Z, Dudek H, Miranti CK, Greenberg ME. Calcium influx via the NMDA receptor induces immediate early gene transcription by a MAP kinase/ERK-dependent mechanism. The Journal of Neuroscience. 1996;**16**:5425-5436

[54] Lau D, Bading H. Synaptic activity-mediated suppression of p53 and induction of nuclear calcium-regulated Neuroprotective genes promote survival through inhibition of mitochondrial permeability transition. The Journal of Neuroscience. 2009;**29**:4420-4429. DOI: 10.1523/JNEUROSCI.0802-09.2009

[55] Leveille F, Papadia S, Fricker M, Bell KFS, Soriano FX, Martel M-A, et al. Suppression of the intrinsic apoptosis pathway by synaptic activity. The Journal of Neuroscience. 2010;**30**:2623-2635. DOI: 10.1523/JNEUROSCI.5115-09.2010

[56] Riedl SJ, Salvesen GS. The apoptosome: Signalling platform of cell death. Nature Reviews. Molecular Cell Biology. 2007;**8**:405-413. DOI: 10.1038/nrm2153

[57] Ivanov A, Pellegrino C, Rama S, Dumalska I, Salyha Y, Ben-Ari Y, et al. Opposing role of synaptic and extrasynaptic NMDA receptors in regulation of the extracellular signal-regulated kinases (ERK) activity in cultured rat hippocampal neurons. The Journal of Physiology. 2006;**572**:789-798. DOI: 10.1113/jphysiol.2006.105510

[58] Myung JK, Dunah AW, Yu TW, Sheng M. Differential roles of NR2A- and NR2B-containing NMDA receptors in Ras-ERK signaling and AMPA receptor trafficking. Neuron. 2005;**46**:745-760. DOI: 10.1016/j.neuron.2005.04.031

[59] Chen HJ, Rojas-Soto M, Oguni A, Kennedy MB. A synaptic Ras-GTPase activating protein (p135 SynGAP) inhibited by CaM kinase II. Neuron. 1998;**20**:895-904. DOI: 10.1016/S0896-6273(00)80471-7

[60] Salih DAM, Brunet A. FoxO transcription factors in the maintenance of cellular homeostasis during aging. Current Opinion in Cell Biology. 2008;**20**:126-136. DOI: 10.1016/j.ceb.2008.02.005.FoxO

[61] Al-Mubarak B, Soriano FX, Hardingham GE. Synaptic NMDAR activity suppresses FOXO1 expression via a cis-acting FOXO binding site: FOXO1 is a FOXO target gene. Channels. 2009;**3**:233-238. DOI: 10.1038/nn2071.Al-Mubarak

[62] Dick O, Bading H. Synaptic activity and nuclear calcium signaling protect hippocampal neurons from death signal-associated nuclear translocation of FoxO3a induced by extrasynaptic N-methyl-D-aspartate receptors. The Journal of Biological Chemistry. 2010;**285**:19354-19361. DOI: 10.1074/jbc.M110.127654

[63] Dieterich DC, Karpova A, Mikhaylova M, Zdobnova I, König I, Landwehr M, et al. Caldendrin-Jacob: A protein liaison that couples NMDA receptor signalling to the nucleus. PLoS Biology. 2008;**6**:0286-0306. DOI: 10.1371/journal.pbio.0060034

[64] Liu J, Liu MC, Wang KKW. Calpain in the CNS: from synaptic function to neurotoxicity. Science Signaling. 2008;**1**:re1. DOI: 10.1126/stke.114re1

[65] Xu J, Kurup P, Zhang Y, Goebel-goody SM, Wu PH, Hawasli AH, et al. Extrasynaptic NMDAR couple preferentially to excitotoxicity via calpain-mediated cleavage of STEP. The Journal of Neuroscience. 2009;**2929**:9330-9343. DOI: 10.1523/JNEUROSCI.2212-09.2009.Extrasynaptic

[66] Nguyen TH, Paul S, Xu Y, Gurd JW, Lombroso PJ. Calcium-dependent cleavage of striatal enriched tyrosine phosphatase (STEP). Journal of Neurochemistry. 1999;**73**:1995-2001

[67] Gurd JW, Bissoon N, Nguyen TH, Lombroso PJ, Rider CC, Beesley PW, et al. Hypoxia-ischemia in perinatal rat brain induces the formation of a low molecular weight isoform of striatal enriched tyrosine phosphatase (STEP). Journal of Neurochemistry. 1999;**73**:1990-1994

[68] Kawasaki H, Morooka T, Shimohama S, Kimura J, Hirano T, Gotoh Y, et al. Activation and involvement of p38 mitogen-activated protein kinase in glutamate-induced apoptosis in rat cerebellar granule cells. The Journal of Biological Chemistry. 1997;**272**:18518-18521

[69] Verkhratsky A, Kirchhoff F. NMDA receptors in glia. The Neuroscientist. 2007;**13**:28-37

[70] Dzamba D, Honsa P, Anderova M. NMDA receptors in glial cells: Pending questions. Current Neuropharmacology. 2013;**11**:250-262. DOI: 10.2174/1570159X11311030002

[71] Krnjevic K, Schwartz S. Some properties of unresponsive cells in the cerebral cortex. Experimental Brain Research. 1967;**3**:306-319

[72] Hösli L, Andrés PF, Hösli E. Depolarization of cultured astrocytes by glutamate and aspartate. Neuroscience. 1979;**4**:1593-1598. DOI: 10.1016/0306-4522(79)90022-8

[73] Constanti A, Galvan M. Amino acid-evoked depolarization of electrically inexcitable (neuroglial?) cells in the guinea pig olfactory cortex slice. Brain Research. 1978;**153**:183-187

[74] Kettenmann H, Schachner M. Pharmacological properties of gamma-aminobutyric acid-, glutamate-, and aspartate-induced depolarizations in cultured astrocytes. The Journal of Neuroscience. 1985;**5**:3295-3301

[75] Bowman CL, Kimelberg HK. Excitatory amino acids directly depolarize rat brain astrocytes in primary culture. Nature. 1984;**311**:656-659

[76] Sontheimer H, Kettenmann H, Backus KH, Schachner M. Glutamate opens Na^+/K^+ channels in cultured astrocytes. Glia. 1988;**1**:328-336. DOI: 10.1002/glia.440010505

[77] Pearce B, Albrecht J, Morrow C, Murphy S. Astrocyte glutamate receptor activation promotes inositol phospholipid turnover and calcium flux. Neuroscience Letters. 1986;**72**:335-340. DOI: 10.1016/0304-3940(86)90537-9

[78] Usowicz MM, Gallo V, Cull-Candy SG. Multiple conductance channels in type-2 cerebellar astrocytes activated by excitatory amino acids. Nature. 1989;**339**:380-383. DOI: 10.1038/340301a0

[79] Backus K, Kettenmann H, Schachner M. Pharmacological characterization of the glutamate receptor in cultured astrocytes. Journal of Neuroscience Research. 1989;**282**:274-282

[80] Cornell-Bell AH, Finkbeiner SM, Cooper MS, Smith SJ. Glutamate induces calcium waves in cultured astrocytes: Long-range glial signaling. Science (80-). 1990;**247**:470-473

[81] Jensen AM, Chiu SY. Fluorescence measurement of changes in intracellular calcium induced by excitatory amino acids in cultured cortical astrocytes. The Journal of Neuroscience. 1990;**10**:1165-1175

[82] Cornell-Bell AH, Thomas PG, Smith SJ. The excitatory neurotransmitter glutamate causes filopodia formation in cultured hippocampal astrocytes. Glia. 1990;**3**:322-334

[83] Dani JW, Chernavsky A, Smith SJ. Neuronal activity triggers calcium waves in hippocampal astrocytic networks. Neuron. 1992;**8**:429-440

[84] Holzwarth JA, Gibbons SJ, Brorson JR, Philipson LH, Miller RJ. Glutamate receptor agonists stimulate diverse calcium responses in different types of cultured rat cortical glial cells. The Journal of Neuroscience 1994;**14**:1879-1891

[85] Seifert G, Steinhäuser C. Glial cells in the mouse hippocampus express AMPA receptors with an intermediate Ca^{2+} permeability. The European Journal of Neuroscience. 1995;**7**:1872-1881. DOI: 10.1111/j.1460-9568.1995.tb00708.x

[86] Steinhauser C, Jabs R, Ket H. Properties of GABA and glutamate responses in identified glial cells of the mouse hippocampal slice. Hippocampus. 1994;**4**:19-36

[87] Porter JT, McCarthy KD. GFAP-positive hippocampal astrocytes in situ respond to glutamatergic neuroligands with increases in $[Ca^{2+}]i$. Glia. 1995;**13**:101-112. DOI: 10.1002/glia.440130204

[88] Conti F, Minelli A, Molnar M, Brecha NC. Cellular localization and laminar distribution of NMDAR1 mRNA in the rat cerebral cortex. The Journal of Comparative Neurology. 1994;**343**:554-565

[89] Gracy KN, Pickel VM. Comparative ultrastructural localization of the NMDAR1 glutamate receptor in the rat basolateral amygdala and bed nucleus of the stria terminalis. Journal of Comparative Neurology. 1995;**362**:71-85

[90] Conti F, DeBiasi S, Minelli A, Melone M. Expression of NR1 and NR2A/B subunits of the NMDA receptor in cortical astrocytes. Glia. 1996;**17**:254-258

[91] Petralia RS, Wang YX, Zhao HM, Wenthold, R.J.Wenthold RJ. Ionotropic and metabotropic glutamate receptors show unique postsynaptic, presynaptic, and glial localizations in the dorsal cochlear nucleus. The Journal of Comparative Neurology 1996;**372**:356-383. DOI: 10.1016/0306-4522(95)00533-1

[92] Van Bockstaele EJ, Colago EEO. Selective distribution of the NMDA-R1 glutamate receptor in astrocytes and presynaptic axon terminals in the nucleus locus coeruleus of the rat brain: An immunoelectron microscopic study. The Journal of Comparative Neurology. 1996;**369**:483-496. DOI: 10.1002/(SICI)1096-9861(19960610)369:4<483::AID-CNE1>3.0.CO;2-0

[93] Farb CR, Aoki C, Ledoux JE. Differential localization of NMDA and AMPA receptor subunits in the lateral and basal nuclei of the amygdala: A light and electron microscopic study. The Journal of Comparative Neurology. 1995;**362**:86-108. DOI: 10.1002/cne.903620106

[94] Pasti L, Volterra A, Pozzan T, Carmignoto G. Intracellular calcium oscillations in astrocytes: A highly plastic, bidirectional form of communication between neurons and astrocytes in situ. The Journal of Neuroscience. 1997;**17**:7817-7830. DOI: 10.1038/nrn1722

[95] Cai Z, Kimelberg HK. Glutamate receptor-mediated calcium responses in acutely isolated hippocampal astrocytes. Glia. 1997;**21**:380-389

[96] Gottlieb M, Matute C. Expression of ionotropic glutamate receptor subunits in glial cells of the hippocampal CA1 area following transient forebrain ischemia. Journal of Cerebral Blood Flow and Metabolism. 1997;**17**:290-300

[97] Nishizaki T, Matsuoka T, Nomura T, Kondoh T, Tamaki N, Okada Y. Store Ca^{2+} depletion enhances NMDA responses in cultured human astrocytes. Biochemical and Biophysical Research Communications. 1999;**259**:661-664

[98] Shelton MK, Mccarthy KEND. Mature hippocampal astrocytes exhibit functional metabotropic and ionotropic glutamate receptors in situ. Glia. 1999;**26**:1-11

[99] Conti F, Barbaresi P, Melone M, Ducati A. Neuronal and glial localization of NR1 and NR2A/B subunits of the NMDA receptor in the human cerebral cortex. Cerebral Cortex. 1999;**9**:110-120. DOI: 10.1093/cercor/9.2.110

[100] Schipke CG, Ohlemeyer C, Matyash M, Nolte C, Kettenmann H, Kirchhoff F. Astrocytes of the mouse neocortex express functional N-methyl-D-aspartate receptors. The FASEB Journal. 2001;**15**:1270-1272

[101] Kondoh T, Nishizaki T, Aihara H, Tamaki N. NMDA-responsible, APV-insensitive receptor in cultured human astrocytes. Life Sciences. 2001;**68**:1761-1767

[102] Krebs C, Fernandes HB, Sheldon C, Raymond LA, Baimbridge KG. Functional NMDA receptor subtype 2B is expressed in astrocytes after ischemia in vivo and anoxia in vitro. The Journal of Neuroscience. 2003;**23**:3364-3372

[103] Zhang Q, Hu B, Sun S, Tong E. Induction of increased intracellular calcium in astrocytes by glutamate through activating NMDA and AMPA receptors. Journal of Huazhong University of Science and Technology. Medical Sciences. 2003;**23**:254-257. DOI: 10.1007/BF02829506

[104] Hu B, Sun S-G, Tong E-T. NMDA and AMPA receptors mediate intracellular calcium increase in rat cortical astrocytes 1. Acta Pharmacologica Sinica. 2004;**25**:714-720

[105] Lalo U, Pankratov Y, Kirchhoff F, North RA, Verkhratsky A. NMDA receptors mediate neuron-to-glia signaling in mouse cortical astrocytes. The Journal of Neuroscience. 2006;**26**:2673-2683

[106] Wang X, Lou N, Xu Q, Tian G-F, Peng WG, Han X, et al. Astrocytic Ca^{2+} signaling evoked by sensory stimulation in vivo. Nature Neuroscience. 2006;**9**:816-823. DOI: 10.1038/nn1703

[107] Serrano A. GABAergic network activation of glial cells underlies hippocampal heterosynaptic depression. The Journal of Neuroscience. 2006;**26**:5370-5382. DOI: 10.1523/JNEUROSCI.5255-05.2006

[108] Kato H, Narita M, Miyatake M, Yajima Y, Suzuki T. Role of neuronal NR2B subunit-containing NMDA receptor-mediated Ca^{2+} influx and astrocytic activation in cultured mouse cortical neurons and astrocytes. Synapse. 2006;**59**:10-17

[109] Edling Y, Ingelman-Sundberg M, Simi A. Glutamate activated c-fos in glial cells via a novel mechanism involving the glutamate receptor subtype mGlu5 and the transcriptional repressor DREAM. Glia. 2007;**55**:328-340. DOI: 10.1002/glia

[110] Cahoy JD, Emery B, Kaushal A, Foo LC, Zamanian JL, Christopherson KS, et al. A transcriptome database for astrocytes, neurons, and oligodendrocytes: A new resource for understanding brain development and function. The Journal of Neuroscience. 2008;**28**:264-278. DOI: 10.1523/JNEUROSCI.4178-07.2008

[111] Serrano A, Robitaille R, Lacaille JC. Differential NMDA-dependent activation of glial cells in mouse hippocampus. Glia. 2008;**56**:1648-1663. DOI: 10.1002/glia.20717

[112] Palygin O, Lalo U, Verkhratsky A, Pankratov Y. Ionotropic NMDA and P2X1/5 receptors mediate synaptically induced Ca^{2+} signalling in cortical astrocytes. Cell Calcium. 2010;**48**:225-231

[113] Lee MC, Ting KK, Adams S, Brew BJ, Chung R, Guillemin GJ. Characterisation of the expression of NMDA receptors in human astrocytes. PLoS One. 2010;**5**:e14123

[114] Jiang J, Yan M, Lv Q, Cheng C, Li X, Guo Z, et al. Inhibition of nitric oxide-induced nuclear localization of CAPON by NMDA receptor antagonist in cultured rat primary astrocytes. Neurochemistry International. 2010;**56**:561-568

[115] Holmes KD, Mattar P, Marsh DR, Jordan V, Weaver LC, Dekaban GA. The C-terminal C1 cassette of the N-methyl-D-aspartate receptor 1 subunit contains a bi-partite nuclear localization sequence. Journal of Neurochemistry. 2002;**81**:1152-1165. DOI: 10.1046/j.1471-4159.2002.00865.x

[116] Jeffrey RA, Ch'ng TH, O'Dell TJ, Martin KC. Activity-dependent anchoring of Importin at the synapse involves regulated binding to the cytoplasmic tail of the NR1-1a subunit of the NMDA receptor. The Journal of Neuroscience. 2009;**29**:15613-15620. DOI: 10.1523/JNEUROSCI.3314-09.2009

[117] Zhou Y, Li HL, Zhao R, Yang LT, Dong Y, Yue X, et al. Astrocytes express N-methyl-D-aspartate receptor subunits in development, ischemia and post-ischemia. Neurochemical Research. 2010;**35**:2124-2134. DOI: 10.1007/s11064-010-0325-x

[118] Palygin O, Lalo U, Pankratov Y. Distinct pharmacological and functional properties of NMDA receptors in mouse cortical astrocytes. British Journal of Pharmacology. 2011;**163**:1755-1766. DOI: 10.1111/j.1476-5381.2011.01374.x

[119] Lalo U, Palygin O, North RA, Verkhratsky A, Pankratov Y. Age-dependent remodelling of ionotropic signalling in cortical astroglia. Aging Cell. 2011;**10**:392-402. DOI: 10.1111/j.1474-9726.2011.00682.x

[120] Martins-De-Souza D, Lebar M, Turck CW. Proteome analyses of cultured astrocytes treated with MK-801 and clozapine: Similarities with schizophrenia. European Archives of Psychiatry and Clinical Neuroscience. 2011;**261**:217-228. DOI: 10.1007/s00406-010-0166-2

[121] Gerard F, Hansson E. Inflammatory activation enhances NMDA-triggered Ca^{2+} signalling and IL-1beta secretion in primary cultures of rat astrocytes. Brain Research. 2012;**1473**:1-8

[122] Orre M, Kamphuis W, Osborn LM, Melief J, Kooijman L, Huitinga I, et al. Acute isolation and transcriptome characterization of cortical astrocytes and microglia from young and aged mice. Neurobiology of Aging. 2014;**35**:1-14. DOI: 10.1016/j.neurobiolaging.2013.07.008

[123] Rusnakova V, Honsa P, Dzamba D, Ståhlberg A, Kubista M, Anderova M. Heterogeneity of astrocytes: From development to injury - single cell gene expression. PLoS One. 2013;**8**. DOI: 10.1371/journal.pone.0069734

[124] Zhang Y, Chen K, Sloan SA, Bennett ML, Scholze AR, O'Keeffe S, et al. An RNA-sequencing transcriptome and splicing database of glia, neurons, and vascular cells of the cerebral cortex. The Journal of Neuroscience. 2014;**34**:11929-11947. DOI: 10.1523/JNEUROSCI.1860-14.2014

[125] Haustein MD, Kracun S, XH L, Shih T, Jackson-Weaver O, Tong X, et al. Conditions and constraints for astrocyte calcium signaling in the hippocampal mossy fiber pathway. Neuron. 2014;**82**:413-429. DOI: 10.1016/j.neuron.2014.02.041

[126] Jimenez-Blasco D, Santofimia-Castaño P, Gonzalez A, Almeida A, Bolaños JP. Astrocyte NMDA receptors' activity sustains neuronal survival through a Cdk5-Nrf2 pathway. Cell Death and Differentiation. 2015;**22**:1877-1889. DOI: 10.1038/cdd.2015.49

[127] Obara-Michlewska M, Ruszkiewicz J, Zielińska M, Verkhratsky A, Albrecht J. Astroglial NMDA receptors inhibit expression of K_{ir} 4.1 channels in glutamate-overexposed astrocytes in vitro and in the brain of rats with acute liver failure. Neurochemistry International. 2015;**88**:20-25. DOI: 10.1016/j.neuint.2014.10.006

[128] Morquette P, Verdier D, Kadala A, Féthière J, Philippe AG, Robitaille R, et al. An astrocyte-dependent mechanism for neuronal rhythmogenesis. Nature Neuroscience. 2015;**18**:844-854. DOI: 10.1038/nn.4013

[129] Otsu Y, Couchman K, Lyons DG, Collot M, Agarwal A, Mallet J, et al. Calcium dynamics in astrocyte processes during neurovascular coupling. Nature Neuroscience. 2015;**18**:210-218. DOI: 10.1038/nn.3906

[130] Srinivasan R, Huang BS, Venugopal S, Johnston AD, Chai H, Zeng H, et al. Ca^{2+} signaling in astrocytes from Ip3r2$^{-/-}$ mice in brain slices and during startle responses in vivo. Nature Neuroscience. 2015;**18**:708-717. DOI: 10.1038/nn.4001

[131] Shigetomi E, Tong X, Kwan KY, Corey DP, Khakh BS. TRPA1 channels regulate astrocyte resting calcium and inhibitory synapse efficacy through GAT-3. Nature Neuroscience. 2011;**15**:70-80. DOI: 10.1038/nn.3000

[132] Dzamba D, Honsa P, Valny M, Kriska J, Valihrach L, Novosadova V, et al. Quantitative analysis of glutamate receptors in glial cells from the cortex of GFAP/EGFP mice following ischemic injury: Focus on NMDA receptors. Cellular and Molecular Neurobiology. 2015;**35**:1187-1202. DOI: 10.1007/s10571-015-0212-8

[133] Yu W, Zhu H, Wang Y, Li G, Wang L, Li H. Reactive transformation and increased bdnf signaling by hippocampal astrocytes in response to mk-801. PLoS One. 2015;**10**:1-13. DOI: 10.1371/journal.pone.0145651

[134] Pinacho R, Vila E, Prades R, Tarragó T, Castro E, Ferrer I, et al. The glial phosphorylase of glycogen isoform is reduced in the dorsolateral prefrontal cortex in chronic schizophrenia. Schizophrenia Research. 2016;**177**:37-43. DOI: 10.1016/j.schres.2016.04.024

[135] Mehina EMF, Murphy-Royal C, Gordon GR. Steady-state free Ca^{2+} in astrocytes is decreased by experience and impacts arteriole tone. The Journal of Neuroscience. 2017;**37**:8150-8165. DOI: 0.1523/JNEUROSCI.0239-17.2017

[136] Lopez-Colome AM, Ortega A, Romo-de-Vivar M. Excitatory amino acid-induced phosphoinositide hydrolysis in Muller glia. Glia. 1993;**9**:127-135

[137] López-Colomé AM, Ortega A, Fragoso G, Trueba E. Excitatory amino acid receptors coupled to the phosphoinositide pathway in Bergmann glia. Neurochemical Research. 1997;**22**:305-312. DOI: 10.1023/A:1022494923084

[138] Rodríguez-Moreno A, Sihra TS. Kainate receptors with a metabotropic modus operandi. Trends in Neurosciences. 2007;**30**:630-637. DOI: 10.1016/j.tins.2007.10.001

[139] Khakh BS, McCarthy KD. Astrocyte calcium signaling: From observations to functions and the challenges therein. Cold Spring Harbor Perspectives in Biology. 2015;**7**:a020404. DOI: 10.1101/cshperspect.a020404

[140] Kettenmann H, Ransom B, editors. Neuroglia. 3rd ed. New York: Oxford; 2013

[141] Nedergaard M, Rodr??guez JJ, Verkhratsky A. Glial calcium and diseases of the nervous system. Cell Calcium. 2010;**47**:140-149. DOI: 10.1016/j.ceca.2009.11.010

[142] Chung CNMDA. Receptor as a newly identified member of the metabotropic glutamate receptor family: Clinical implications for neurodegenerative diseases. Molecules and Cells. 2013;**36**:99-104. DOI: 10.1007/s10059-013-0113-y

[143] Gonzalez-Hernandez JR, Montes de Oca Balderas P. Mitochondrial Membrane Potential Response to NMDA and MK-801 in rat cultured cortical astrocytes. In: 2nd Congress of the Neurobiology Branch de la Sociedad Mexicana de Bioquímica. October 15-18, Querétaro, México. 2017

[144] Montes de Oca Balderas P, Aguilera P, Santamaria A. N-Methyl D-Aspartate Receptor is expressed by Rat Cultured Cortical Astrocytes and Regulates their Mitochondrial Membrane Potential. Congress of the Society of Neuroscience. November 9-13 San Diego, CA. USA. 2013

[145] Khakh BS, Sofroniew MV. Diversity of astrocyte functions and phenotypes in neural circuits. Nature Neuroscience. 2015;**18**:942-952. DOI: 10.1038/nn.4043

[146] Matyash V, Kettenmann H. Heterogeneity in astrocyte morphology and physiology. Brain Research Reviews. 2010;**63**:2-10

[147] Clements JD, Lester RA, Tong G, Jahr CE, Westbrook GL. The time course of glutamate in the synaptic cleft. Science (80-). 1992;**258**:1498-1501

[148] Leibowitz A, Boyko M, Shapira Y, Zlotnik A. Blood glutamate scavenging: Insight into neuro protection. International Journal of Molecular Sciences. 2012;**13**:10041-10066. DOI: 10.3390/ijms130810041

[149] Lee FJS, Liu F. Direct interactions between NMDA and D1 receptors: A tale of tails. Biochemical Society Transactions. 2004;**32**:1032-1036. DOI: 10.1042/BST0321032

[150] Pauly T, Ratliff M, Pietrowski E, Neugebauer R, Schlicksupp A, Kirsch J, et al. Activity-dependent shedding of the NMDA receptor glycine binding site by matrix metalloproteinase 3: A PUTATIVE mechanism of postsynaptic plasticity. PLoS One. 2008;**3**:e2681

[151] Montes de Oca BP. Ectdomain shedding and regulated intracellular proteolysis in the central nervous system. Central Nervous System Agents in Medicinal Chemistry. 2010;**10**:337-359

[152] Meisenbock G, De Angelis DA, Rothman JE. Visualizing sectretion and synaptic transmission with pH-sensitive green fluorescent proteins. Nature. 1998;**394**:192-195. DOI: 10.1038/nature00909.1

[153] Chesler M. Regulation and modulation of pH in the brain. Physiological Reviews. 2003;**83**:1183-1221. DOI: 10.1152/physrev.00010.2003

[154] Bernardinelli Y, Randall J, Janett E, Nikonenko I, König S, Jones EV, et al. Activity-dependent structural plasticity of perisynaptic astrocytic domains promotes excitatory synapse stability. Current Biology. 2014;**24**:1679-1688. DOI: 10.1016/j.cub.2014.06.025

[155] Heller JP, Rusakov DA. Morphological plasticity of astroglia: Understanding synaptic microenvironment. Glia. 2015;**63**:2133-2151. DOI: 10.1002/glia.22821

[156] Patrushev I, Gavrilov N, Turlapov V, Semyanov A. Subcellular location of astrocytic calcium stores favors extrasynaptic neuron-astrocyte communication. Cell Calcium. 2013;**54**:343-349. DOI: 10.1016/j.ceca.2013.08.003

[157] Montes de Oca Balderas P, Montes de Oca Balderas H. Synaptic neuron-astrocyte communication is supported by an order of magnitude analysis of inositol tris-phosphate diffusion at the nanoscale in a model of peri-synaptic astrocyte projection. BMC Biophysics. 2018. Accepted with minor reviews

Section 3

Astrocytes in Pathology

Chapter 5

Astrocytes in Pathogenesis of ALS Disease and Potential Translation into Clinic

Izrael Michal, Slutsky Shalom Guy,
Joseph Itskovitz-Eldor and Revel Michel

Additional information is available at the end of the chapter

http://dx.doi.org/10.5772/intechopen.72862

Abstract

Astrocytes are the major cell population in the central nervous system (CNS) and play pivotal role in CNS homeostasis and functionality. Malfunction of astrocytes were implicated in multiple neurodegenerative diseases and disorders, including amyotrophic lateral sclerosis (ALS), spinal cord injury (SCI), brain stroke, Parkinson's disease (PD), and Alzheimer disease (AD). These new insights led to the rationale that transplantation of healthy and functional human astrocytes could support survival of neurons and be of therapeutic value in treating neurodegenerative diseases. Here, we will mainly focus on the role of astrocytes in ALS disease, the major cell sources for generation of human astrocytes, or astrocyte like cells and show how multiple preclinical studies demonstrate the efficacy of these cells in animal models. In addition, we will cover immerging early stage clinical trials that are currently being conducted using human astrocytes or human astrocyte like cell population.

Keywords: astrocytes, amyotrophic lateral sclerosis (ALS), hSOD1^{G93A}, neurodegenerative diseases, mesenchymal stem cells (MSCs), glial cells

1. Introduction

Amyotrophic lateral sclerosis (ALS) is a progressive and fatal neurodegenerative disease that affects upper and lower motor neurons (MN) in the brain and spinal cord, respectively, this leads to paralysis and eventually death, mainly due to respiratory failure [1, 2]. The disease is incurable and fatal within 3–5 years of first symptoms. About 90% of ALS cases are sporadic, and about 10% of ALS cases are familial (with genetic background). Around 45% of familial ALS cases are caused by hexanucleotide expansion in the C9orf72 gene [3], while approximately 20% of the cases are associated with mutations in the Cu/Zu superoxide dismutase

(SOD1) gene [4]. Other mutations consist of RNA/DNA binding proteins FUS, TAR DNA binding protein-43 [5, 6]. hSOD1^{G93A} high copy number transgenic rats and mice recapitulate the disease phenotype and serve as an animal model for ALS [7, 8].

In ALS, the motor neuron degeneration process is accompanied by signs of oxidative stress and mitochondrial dysfunction, inclusion bodies, impairment of RNA processing, neurofilament aggregation, loss of axonal transport, disruption of the neuromuscular junction, and axon demyelination [9]. In the extracellular environment, there are signs of toxicity, resulting from glutamate accumulation, neuroinflammation, and blood barrier disruption. Astrocytes are the most abundant cells in the central nervous system (CNS) and are necessary for the protection and regeneration of neurons, as they promote axonal growth, deliver essential neurotrophic factors, and control blood-brain barrier integrity. Through their surface receptors and transporters, they control neurotransmitter levels at the synaptic cleft and regulate synapse formation [10, 11]. Thus, astrocytes regulate glutamate homeostasis by two major CNS glutamate transporters, GLT-1/EAAT2 and GLAST/EAAT1, which are expressed almost exclusively by astrocytes in adult mammals. In addition, astrocyte dysfunction may be the reason for the observed decrease in neurotrophic factors [12, 13], as well as for the oxidative stress [14] and neuroinflammation [15].

These observations led many academic groups and biotech companies, including Kadimastem to the rationale that ALS could be treated by implantation of normal astrocytes or cells with similar astrocytic characteristics from an external source, to support or replace dysfunctional ALS astrocytes [16]. Following encouraging preclinical proof-of-concept studies with various cell-based therapies in ALS rodent models, some of the cell therapies were next evaluated in clinical trials in ALS patients.

2. Pathophysiology of astrocytes in amyotrophic lateral sclerosis disease

The pathological mechanisms for ALS are still not well understood and the proposed mechanisms include inflammation, oxidative stress, cytotoxicity by glutamate, and protein aggregation. Though MNs are the main affected cells in the disease, growing body of evidence suggests the involvement of astrocytes in the pathology of ALS in a noncell autonomous pathway. The contribution of astrocytes to the pathology of ALS is probably a combination of loss of homeostatic functions and/or gain of toxic functions.

2.1. Toxicity of astrocytes from ALS patients

Astrocytes that were isolated from sporadic and familial postmortem ALS patients and astrocytes derived from iPSC of ALS patients have been shown to be toxic to healthy (WT) motor neurons [17, 18]. Similar results were obtained by primary astrocytes isolated from hSOD1^{G93A} mouse model [19, 20]. The toxic effect of astrocytes on MNs was demonstrated also by addition of astrocyte condition medium [21, 22]. This lead to the notion that astrocytes of ALS patients secrete toxic/mutated proteins that cause specific death of MNs. This hypothesis is supported by data from in vivo studies in ALS models. Intraspinal transplantation in WT rats of mutated SOD1 astrocytes, but not WT astrocytes, led to deterioration of MNs. MN death was suggested to be mediated by microglia activation since no activation of microglia was observed with WT astrocyte injection [23]. In addition, in ALS mouse models where SOD1 transgene was deleted specifically in astrocytes, the animals exhibited a delay in disease onset and slower progression [24–26]. Another study demonstrated that selective expression of mutant Tar DNA-binding protein 43 (TDP-43, found in ALS) in astrocytes causes a progressive loss of motor neurons and the denervation atrophy of skeletal muscles, resulting in progressive paralysis [27]. In addition, spinal cord astrocytes were found to degenerate in the microenvironment of motor neurons in hSOD1^{G93A} mouse model [28] and ubiquitin-positive inclusions were shown in MN microenvironment close to disease onset [29].

2.2. Failure in supporting MNs

Excessive stimulation of glutamate receptors causes excitotoxicity to neurons [30]. Reduction of functional astrocytic glutamate transporters is suggested to contribute to glutamate excitotoxicity found in ALS patients [31]. GLT-1, a glutamate transporter (a.k.a EAAT2) was found impaired in ALS patients [32, 33]. In vivo studies have demonstrated that focal loss of GLT-1 in the ventral horn of the spinal cord precedes disease onset in transgenic rat model for ALS overexpressing Cu(+2)/Zn(+2) superoxide dismutase 1 (SOD1) [34]. Transplantation of SOD1^{G93A} (glial-restricted precursor cells-glial progenitors that are capable to differentiate into astrocytes) in the cervical spinal cord of WT rats induced host MN ubiquitination and death, forelimb motor and respiratory dysfunction, reactive astrocytosis, as well as reduced GLT-1 transporter expression [23]. Mutating the caspase-3 cleavage consensus site in the GLT-1 sequence (D504N), inhibits caspase-3 deactivation of GLT-1. GLT-1^{D504N} mutation in SOD1-^{G93A} mice slowed down disease progression time, delayed the development of hindlimb and forelimb muscle weakness, and significantly increased the lifespan of the diseased mice [35]. Activation of mGlu3 metabotropic glutamate receptors in hSOD1^{G93A} mice enhances GLT-1 formation as well as secretion of glial-derived growth factor (GDNF) in the spinal cord and rescues motor neurons [36]. Several lines of evidence indicate that strategies designed to increase GLT-1 expression have a potential to prevent excitotoxicity; for example, the pyridazine derivative LDN/OSU-0212320 promotes GLT-1 translation [37], ceftriaxone increases GLT-1 expression by triggering NF-kB activity [38], and immunophilin ligand GPI-1046 also increases expression of GLT-1 [39]; all have been found to delay disease development and death of SOD1^{G93A} mice. However, a clinical trial evaluating ceftriaxone in ALS has been prematurely stopped because of lack of efficacy [40]. Nevertheless, Riluzole the first FDA-approved drug for ALS was found to increase glutamate uptake by C6 astroglial cells [41] shedding light on its therapeutic mechanism.

2.3. Cytotoxic cytokines

Inflammation-mediated neuronal injury is also recognized as a major factor to promote ALS disease progression and amplifies MN death-inducing processes. The neuroimmune activation is not only a physiological reaction to cell-autonomous death, but also an active component of nonautonomous cell death. Astrocytes participate in the cellular response to damage and danger signals by releasing inflammation-related molecules like NO, IL-6, INF-γ, prostaglandin D2, TGF-β, and TNF-α that can induce the apoptosis of neurons observed in ALS disease [21, 42–46]. INF-γ, for instance, was found to be expressed in GFAP-positive cells in the CNS [47] that possess a neurotoxic activity [48]. INF-γ was shown to induce selective death of motor neurons through activation of lymphotoxin-β receptor via LIGHT. The ablation of LIGHT was shown to slow down disease progression and prolonged animals' life span [49, 50]. Cerebrospinal fluid-targeted delivery of neutralizing anti-IFNγ antibody delays motor decline in an ALS mouse model [51]. Other example of a key proinflammatory mediator is prostaglandin E2 (PGE2). High levels of PGE2 were found in postmortem brain tissue, cerebrospinal fluid, and serum from patients with sporadic ALS [52, 53]. PGE2 levels were also elevated in both the cerebral cortex and spinal cord of $SOD1^{G93A}$ mice [54]. Moreover, the expression of cyclooxygenase (COX)-2, a key enzyme in the synthesis of prostaglandins, is higher in the spinal cord of ALS patients and model mice [55]. In addition, the level of microsomal PGE synthase-1 (mPGES-1), the final regulatory enzyme for PGE2 production, is up-regulated in the motor neurons of G93A mice [56]. Recently, it was found that PGE2 induced an upregulation of the EP2 receptor in motor neuron-like NSC-34 cells and lumbar motor neurons of ALS model mice [57].

2.4. Necroptosis

Astrocytes from both ALS patients and animal models were also found to induce MN death by activation of necroptosis [58]. Necroptosis is a form of programmed necrosis that is independent from the activation of caspases and involves loss of the plasma membrane integrity. The receptor-interacting serine/threonine-protein kinase 1 (RIPK1) and mixed lineage kinase domain-like (MLKL) have been identified as effector proteins of necroptosis. In vitro inhibition of the necroptosis pathway by the RIPK1 antagonist necrostatin-1 (Nec-1) or by direct silencing of RIPK1 via a short hairpin RNA (shRNA) has been reported to protect MNs from astrocyte-induced toxicity [59, 60]. Necrosulfonamide that inhibits MLKL was shown to almost completely rescue MNs from astroglial toxicity. The mechanism by which astrocytes induce necroptosis is still not understood. However, the factors TNF-α, TRAIL, and FasL were suggested to play a role in induction of necroptosis.

2.5. Mitochondrial alterations

Mitochondrial alterations have been observed in both neuronal and glial cells of ALS patients as well as in ALS animal models [61–63]. As mitochondria are both the main producers and target of reactive oxygen species (ROS), increased mitochondrial ROS production in ALS may lead to mitochondrial dysfunction and cell death. Mitochondrial dysfunction in $SOD1^{G93A}$-bearing astrocytes resulted in enhanced generation of reactive oxygen species (ROS) that promoted motor neuron degeneration [64, 65]. Mitochondria from rat $SOD1^{G93A}$-bearing astrocytes are defective in respiratory function and show an elevation in superoxide radical formation [64]. Thus, restoring mitochondrial dysfunction or reducing oxidative stress is an attractive therapeutic approach to treat ALS. For example, blocking the interaction of mutant SOD1 with one of its mitochondrial targets, Bcl-2, restores mitochondrial function in ALS mice [66]. In addition, Edaravone (a.k.a Radicava) that was recently approved by the FDA for the treatment of ALS possess a broad free radical scavenging activity and protects neurons, glia, and vascular endothelial cells against oxidative stress [67].

2.6. Neurotrophic factors

In both physiological and pathological conditions, astrocytes secrete a wide range of factors with multiple influences on their cellular neighbors. A well-known factor that is secreted by astrocytes is the glial cell line-derived neurotrophic factor (GDNF), one of the most potent protective agents for motor neurons. Disruption of the astrocytic TNFR1-GDNF axis accelerates motor neuron degeneration and disease progression [68]. Astrocytes in ALS rat model acquire an accelerated senescent phenotype and show a reduced support in motor neurons, which can be partially reversed by glial cell line-derived neurotrophic factor (GDNF) [69]. Another factor that plays a role in ALS pathology is vascular endothelial growth factor (VEGF), originally described as a factor with a regulatory role in vascular growth and development, but which also directly affects neuronal cells [70, 71]. Transgenic mice expressing reduced levels of VEGF develop late-onset MN pathology, similar to that of ALS [72]. VEGF is secreted by astrocytes and has been shown to protect MNs from excitotoxic death, which occurs in ALS [72]. VEGF delays MN degeneration and increases survival in animal models of ALS [73, 74]. In line with these results, low levels of VEGF and GDNF were reported in the CSF of ALS patients [75]. VEGF exerts its antiexcitotoxic effects on MNs through mechanisms involving VEGF receptor-2 and activation of the PI3-K/Akt signaling pathway [72].

Thus, astrocytes play a pivotal role in the pathology of ALS and contribute to MN loss. A therapeutic approach would therefore be a replacement, or support, malfunctioning astrocytes in ALS with wild-type healthy astrocytes or modified cells with astrocytic characteristics. Such cells can mitigate the toxic CNS environment, modulate neuroinflammation, secrete neuroprotective factors, and foster MN repair process.

3. Cell sources for derivation of astrocytes

3.1. Glial restricted progenitors (GRP)-derived astrocytes

Glial restricted progenitors (GRP) are early cell population of the CNS that can self-renew and give rise to astrocytes and oligodendrocytes [76, 77]. Isolation of GRPs from human fetal tissues (i.e., 20-week-old fetal cadaveric brain tissue) [78] was described. In vitro studies demonstrated the capacity of these cells to differentiate toward astrocytes by using platelet-derived growth factor (PDGF), epidermal growth factor (EGF), basic fibroblast growth factor (bFGF), T3 thyroid hormone, and ciliary growth factors (CNTF) as well as bone morphogenic proteins (BMPs) [78–81]. Yet, in vitro, only a subset of GRPs give rise to mature astrocytes [82]. In vivo transplantation of human GRPs into the spinal cord-injured animals demonstrated survival and differentiation toward astrocytes [83]. Moreover, intraspinal transplantation of GRPs overexpressing GLT-1 into ventral horn following cervical hemicontusion (injured spinal cord) significantly increased GLT1 protein expression and functional glutamate uptake following astrocyte differentiation. Transplantation into C4 hemicontusion compared to sham-injected animals demonstrated the paradigm that transplantation of GRPs might be a promising approach in cell therapy [79]. Yet, investigating human astrocyte maturation using a primary brain tissue obtained from cadaveric donors is challenging. Sample availability is limited, particularly for critical developmental time periods such as late gestation or early postnatal stages. In addition, derivation of homogenous astrocyte populations from GRPs is still a great challenge.

3.2. Derivation of astrocytes from embryonic stem cells or induced pluripotent stem cells

Two main pluripotent stem cells (PSC) sources for derivation of human astrocytes are embryonic stem cells and induced pluripotent stem cells (iPSCs), which are generated from adult human somatic cells that are reprogrammed into pluripotent stem cells using multiple technologies [84]. Both cell sources possess astonishing capacity to undergo unlimited self-renewal and to differentiate into all cell types present in the adult body. These sources potentially provide unlimited supply of cells for cell-based therapy and drug screening platforms. Methods for producing neural precursor cells from PSC and their further differentiation toward glial lineage were demonstrated in pioneering studies in animal models of neurodevelopment [85–92]. In these studies, the key steps in neural commitment in vivo were identified and were recapitulated in a stepwise process of neural commitment in vitro that results in specific commitment of pluripotent stem cells toward neural and glial lineage. The differentiation process is usually done by exposing iPSC as well as hESC to different morphogens and mitogens [93] and specifying the different subtypes of neural and glial cells. Examples for such mitogens include sonic hedgehog (SHH) [94], which was found to be secreted in vivo from the notochord and neural tube, and WNT proteins [95] and bone morphogenetic protein (BMP) [96] that are secreted from the dorsal regions. This allowed specifying different subtypes of neural and glial cells. Other key factors, which are often used for the differentiation into neural progenitor fate, include fibroblast growth factors (FGFs), epidermal growth factors (EGFs), and retinoic acid (RA) [97, 98].

Recently, formation of organoids, a simplified version of an organ produced in vitro in three dimensions (3D), is being used as an alternative method for deriving glial cells from hPSC. This 3D structure allows spontaneous recapitulation of morphogenic and mitogenic features that occurs during neurodevelopment [99, 100]. This platform allows to study neural development and model various neurodegenerative diseases.

3.3. Direct conversion of somatic cells into astrocytes (iAstrocytes) or astrocyte-like cells

Direct cell-reprogramming principle that was applied for derivation of iPSC (i.e., by transduction of specified transcription factors or by using a defined chemical cocktail [84] are now being applied for a direct conversion of somatic cells into neural cells and astrocytes. Although rapid progress has been made in converting somatic cells into neural stem cells, neurons, and oligodendrocytes, direct reprogramming of somatic cells into astrocytes remains largely behind. Recently, Caiazzo et al. described for the first time conversion of mouse fibroblast into astrocytes (iAstrocytes), comparable to endogenous brain astrocytes. This was carried out by transducing the transcription factors NFIA, NFIB, and SOX9, and these factors were found to be involved in astroglial commitment and enabled direct conversion into astrocytes [101]. Another approach for direct conversion or reprogramming of mammalian fibroblasts into astrocytes is culturing the cells in the presence of a small molecules cocktail that includes histone deacetylase inhibitor VPA and GSK3β inhibitor CHIR99021, among other factors. TGFβ Inhibitor was found to be the critical factor in this cocktail [102].

3.4. Mesenchymal stem cells

Mesenchymal stem cells (MSC) are adult multipotent precursors derived from various adult tissues and differentiate in vivo or in vitro into osteocytes, chondrocytes, fibroblasts, and adipocytes [103]. Recently, it was reported by several groups that MSC can also adopt a neural fate in appropriate in vivo or in vitro experimental conditions [104]. Recently, several laboratories have managed to differentiate MSC into astrocytes-like cells; for example, addition of cAMP-elevating agents, forskolin and 3-isobutyl-1-methylxanthine (IBMX), resulted in the expression of neural markers including β-tubulin III (Tuj-1), neuron-specific enolase (NSE), microtubule-associated protein-2 (MAP-2), nestin, and glial fibrillary acidic protein (GFAP) [105]. Another study showed that by using subsonic vibration (SSV) on MSC promoted their differentiation into neural-like cells in vitro [106]. Other studies developed protocols that induce adult human bone marrow-derived mesenchymal stem cells (MSCs) into becoming neurotrophic factor secreting astrocyte-like cells and attenuated clinical symptoms in animal model of multiple sclerosis and ALS [107–109].

4. Preclinical studies using cell-based therapies in ALS rodent models

4.1. Transgenic rodents overexpressing the mutant gene hSOD1G93A as a model for ALS

Several mutated genes have been identified as ALS causing mutations including C9ORF72, Cu/Zn superoxide dismutase 1 (SOD1), TAR DNA-binding protein 43 (TDP-43), UBQLN2, p62, VCP, Profilin1, and Matrin 3 [110]. Mutated SOD1 is the second most abundant ALS causing gene after gene encoding C9ORF72 and found in about 15% of the familial ALS cases [4, 111]. Several genetic mouse models expressing various ALS mutant genes were developed in order to mimic the human disease [7, 34, 112–115]; however, overexpression of the mutant SOD1 gene was shown to best recapitulate the pathology of the human disease [116]. Among SOD1 mutations, transgenic mice and rats overexpressing the human mutated gene $SOD1^{G93A}$ is the most used model of ALS in preclinical in vivo studies toward clinical trials [116]. Transgenic $hSOD1^{G93A}$ mice and rats exhibit histopathological hallmarks similar to those associated with ALS in humans with a massive degradation of motor neurons [7, 34]. The transgenic rodents show a clear disease pathology, including selective death of spinal cord motor neurons and muscle atrophy in both hind and forelimbs, early astrogliosis and microgliosis, glutamate-mediated excitotoxicity, protein aggregation, mitochondrial dysfunction, and impaired axonal transport [116–118]. Upon disease onset, $hSOD1^{G93A}$ mice progressively develop symptoms that include hyperreflexia and shaking of the limbs, decrease in locomotor activity, impairment in walking patterns, decreased grip strength, and impaired coordination. In the late stage of the disease, the mice develop a severe paralysis [7, 34].

4.2. Preclinical studies using human neural stem cells

Neural stem cells (NSC) are derived from CNS tissue at various developmental stages of embryogenesis, fetal and in adults. NSCs can potentially form all neural types of cells of the CNS including astrocytes, neurons, and oligodendrocytes [119]. The differentiation capacity of NSCs depends on the developmental stage from which the cells are isolated and might be wider when cells are isolated at early stage [120]. The NSC features of multipotency, homing, neurotrophism, immunomodulation, and neuroprotection make them a promising therapeutic candidate for ALS [121–126]. Several studies reported a beneficial effect on disease progression and survival of ALS rodent models following a direct injection of NSCs into the spinal cord parenchyma. Fetal spinal cord NSCs that were injected into the lumbar spinal cord of $SOD1^{G93A}$ rats completed their differentiation and secreted neurotrophic factors to the proximate areas. The transplanted cells also formed synaptic contacts with host motor neurons. Transplantation of the cells delayed the disease onset, attenuated the progression, and moderately expanded life expectancy of the diseased rats by 10 days [127]. In order to support more muscle groups in SOD ^{G93A} rats, including muscles of hind- and forelimbs and respiratory, NSCs were injected into the ventral horn of both the lumbar and cervical spinal segments of presymptomatic animals. The dual treatment extended the survival of the rats by 17 days and delayed disease onset by 10 days compared to control animals, demonstrating the advantage of multiple injections [128]. A different study involving injection of NSCs to the lumbar ventral horn of presymptomatic SOD1 ^{G93A} rats did not demonstrate similar improvement in survival. However, the study still showed a limited and transient protection of motor function in the experimental animals [129]. The study has also demonstrated that the graft provided a neuroprotective effect, which was limited to the motor neurons of the lumbar segment. The grafted cells expressed markers of early mitotic neurons, including human neuron-specific enolase and doublecortin. In addition, the hNSCs reduced astrogliosis and numbers of activated microglia at the site of injection. Knippenberg et al. showed that intraspinal transplantation of human spinal cord-derived neural progenitor cells into the lumbar spinal cord of hSOD1^{G93A} mice delayed accumulation of motor deficiencies in a narrow time window during disease progression and moderately increased the life span by 5 days. Interestingly, female mice responded slightly better to the cell treatment, as observed in other studies in transgenic mutant hSOD1 mice [130, 131]. Characterization of the graft 6 weeks post-transplantation revealed that the cells were positive for the early neural marker nestin and rarely expressed the glial marker GFAP. Elevation of endogenous neurotrophic factors, but not human-derived factors, was measured in the spinal cord parenchyma [132]. A meta-analysis of intraspinal NSC transplantations in SOD1^{G93A} transgenic mice of 11 independent studies, performed by a consortium of ALS investigators, suggests that transplantation of NSCs from either human or mouse source delays disease onset, slows down symptom progression and prolongs survival of the mutated mice (e.g., the more than 1 year life extension in 25% of the mice that were injected at 4 sites). The authors proposed several mechanisms by which NSCs exert their therapeutic effects, including production of neurotrophic factors, preservation of motor function, and attenuation of inflammation and astrogliosis processes [133].

4.3. Preclinical studies using human mesenchymal stem cells

Mesenchymal stem cells (MSC) can be isolated from the placenta and from adult bone marrow and adipose tissues [134]. Although MSCs are of mesoderm origin, they maintain the potential to differentiate to cells types other than mesoderm derivatives including neurons-like cells and glial-like cells [135, 136].

MSC availability, well-established methods for harvesting and expansion, immunomodulatory features, ability to release neurotrophic factors, and lack of ethical issues make them attractive candidates for cell therapy applications [137, 138]. Several studies explored the therapeutic potential of MSCs in ALS models. These studies delivered MSCs to diseased animal through various routes, local and systemic, including intraspinal, intrathecal, intramuscular, and intravenous [137–140].

Transplantation of hMSCs into the lumbar spinal cord of asymptomatic SOD1^{G93A} mice reduced astrogliosis microglial reactivity and improved motor neuron counts. However, changes were gender dependent and observed only in female mice. On the other hand, behavioral tests demonstrated that the improvement in motor performance was restricted to transplanted males [141]. Boucherie et al. reported an alternative delivery approach of rat MSCs by intrathecal injection to the cerebrospinal fluid of symptomatic hSOD1^{G93A} rats [142]. The transplantation led to infiltration of the injected cells into the CNS parenchyma including to the ventral horn. Transplantation of MSCs partially rescued motor neurons in the ventral horn, prolonged animal survival and improved motor performance over sham-injected rats [142].

A systemic administration of murine adipose-derived MSCs to hSOD1G93A mice by intravenous injection upon onset of disease symptom showed that a restricted number of labeled cells were able to reach the parenchyma of the spinal cord, with no evidence of neural differentiation. Upon transplantation, an increase in GDNF and bFGF levels was measured in the spinal cord. Researchers reported a better MN survival and a reduced reactive astrogliosis in the spinal cord in addition to amelioration of the course of disease progression [143]. A different study using an intravenous delivery of murine MSCs to SOD1G93A mice also prolonged survival and increased motor functions, in addition to improvement in histological pathology traits [144].

Another promising approach to rescue motor neurons in ALS is secretion of neurotrophic factors at the site of the damage by grafted cells. Human MSCs overexpressing the neurotrophic factor GDNF were injected into three muscle groups of presymptomatic SOD1G93A rats. The cells survived in the muscle and helped to preserve neuromuscular junction innervations. While engineered-MSC injection did not affect disease onset, it delayed disease progression and profoundly increased overall lifespan by up to 2 weeks [145]. Additional study demonstrated the advantage of combined delivery of hMSCs expressing both GDNF and VEGF. The NTF combination synergistically prolonged survival and attenuated disease progression in SOD1G93A rats [146].

4.4. Preclinical studies using human glial-restricted cells derived aborted human fetuses

Glial-restricted precursors (GRP) can be isolated from embryonic CNS tissue. These cells maintain a limited differentiation capacity to form only glial cells including astrocytes and oligodendrocytes [147, 148]. Endogenous glial cells in ALS experimental models and in patients were shown to be malfunctioning and even toxic to motor neurons, contributing to disease progression. Thus, introduction of healthy functional astrocytes to damaged areas in the CNS can potentially compensate for diseased astrocytes. Transplantation of rat GRPs into the cervical spinal cord of SOD1^{G93A} rats was found to maintain respiratory motor function. In this study, the cells robustly survived, migrated within the cervical spinal cord, and specifically localized in the ventral horn. At the time of transplantation, most of GRPs were nestin+, but they efficiently completed their differentiation into GFAP+ astrocytes by end-stage disease (87% GFAP+ astrocytes). At this stage, approximately only 10% of the cells remained as undifferentiated nestin + cells. During the course of disease, the transplanted astrocytes developed mature astrocyte morphologies and spatially interacted with host MNs in the spinal cord. GRP transplants slowed cervical spinal cord motor neuron loss and reduced microgliosis in the cervical segment. Overall, the cell transplantation extended animals' survival and attenuated declines in motor performance [149]. The authors tried to reproduce these results by the injection of human GRP to SOD1^{G93A} mouse model. However, although the cells could survive in the cervical spinal cord under intensive immune suppression regimen and differentiate into GFAP+ astrocytes, the graft did not protect motor neuron loss or motor function and did not extent life expectancy. The difference between the outcomes of the two studies might be attributed to the different rodent models, cell dose, and number of injection sites [80].

4.5. Preclinical studies using human glial progenitors derived from ESCs and IPSCs

Embryonic stem cells are isolated from the inner-cell mass of a blastocyst and can be expanded in culture without losing their self-renewal capacity [150]. The cells can give rise to any cell type of the body. Induced pluripotent stem cells (iPSCs) are derived from somatic cells, mostly fibroblasts, which acquire an ESC-like pluripotent state after reprograming by induction of specific transcription factors. iPSCs can be generated from the patient's own cells. Transplantation of cells derived from such autologous iPSCs reduces the risk of immune rejection without the need of immunosuppression [151]. Kondo et al. differentiated human iPSCs into glial-rich neural progenitors (hiPSC-GRNP), highly enriched with GFAP+ cells. hiPSC-GRNPs were injected bilaterally into the lumbar spinal cord of transgenic $SOD1^{G93A}$ mice after disease onset. Treated mice showed an improvement in motor function and a prolonged survival of 12 days over sham-injected group. Transplanted cells survived in the spinal cord and differentiated mainly into $GFAP^+$, $ALDH1L1^+$, and $GLT\text{-}1^+$ astrocytes. Analysis of NTFs expression at the lumbar spinal cord reveled upregulation in mouse-originated VEFF, NT3, and GDNF [152].

We developed a protocol to produce large quantities of highly enriched astrocyte progenitors (APC; >90% GFAP+ cells) from human embryonic stem cells (hESC) according to GMP standards (unpublished data by the authors). In vitro, these cells express astrocyte markers including GFAP, S100β, GLAST, GLT-1, and Aquaporin- 4, and possess the activities of functional healthy astrocytes upon differentiation into mature astrocytes. These astrocytes are shown in vitro to have multiple activities including (1) protection of spinal cord motor neurons from oxidative stress produced by H_2O_2, (2) efficient glutamate uptake, which is in part due to GLT-1 (as shown by GLT-1 inhibitors), (3) stimulation of axonal growth in neurons seen in co-cultures with hES-AS, and (4) secretion of many factors with neuron protecting and stimulating activities. Intrathecal transplantation of hESC-derived APCs to the cerebrospinal fluid (CSF) of $SOD1^{G93A}$ transgenic rats and mice showed that the cells distribute along the neural axis and attach to the spinal cord and brain meninges, mainly to pia mater. In these studies, intrathecal transplantation of hESC-derived APCs significantly delayed disease onset and improved motor performance compared to sham-injected animals. The cells were shown to be safe and express markers of mature astrocytes including GFAP, GLAST, GLT-1, and Aquaporinn-4 in vivo. The cells did not express pluripotent markers and did not form teratomas or other tumors after a follow-up duration of 9 months. These cells are now the basis for a planned clinical trial.

5. Translation into the clinic

Following encouraging preclinical proof-of-concept studies with various cell-based therapies in ALS rodent models, demonstrating the safety and efficacy of the treatments, some of the cell therapies were already evaluated in clinical trials in ALS patients.

5.1. Route of cell administration

Several aspects of route of administration of cell therapies to ALS patients should be considered to ensure long-term survival, homing, and functionality of the cells in the target organ after transplantation. Cells for ALS treatment can be delivered by several routes, local or systemic, including intraspinal, intrathecal, intraventricular, intramuscular, and intravenous injections. Among these routes, intraspinal and intrathecal cell delivery routes were mostly used in ALS clinical studies [153, 154]. Intraspinal injection allows delivery of cells to the region of ventral horn in close proximity of motor neurons. However, migration of cells distal to injection site along the spinal cord is limited [80, 155] and therefore, only neural projections at the vicinity of the injected site are expected to be affected. Although intraspinal injection of cell was demonstrated to be a relatively safe procedure in animal models and in humans [156, 157], it is still a very challenging invasive procedure that requires an expertise and unique surgery instruments [158]. In addition, in order to support several groups of muscles in the patient's body, multiple independent injections along the spinal cord are required, increasing the complexity of the surgical procedure [159]. An alternative delivery of cells to the CNS is intrathecal injection to the subarachnoid space. Intrathecal injection is a routine procedure performed in humans by lumbar puncture. The intrathecal delivery is considered as a safe and simple method and does not require high level of expertise or instruments. IT injection allows the cell to distribute along the neuroaxis, distal from the injection site (unpublished data by the authors). Studies in animal models demonstrated a limited infiltration of engrafted cells from the CSF into the neural parenchyma [107, 160, 161]. Nevertheless, secreted factors such as NTFs, and anti-inflammatory/immunomodulatory cytokines circulate with the CSF and can diffuse into the parenchyma. In addition, the transplanted cells can remove from CSF circulating toxic factors such as excess glutamate and ROS. Therefore, the biodistribution of the cells in the CSF by IT injection is expected to exert systemic effect in the CNS, affecting both upper and lower MNs.

5.2. Clinical trials using cell-based therapies for the treatment of ALS

Cell therapy for ALS is considered as an innovative approach and many of the trials tested the cell therapy for the first time in humans. The primary endpoint of most studies was safety and the secondary endpoint included efficacy measurements. However, due to the small size studies and lack of placebo groups, the interpretation of the efficacy outcomes is difficult. Two, phase I and phase II, clinical trials (NCT01348451 and NCT 01730716) in ALS patients were conducted by Neuralstem Inc. [157, 162, 163]. The source of the human NSCs was a stem cell line generated from cervico-thoracic segments of spinal cord of a single 8-week-old aborted fetus. The cells were transplanted by an intraparenchymal injection procedure, performed using a spinal-mounted stabilization surgical device following laminectomy. Various concentrations of $0.5–16 \times 10^6$ cells were delivered to the lumbar and/or cervical vertebral levels. The primary endpoint of the two studies was safety. Adverse events were associated mainly with transient pain from the surgery procedure and to side effects of the immunosuppressive drugs. The efficacy of the treatment was evaluated by measuring ALSFRS-R, %, predicated forced vital capacity (FVC) and grip strength. Since the study did not include a randomized placebo group, the efficacy outcomes were compared to historical data. Although the efficacy data did not show an advantage of the treatment over historical controls, the small size groups, lack of placebo arms and variability in disease progression between participants, make it difficult to draw a conclusion about the therapeutic benefits of the treatment. Graft survival was analyzed in six autopsy cases. Transplanted cells were identified in all cases by qPCR at the injection site in all cases, up to 2.5 years after cell injection. The presence of donor cells represented 0.67–5.4% of total tissue DNA. In one female patient, the injected cells, which were of male origin, were identified in histological sections 196 days post-transplantation by FISH targeting the Y chromosome. Some cells in the graft of this female patient completed their neural differentiation and expressed the neuronal marker NeuN, while other remained positive to the neural progenitor marker SOX2. However, many of the XY donor cells were negative to both markers with an unknown identity. These results demonstrate the survival of the graft in the patient under immune suppression. Yet, the interaction of the cells with the surrounding tissue and their effect of MNs in the spinal cord were not explored [164]. Another clinical trial using hNSCs for the treatment of ALS was conducted by Mazzini et al.. Under this trial, hNSCs were injected into the thoracic spinal cord segment of ALS patients (EudraCT:2009–014484-39). The NSCs were isolated from the forebrain of aborted fetuses and expanded in culture under GMP conditions. Upon laminectomy, 2.25–5.5 × 10^6 cells were injected unilaterally or bilaterally into the T8-T11 ventral horn of six ALS patients. No severe adverse events were related to the treatment, and the most common reported adverse event was transient postsurgical pain. Patients were monitored for 1 year on a monthly basis and then for every 3 months. Clinical assessments up to 18 months after transplantation showed no acceleration in the disease progression that could be related to the treatment. A transitory improvement of the ambulation abilities was reported in two patients and one patient demonstrated a transient improvement in muscle power of lower limbs [156].

The safety and efficacy of MSC transplantation for treating ALS was conducted by Mazzini et al. In total, 10 ALS patients were injected intraspinally at T4-T6 with 11–120 × 10^6 autologous MSCs (Italian registration number: 16,454-pre21–823). The cells were isolated from bone marrow and expanded ex vivo under GMP conditions. The patients have been monitored for at least a 24-month follow-up period after transplantation. No serious treatment-related adverse events were reported. Overall, the procedure was demonstrated to be safe with only transient adverse events that were associated with the surgery procedure. Yet, no significant changes in the progression of the disease were reported in the follow-up period [165]. In separate long-term consecutive phase I studies, 19 patients were followed for up to 9 years after intraspinal transplantation of autologous MSCs. The procedure was demonstrated to be safe and did not accelerate the progression of the disease. MRI analysis showed no structural changes from baseline and lack of tumor formation. However, no clinical benefits were observed in the patients during the follow-up phase [153, 166].

In order to improve the potential of MSCs to support motor neurons, Brainstorm cell therapeutics Inc. developed an in vitro procedure to expand autologous MSCs and induced them to secrete neurotrophic factors including GDNF, BDNF, VEGF and HGF. These NTF secreting cells were delivered to the cerebrospinal fluid by intrathecal administration and/or to motor end-plates by intramuscular (IM) administration [167].

The company conducted Phase I/II clinical trials in 26 ALS patients (NCT01051882 and NCT01777646). One million cells/sites at 24–48 separate sites were injected to the biceps and triceps, and 1–2 × 10^6 cells/kg were injected intrathecally. Overall, the treatment was found to be safe and tolerable by patients with only transient and mild adverse events appearing after the administration of cells. The authors also reported an improvement in the decline of ALSFRS-R within 6 month of follow-up period compared to the run-in period, from −1.2 to 0.6 points/month, and also a decline from −5.1% to −1.2%/month in the predicted forced vital capacity [168]. The safety and efficacy of MSC-NTF cells were further tested in a randomized, double-blinded phase IIb clinical trial in 48 ALS patients, divided in a ratio of 3:1 between treatment and placebo arms, respectively (NCT02017912). According to the sponsor's website, the cells were injected both intramuscularly (48×10^6 cells at 24 sites) and intrathecally (125×10^6 cells), and patients were monitored for 24 weeks. Treatment was shown to be safe and well tolerated. A responder in the analysis of the trial was defined as a subject that who improved post-treatment compared with pretreatment run-in period. Data analysis demonstrated higher percentage of responders in the treatment arm subjects over placebo in most time points of the analysis. The responder analysis also revealed a subgroup of more rapidly progressing patients that were more likely to benefit from the treatment. The sponsor reported that the concentration of neurotrophic factors in the CSF including VEGF, HGF, and LIF elevated in the cell-treated arm after transplantation, but not in the placebo arm. These results were observed in parallel with a reduction in inflammatory markers in the CSF of cell-treated patients. According to the company's announcement, the efficacy of the therapy will be evaluated under a prospective placebo-controlled, multidose phase III trial in approximately 200 rapidly progressing ALS patients (NCT03280056).

Administration of autologous bone-marrow-derived MSCs by intrathecal injection to ALS patients was conducted by Corestem Inc., in a two-stage phase I/II clinical trial (NCT01363401). In the first stage of the study, cultured MSC expressing the markers CD29, CD44, CD73, and CD105 were administrated to the seven patients by two repeated LP injections (1 × 106 cells/kg), one monte apart. The patients were monitored for a period of 12 months. During the follow-up period, the treatment was shown to be tolerable and generally safe. Although the first stage of the study did not include a control group and was not powered to detect meaningful efficacy changes, the study showed encouraging results of stabilization of the ALSFRS-R score in all patients over a period of 6 months after first cell injection. In addition, levels of the immune response cytokines IL-10, TGF-β, and IL-6 were increased in the CSF after MSC injection, suggesting that of the effect of MSC injection on ALS patients is mediated, at least partially, by an immune response [169].

6. Conclusion

ALS is a multifactorial disease involving both genetic mutations and dysregulation of molecular pathways. Several mechanisms were identified in the pathophysiology of the disease, among them, glutamate excitoxicity, accumulation of free radicals, protein aggregation, mitochondrial dysfunction and impaired axonal transport and inflammation. In addition, during the last few years, growing evidence shows that astrocytes of both ALS animal models and ALS patients are malfunctional and even toxic. These astrocytes cannot support MNs and therefore contribute to the progression of the disease. Transplantation of healthy functional cells that can replace diseased astrocytes is, therefore, a promising strategy to treat ALS. Although different types of cells were proposed as a therapy for ALS, they all share mechanisms of action including, anti-inflammation/immunomodulation, clearing of toxic environment, and secretion of neurotrophic factors. The combined mechanism of action provided by cell transplantation is postulated to better cope with the multifactorial nature of the disease compared to a single pathway-based drug. Preclinical studies in ALS animal models showed the high safety profile of cell-based treatments in addition to their benefits in delaying disease onset, slowing down clinical symptoms and in many cases also to extend survival. Besides behavioral measurements, many of the studies also demonstrated graft survival, decline in inflammation, and improvement in histopathological attributes of the disease. Translation of the preclinical studies into clinical trials confirmed the safety of the procedures. Efficacy in most of these trials was a secondary endpoint, and some studies showed moderate and/or transient beneficial effects. Yet, since most of the clinical trials were at early stage, with small-size groups without a control arm, it is difficult to evaluate the efficacy of the treatments. Late-stage, placebo-controlled clinical studies with greater number of patients will prove whether any of the cell-based therapies indeed change the course of the disease.

Author details

Izrael Michal[1*], Slutsky Shalom Guy[1], Joseph Itskovitz-Eldor[1] and Revel Michel[1,2]

*Address all correspondence to: m.izrael@kadimastem.com

1 Neurodegenerative Diseases Department at Kadimastem Ltd., Nes-Ziona, Israel

2 Department of Molecular Genetics, Weizmann Institute of Science, Rehovot, Israel

References

[1] Hardiman O, van den Berg LH, Kiernan MC. Clinical diagnosis and management of amyotrophic lateral sclerosis. Nature Reviews Neurology. 2011;**7**(11):639-649

[2] Kiernan MC, Vucic S, Cheah BC, et al. Amyotrophic lateral sclerosis. Lancet. 2011; **377**(9769):942-955

[3] Renton AE, Majounie E, Waite A, et al. A hexanucleotide repeat expansion in C9ORF72 is the cause of chromosome 9p21-linked ALS-FTD. Neuron. 2011;**72**(2):257-268

[4] Rosen DR. Mutations in cu/Zn superoxide dismutase gene are associated with familial amyotrophic lateral sclerosis. Nature. 1993;**364**(6435):362

[5] Lagier-Tourenne C, Polymenidou M, Hutt KR, et al. Divergent roles of ALS-linked proteins FUS/TLS and TDP-43 intersect in processing long pre-mRNAs. Nature Neuroscience. 2012;**15**(11):1488-1497

[6] Guerrero EN, Wang H, Mitra J, et al. TDP-43/FUS in motor neuron disease: Complexity and challenges. Progress in Neurobiology. 2016;**145-146**:78-97

[7] Gurney ME, Pu H, Chiu AY, et al. Motor neuron degeneration in mice that express a human cu,Zn superoxide dismutase mutation. Science. 1994;**264**(5166):1772-1775

[8] Nagai M, Aoki M, Miyoshi I, et al. Rats expressing human cytosolic copper-zinc superoxide dismutase transgenes with amyotrophic lateral sclerosis: Associated mutations develop motor neuron disease. The Journal of Neuroscience: The Official Journal of the Society for Neuroscience. 2001;**21**(23):9246-9254

[9] Robberecht W, Philips T. The changing scene of amyotrophic lateral sclerosis. Nature Reviews Neuroscience. 2013;**14**(4):248-264

[10] Haim LB, Rowitch DH. Functional diversity of astrocytes in neural circuit regulation. Nature Reviews Neuroscience. 2017;**18**(1):31-41

[11] Liddelow S, Barres B. SnapShot: Astrocytes in health and disease. Cell. 2015;**162**(5):1170-11e1

[12] Deepa P, Shahani N, Alladi PA, et al. Down regulation of trophic factors in neonatal rat spinal cord after administration of cerebrospinal fluid from sporadic amyotrophic lateral sclerosis patients. Journal of Neural Transmission. 2011;**118**(4):531-538

[13] Devos D, Moreau C, Lassalle P, et al. Low levels of the vascular endothelial growth factor in CSF from early ALS patients. Neurology. 2004;**62**(11):2127-2129

[14] Lee J, Hyeon SJ, Im H, Ryu H, Kim Y, Ryu H. Astrocytes and microglia as non-cell autonomous players in the pathogenesis of ALS. Experimental neurobiology. 2016;**25**(5):233-240

[15] Gimsa U, Mitchison NA, Brunner-Weinzierl MC. Immune privilege as an intrinsic CNS property: Astrocytes protect the CNS against T-cell-mediated neuroinflammation. *Mediators of Inflammation*. 2013;**2013**:320519

[16] Nicaise C, Mitrecic D, Falnikar A, Lepore AC. Transplantation of stem cell-derived astrocytes for the treatment of amyotrophic lateral sclerosis and spinal cord injury. World J Stem Cells. 2015;**7**(2):380-398

[17] Haidet-Phillips AM, Hester ME, Miranda CJ, et al. Astrocytes from familial and sporadic ALS patients are toxic to motor neurons. Nature Biotechnology. 2011;**29**(9):824-828

[18] Meyer K, Ferraiuolo L, Miranda CJ, et al. Direct conversion of patient fibroblasts demonstrates non-cell autonomous toxicity of astrocytes to motor neurons in familial and sporadic ALS. Proceedings of the National Academy of Sciences of the United States of America. 2014;**111**(2):829-832

[19] Di Giorgio FP, Carrasco MA, Siao MC, Maniatis T, Eggan K. Non-cell autonomous effect of glia on motor neurons in an embryonic stem cell-based ALS model. Nature Neuroscience. 2007;**10**(5):608-614

[20] Nagai M, Re DB, Nagata T, et al. Astrocytes expressing ALS-linked mutated SOD1 release factors selectively toxic to motor neurons. Nature Neuroscience. 2007;**10**(5):615-622

[21] Di Giorgio FP, Boulting GL, Bobrowicz S, Eggan KC. Human embryonic stem cell-derived motor neurons are sensitive to the toxic effect of glial cells carrying an ALS-causing mutation. Cell Stem Cell. 2008;**3**(6):637-648

[22] Marchetto MC, Muotri AR, Mu Y, Smith AM, Cezar GG, Gage FH. Non-cell-autonomous effect of human SOD1 G37R astrocytes on motor neurons derived from human embryonic stem cells. Cell Stem Cell. 2008;**3**(6):649-657

[23] Papadeas ST, Kraig SE, O'Banion C, Lepore AC, Maragakis NJ. Astrocytes carrying the superoxide dismutase 1 (SOD1G93A) mutation induce wild-type motor neuron degeneration in vivo. Proceedings of the National Academy of Sciences of the United States of America. 2011;**108**(43):17803-17808

[24] Yamanaka K, Boillee S, Roberts EA, et al. Mutant SOD1 in cell types other than motor neurons and oligodendrocytes accelerates onset of disease in ALS mice. Proceedings of the National Academy of Sciences of the United States of America. 2008;**105**(21):7594-7599

[25] Yamanaka K, Chun SJ, Boillee S, et al. Astrocytes as determinants of disease progression in inherited amyotrophic lateral sclerosis. Nature Neuroscience. 2008;**11**(3):251-253

[26] Wang R, Yang B, Zhang D. Activation of interferon signaling pathways in spinal cord astrocytes from an ALS mouse model. Glia. 2011;**59**(6):946-958

[27] Tong J, Huang C, Bi F, et al. Expression of ALS-linked TDP-43 mutant in astrocytes causes non-cell-autonomous motor neuron death in rats. The EMBO Journal. 2013; **32**(13):1917-1926

[28] Martorana F, Brambilla L, Valori CF, et al. The BH4 domain of Bcl-X(L) rescues astrocyte degeneration in amyotrophic lateral sclerosis by modulating intracellular calcium signals. Human Molecular Genetics. 2012;**21**(4):826-840

[29] Rossi D, Brambilla L, Valori CF, et al. Focal degeneration of astrocytes in amyotrophic lateral sclerosis. Cell Death and Differentiation. 2008;**15**(11):1691-1700

[30] Zou J, Wang YX, Dou FF, et al. Glutamine synthetase down-regulation reduces astrocyte protection against glutamate excitotoxicity to neurons. Neurochemistry International. 2010;**56**(4):577-584

[31] Foran E, Trotti D. Glutamate transporters and the excitotoxic path to motor neuron degeneration in amyotrophic lateral sclerosis. Antioxidants & Redox Signaling. 2009;**11**(7):1587-1602

[32] Rothstein JD, Van Kammen M, Levey AI, Martin LJ, Kuncl RW. Selective loss of glial glutamate transporter GLT-1 in amyotrophic lateral sclerosis. Annals of Neurology. 1995;**38**(1):73-84

[33] Lin CL, Bristol LA, Jin L, et al. Aberrant RNA processing in a neurodegenerative disease: The cause for absent EAAT2, a glutamate transporter, in amyotrophic lateral sclerosis. Neuron. 1998;**20**(3):589-602

[34] Howland DS, Liu J, She Y, et al. Focal loss of the glutamate transporter EAAT2 in a transgenic rat model of SOD1 mutant-mediated amyotrophic lateral sclerosis (ALS). Proceedings of the National Academy of Sciences of the United States of America. 2002;**99**(3):1604-1609

[35] Rosenblum LT, Shamamandri-Markandaiah S, Ghosh B, et al. Mutation of the caspase-3 cleavage site in the astroglial glutamate transporter EAAT2 delays disease progression and extends lifespan in the SOD1-G93A mouse model of ALS. Experimental Neurology. 2017;**292**:145-153

[36] Battaglia G, Riozzi B, Bucci D, et al. Activation of mGlu3 metabotropic glutamate receptors enhances GDNF and GLT-1 formation in the spinal cord and rescues motor neurons in the SOD-1 mouse model of amyotrophic lateral sclerosis. Neurobiology of Disease. 2015;**74**:126-136

[37] Kong Q, Chang LC, Takahashi K, et al. Small-molecule activator of glutamate transporter EAAT2 translation provides neuroprotection. The Journal of Clinical Investigation. 2014; **124**(3):1255-1267

[38] Rothstein JD, Patel S, Regan MR, et al. Beta-lactam antibiotics offer neuroprotection by increasing glutamate transporter expression. Nature. 2005;**433**(7021):73-77

[39] Ganel R, Ho T, Maragakis NJ, Jackson M, Steiner JP, Rothstein JD. Selective up-regulation of the glial Na+-dependent glutamate transporter GLT1 by a neuroimmunophilin ligand results in neuroprotection. Neurobiology of Disease. 2006;**21**(3):556-567

[40] Berry JD, Shefner JM, Conwit R, et al. Design and initial results of a multi-phase randomized trial of ceftriaxone in amyotrophic lateral sclerosis. PLoS One. 2013;**8**(4):e61177

[41] Dall'igna OP, Bobermin LD, Souza DO, Quincozes-Santos A. Riluzole increases glutamate uptake by cultured C6 astroglial cells. Int J Dev Neurosci. 2013;**31**(7):482-486

[42] Raoul C, Estevez AG, Nishimune H, et al. Motoneuron death triggered by a specific pathway downstream of Fas. Potentiation by ALS-linked SOD1 mutations. Neuron. 2002; **35**(6):1067-1083

[43] Barbeito LH, Pehar M, Cassina P, et al. A role for astrocytes in motor neuron loss in amyotrophic lateral sclerosis. Brain Research. Brain Research Reviews. 2004;**47**(1-3):263-274

[44] Endo F, Komine O, Fujimori-Tonou N, et al. Astrocyte-derived TGF-beta1 accelerates disease progression in ALS mice by interfering with the neuroprotective functions of microglia and T cells. Cell Reports. 2015;**11**(4):592-604

[45] Tripathi P, Rodriguez-Muela N, Klim JR, et al. Reactive astrocytes promote ALS-like degeneration and intracellular protein aggregation in human motor neurons by disrupting autophagy through TGF-beta1. Stem Cell Reports. 2017;**9**(2):667-680

[46] Phatnani HP, Guarnieri P, Friedman BA, et al. Intricate interplay between astrocytes and motor neurons in ALS. Proceedings of the National Academy of Sciences of the United States of America. 2013;**110**(8):E756-E765

[47] Hashioka S, Klegeris A, Schwab C, Yu S, McGeer PL. Differential expression of interferon-gamma receptor on human glial cells in vivo and in vitro. Journal of Neuroimmunology. 2010;**225**(1-2):91-99

[48] Hashioka S, Klegeris A, McGeer PL. Proton pump inhibitors exert anti-inflammatory effects and decrease human microglial and monocytic THP-1 cell neurotoxicity. Experimental Neurology. 2009;**217**(1):177-183

[49] Aebischer J, Cassina P, Otsmane B, et al. IFNgamma triggers a LIGHT-dependent selective death of motoneurons contributing to the non-cell-autonomous effects of mutant SOD1. Cell Death and Differentiation. 2011;**18**(5):754-768

[50] Otsmane B, Moumen A, Aebischer J, et al. Somatic and axonal LIGHT signaling elicit degenerative and regenerative responses in motoneurons, respectively. EMBO Reports. 2014;**15**(5):540-547

[51] Otsmane B, Aebischer J, Moumen A, Raoul C. Cerebrospinal fluid-targeted delivery of neutralizing anti-IFNgamma antibody delays motor decline in an ALS mouse model. Neuroreport. 2014;**25**(1):49-54

[52] Ilzecka J. Prostaglandin E2 is increased in amyotrophic lateral sclerosis patients. Acta Neurologica Scandinavica. 2003;**108**(2):125-129

[53] Almer G, Teismann P, Stevic Z, et al. Increased levels of the pro-inflammatory prostaglandin PGE2 in CSF from ALS patients. Neurology. 2002;**58**(8):1277-1279

[54] Miyagishi H, Kosuge Y, Takano A, et al. Increased expression of 15-Hydroxyprostaglandin dehydrogenase in spinal astrocytes during disease progression in a model of amyotrophic lateral sclerosis. Cellular and Molecular Neurobiology. 2017;**37**(3):445-452

[55] Almer G, Guegan C, Teismann P, et al. Increased expression of the pro-inflammatory enzyme cyclooxygenase-2 in amyotrophic lateral sclerosis. Annals of Neurology. 2001; **49**(2):176-185

[56] Miyagishi H, Kosuge Y, Ishige K, Ito Y. Expression of microsomal prostaglandin E synthase-1 in the spinal cord in a transgenic mouse model of amyotrophic lateral sclerosis. Journal of Pharmacological Sciences. 2012;**118**(2):225-236

[57] Kosuge Y, Miyagishi H, Yoneoka Y, et al. Pathophysiological role of prostaglandin E2-induced up-regulation of the EP2 receptor in motor neuron-like NSC-34 cells and lumbar motor neurons in ALS model mice. Neurochemistry International. 2017

[58] Re DB, Le Verche V, Yu C, et al. Necroptosis drives motor neuron death in models of both sporadic and familial ALS. Neuron. 2014;**81**(5):1001-1008

[59] Degterev A, Hitomi J, Germscheid M, et al. Identification of RIP1 kinase as a specific cellular target of necrostatins. Nature Chemical Biology. 2008;**4**(5):313-321

[60] Hitomi J, Christofferson DE, Ng A, et al. Identification of a molecular signaling network that regulates a cellular necrotic cell death pathway. Cell. 2008;**135**(7):1311-1323

[61] Wiedemann FR, Manfredi G, Mawrin C, Beal MF, Schon EA. Mitochondrial DNA and respiratory chain function in spinal cords of ALS patients. Journal of Neurochemistry. 2002;**80**(4):616-625

[62] Hirano A, Nakano I, Kurland LT, Mulder DW, Holley PW, Saccomanno G. Fine structural study of neurofibrillary changes in a family with amyotrophic lateral sclerosis. Journal of Neuropathology and Experimental Neurology. 1984;**43**(5):471-480

[63] Sasaki S, Horie Y, Iwata M. Mitochondrial alterations in dorsal root ganglion cells in sporadic amyotrophic lateral sclerosis. Acta Neuropathologica. 2007;**114**(6):633-639

[64] Cassina P, Cassina A, Pehar M, et al. Mitochondrial dysfunction in SOD1G93A-bearing astrocytes promotes motor neuron degeneration: Prevention by mitochondrial-targeted

antioxidants. The Journal of Neuroscience: The Official Journal of the Society for Neuroscience. 2008;**28**(16):4115-4122

[65] Vargas MR, Johnson DA, Johnson JA. Decreased glutathione accelerates neurological deficit and mitochondrial pathology in familial ALS-linked hSOD1(G93A) mice model. Neurobiology of Disease. 2011;**43**(3):543-551

[66] Tan W, Naniche N, Bogush A, Pedrini S, Trotti D, Pasinelli P. Small peptides against the mutant SOD1/Bcl-2 toxic mitochondrial complex restore mitochondrial function and cell viability in mutant SOD1-mediated ALS. The Journal of Neuroscience: The Official Journal of the Society for Neuroscience. 2013;**33**(28):11588-11598

[67] Takei K, Watanabe K, Yuki S, Akimoto M, Sakata T, Palumbo J. Edaravone and its clinical development for amyotrophic lateral sclerosis. Amyotrophic Lateral Sclerosis & Frontotemporal Degeneration. 2017;**18**(sup1):5-10

[68] Brambilla L, Guidotti G, Martorana F, et al. Disruption of the astrocytic TNFR1-GDNF axis accelerates motor neuron degeneration and disease progression in amyotrophic lateral sclerosis. Human Molecular Genetics. 2016;**25**(14):3080-3095

[69] Das MM, Svendsen CN. Astrocytes show reduced support of motor neurons with aging that is accelerated in a rodent model of ALS. Neurobiology of Aging. 2015;**36**(2):1130-1139

[70] Oosthuyse B, Moons L, Storkebaum E, et al. Deletion of the hypoxia-response element in the vascular endothelial growth factor promoter causes motor neuron degeneration. Nature Genetics. 2001;**28**(2):131-138

[71] Van Den Bosch L, Storkebaum E, Vleminckx V, et al. Effects of vascular endothelial growth factor (VEGF) on motor neuron degeneration. Neurobiology of Disease. 2004;**17**(1):21-28

[72] Llado J, Tolosa L, Olmos G. Cellular and molecular mechanisms involved in the neuroprotective effects of VEGF on motoneurons. Frontiers in Cellular Neuroscience. 2013;**7**:181

[73] Bogaert E, Van Damme P, Poesen K, et al. VEGF protects motor neurons against excitotoxicity by upregulation of GluR2. Neurobiology of Aging. 2010;**31**(12):2185-2191

[74] Gros-Louis F, Laurent S, Lopes AA, et al. Absence of mutations in the hypoxia response element of VEGF in ALS. Muscle & Nerve. 2003;**28**(6):774-775

[75] Mishra PS, Dhull DK, Nalini A, et al. Astroglia acquires a toxic neuroinflammatory role in response to the cerebrospinal fluid from amyotrophic lateral sclerosis patients. Journal of Neuroinflammation. 2016;**13**(1):212

[76] Wu YY, Mujtaba T, Han SS, Fischer I, Rao MS. Isolation of a glial-restricted tripotential cell line from embryonic spinal cord cultures. Glia. 2002;**38**(1):65-79

[77] Dietrich J, Noble M, Mayer-Proschel M. Characterization of A2B5+ glial precursor cells from cryopreserved human fetal brain progenitor cells. Glia. 2002;**40**(1):65-77

[78] Haas C, Fischer I. Human astrocytes derived from glial restricted progenitors support regeneration of the injured spinal cord. Journal of Neurotrauma. 2013;**30**(12):1035-1052

[79] Li K, Javed E, Hala TJ, et al. Transplantation of glial progenitors that overexpress glutamate transporter GLT1 preserves diaphragm function following cervical SCI. Molecular therapy: The journal of the American Society of Gene Therapy. 2015;**23**(3):533-548

[80] Lepore AC, O'Donnell J, Kim AS, et al. Human glial-restricted progenitor transplantation into cervical spinal cord of the SOD1 mouse model of ALS. PLoS One. 2011;**6**(10):e25968

[81] Sandrock RW, Wheatley W, Levinthal C, et al. Isolation, characterization and preclinical development of human glial-restricted progenitor cells for treatment of neurological disorders. Regenerative Medicine. 2010;**5**(3):381-394

[82] Davies SJ, Shih CH, Noble M, Mayer-Proschel M, Davies JE, Proschel C. Transplantation of specific human astrocytes promotes functional recovery after spinal cord injury. PLoS One. 2011;**6**(3):e17328

[83] Jin Y, Neuhuber B, Singh A, et al. Transplantation of human glial restricted progenitors and derived astrocytes into a contusion model of spinal cord injury. Journal of Neurotrauma. 2011;**28**(4):579-594

[84] Chhabra A. Derivation of human induced pluripotent stem cell (iPSC) lines and mechanism of pluripotency: Historical perspective and recent advances. Stem Cell Reviews. 2017;**13**(6): 757-773

[85] Haidet-Phillips AM, Roybon L, Gross SK, et al. Gene profiling of human induced pluripotent stem cell-derived astrocyte progenitors following spinal cord engraftment. Stem Cells Translational Medicine. 2014;**3**(5):575-585

[86] Krencik R, Weick JP, Liu Y, Zhang ZJ, Zhang SC. Specification of transplantable astroglial subtypes from human pluripotent stem cells. Nature Biotechnology. 2011;**29**(6):528-534

[87] Krencik R, Zhang SC. Directed differentiation of functional astroglial subtypes from human pluripotent stem cells. Nature Protocols. 2011;**6**(11):1710-1717

[88] Izrael M, Zhang P, Kaufman R, et al. Human oligodendrocytes derived from embryonic stem cells: Effect of noggin on phenotypic differentiation in vitro and on myelination in vivo. Molecular and Cellular Neurosciences. 2007;**34**(3):310-323

[89] Zhang PW, Haidet-Phillips AM, Pham JT, et al. Generation of GFAP::GFP astrocyte reporter lines from human adult fibroblast-derived iPS cells using zinc-finger nuclease technology. Glia. 2016;**64**(1):63-75

[90] Gorris R, Fischer J, Erwes KL, et al. Pluripotent stem cell-derived radial glia-like cells as stable intermediate for efficient generation of human oligodendrocytes. Glia. 2015; **63**(12):2152-2167

[91] Tcw J, Wang M, Pimenova AA, et al. An efficient platform for astrocyte differentiation from human induced pluripotent stem cells. Stem Cell Reports. 2017;**9**(2):600-614

[92] Fasano CA, Chambers SM, Lee G, Tomishima MJ, Studer L. Efficient derivation of functional floor plate tissue from human embryonic stem cells. Cell Stem Cell. 2010; **6**(4):336-347

[93] Peljto M, Wichterle H. Programming embryonic stem cells to neuronal subtypes. Current Opinion in Neurobiology. 2011;**21**(1):43-51

[94] Fuccillo M, Joyner AL, Fishell G. Morphogen to mitogen: The multiple roles of hedgehog signalling in vertebrate neural development. Nature Reviews Neuroscience. 2006; **7**(10):772-783

[95] Ciani L, Salinas PCWNT. In the vertebrate nervous system: From patterning to neuronal connectivity. Nature Reviews Neuroscience. 2005;**6**(5):351-362

[96] Liu A, Niswander LA. Bone morphogenetic protein signalling and vertebrate nervous system development. Nature Reviews Neuroscience. 2005;**6**(12):945-954

[97] Maden M. Retinoic acid in the development, regeneration and maintenance of the nervous system. Nature Reviews Neuroscience. 2007;**8**(10):755-765

[98] Mason I. Initiation to end point: The multiple roles of fibroblast growth factors in neural development. Nature Reviews Neuroscience. 2007;**8**(8):583-596

[99] Sloan SA, Darmanis S, Huber N, et al. Human astrocyte maturation captured in 3D cerebral cortical spheroids derived from pluripotent stem cells. Neuron. 2017;**95**(4):779-790 e6

[100] Pasca AM, Sloan SA, Clarke LE, et al. Functional cortical neurons and astrocytes from human pluripotent stem cells in 3D culture. Nature Methods. 2015;**12**(7):671-678

[101] Caiazzo M, Giannelli S, Valente P, et al. Direct conversion of fibroblasts into functional astrocytes by defined transcription factors. Stem Cell Reports. 2015;**4**(1):25-36

[102] Tian E, Sun G, Sun G, et al. Small-molecule-based lineage reprogramming creates functional astrocytes. Cell Reports. 2016;**16**(3):781-792

[103] Pittenger MF, Mackay AM, Beck SC, et al. Multilineage potential of adult human mesenchymal stem cells. Science. 1999;**284**(5411):143-147

[104] Wislet-Gendebien S, Wautier F, Leprince P, Rogister B. Astrocytic and neuronal fate of mesenchymal stem cells expressing nestin. Brain Research Bulletin. 2005;**68**(1-2):95-102

[105] Shahbazi A, Safa M, Alikarami F, et al. Rapid induction of neural differentiation in human umbilical cord matrix Mesenchymal stem cells by cAMP-elevating agents. International Journal of Molecular and Cellular Medicine. 2016;**5**(3):167-177

[106] Choi YK, Cho H, Seo YK, Yoon HH, Park JK. Stimulation of sub-sonic vibration promotes the differentiation of adipose tissue-derived mesenchymal stem cells into neural cells. Life Sciences. 2012;**91**(9-10):329-337

[107] Kim H, Kim HY, Choi MR, et al. Dose-dependent efficacy of ALS-human mesenchymal stem cells transplantation into cisterna magna in SOD1-G93A ALS mice. Neuroscience Letters. 2010;**468**(3):190-194

[108] Sadan O, Melamed E, Offen D. Intrastriatal transplantation of neurotrophic factor-secreting human mesenchymal stem cells improves motor function and extends survival in R6/2 transgenic mouse model for Huntington's disease. PLoS currents. 2012;**4**:e4f7f6dc013d4e

[109] Barhum Y, Gai-Castro S, Bahat-Stromza M, Barzilay R, Melamed E, Offen D. Intracerebroventricular transplantation of human mesenchymal stem cells induced to secrete neurotrophic factors attenuates clinical symptoms in a mouse model of multiple sclerosis. Journal of Molecular Neuroscience: MN. 2010;**41**(1):129-137

[110] Boylan K. Familial amyotrophic lateral sclerosis. Neurologic Clinics. 2015;**33**(4):807-830

[111] DeJesus-Hernandez M, Mackenzie IR, Boeve BF, et al. Expanded GGGGCC hexanucleotide repeat in noncoding region of C9ORF72 causes chromosome 9p-linked FTD and ALS. Neuron. 2011;**72**(2):245-256

[112] Neumann M, Sampathu DM, Kwong LK, et al. Ubiquitinated TDP-43 in frontotemporal lobar degeneration and amyotrophic lateral sclerosis. Science. 2006;**314**(5796):130-133

[113] Joyce PI, Fratta P, Fisher EM, Acevedo-Arozena A. SOD1 and TDP-43 animal models of amyotrophic lateral sclerosis: recent advances in understanding disease toward the development of clinical treatments. Mammalian Genome: Official Journal of The International Mammalian Genome Society. 2011;**22**(7-8):420-448

[114] Koppers M, Blokhuis AM, Westeneng HJ, et al. C9orf72 ablation in mice does not cause motor neuron degeneration or motor deficits. Annals of Neurology. 2015;**78**(3):426-438

[115] Fil D, DeLoach A, Yadav S, et al. Mutant Profilin1 transgenic mice recapitulate cardinal features of motor neuron disease. Human Molecular Genetics. 2017;**26**(4):686-701

[116] Philips T, Rothstein JD. Rodent Models of Amyotrophic Lateral Sclerosis. Current Protocols In Pharmacology. 2015;**69**:5 67 1-5 21

[117] Boillee S, Vande Velde C, Cleveland DWALS. A disease of motor neurons and their nonneuronal neighbors. Neuron. 2006;**52**(1):39-59

[118] Nardo G, Trolese MC, Tortarolo M, et al. New insights on the mechanisms of disease course variability in ALS from mutant SOD1 mouse models. Brain Pathology. 2016;**26**(2):237-247

[119] Temple S, Alvarez-Buylla A. Stem cells in the adult mammalian central nervous system. Current Opinion in Neurobiology. 1999;**9**(1):135-141

[120] Gage FH, Ray J, Fisher LJ. Isolation, characterization, and use of stem cells from the CNS. Annual Review of Neuroscience. 1995;**18**:159-192

[121] Gincberg G, Arien-Zakay H, Lazarovici P, Lelkes PI. Neural stem cells: Therapeutic potential for neurodegenerative diseases. British Medical Bulletin. 2012;**104**:7-19

[122] Wei P, Liu J, Zhou HL, et al. Effects of engrafted neural stem cells derived from GFP transgenic mice in Parkinson's diseases rats. Neuroscience Letters. 2007;**419**(1):49-54

[123] Lu P, Jones LL, Snyder EY, Tuszynski MH. Neural stem cells constitutively secrete neurotrophic factors and promote extensive host axonal growth after spinal cord injury. Experimental Neurology. 2003;**181**(2):115-129

[124] Aharonowiz M, Einstein O, Fainstein N, Lassmann H, Reubinoff B, Ben-Hur T. Neuroprotective effect of transplanted human embryonic stem cell-derived neural precursors in an animal model of multiple sclerosis. PLoS One. 2008;**3**(9):e3145

[125] Ben-Hur T. Immunomodulation by neural stem cells. Journal of the Neurological Sciences. 2008;**265**(1-2):102-104

[126] Barnabe-Heider F, Miller FD. Endogenously produced neurotrophins regulate survival and differentiation of cortical progenitors via distinct signaling pathways. The Journal of Neuroscience: The Official Journal of the Society for Neuroscience. 2003;**23**(12):5149-5160

[127] Xu L, Yan J, Chen D, et al. Human neural stem cell grafts ameliorate motor neuron disease in SOD-1 transgenic rats. Transplantation. 2006;**82**(7):865-875

[128] Xu L, Shen P, Hazel T, Johe K, Koliatsos VE. Dual transplantation of human neural stem cells into cervical and lumbar cord ameliorates motor neuron disease in SOD1 transgenic rats. Neuroscience Letters. 2011;**494**(3):222-226

[129] Hefferan MP, Galik J, Kakinohana O, et al. Human neural stem cell replacement therapy for amyotrophic lateral sclerosis by spinal transplantation. PLoS One. 2012;**7**(8):e42614

[130] Habisch HJ, Janowski M, Binder D, et al. Intrathecal application of neuroectodermally converted stem cells into a mouse model of ALS: Limited intraparenchymal migration and survival narrows therapeutic effects. Journal of Neural Transmission. 2007;**114**(11):1395-1406

[131] Morita E, Watanabe Y, Ishimoto M, et al. A novel cell transplantation protocol and its application to an ALS mouse model. Experimental Neurology. 2008;**213**(2):431-438

[132] Knippenberg S, Rath KJ, Boselt S, et al. Intraspinal administration of human spinal cord-derived neural progenitor cells in the G93A-SOD1 mouse model of ALS delays symptom progression, prolongs survival and increases expression of endogenous neurotrophic factors. Journal of Tissue Engineering and Regenerative Medicine. 2017;**11**(3):751-764

[133] Teng YD, Benn SC, Kalkanis SN, et al. Multimodal actions of neural stem cells in a mouse model of ALS: a meta-analysis. Science Translational Medicine. 2012;**4**(165):165ra4

[134] Beyer Nardi N, da Silva Meirelles L. Mesenchymal stem cells: Isolation, in vitro expansion and characterization. Handbook of Experimental Pharmacology. 2006;(174):249-282

[135] Mareschi K, Novara M, Rustichelli D, et al. Neural differentiation of human mesenchymal stem cells: Evidence for expression of neural markers and eag K+ channel types. Experimental Hematology. 2006;**34**(11):1563-1572

[136] Bahat-Stroomza M, Barhum Y, Levy YS, et al. Induction of adult human bone marrow mesenchymal stromal cells into functional astrocyte-like cells: Potential for restorative treatment in Parkinson's disease. Journal of Molecular Neuroscience: MN. 2009;**39**(1-2):199-210

[137] de Girolamo L, Lucarelli E, Alessandri G, et al. Mesenchymal stem/stromal cells: A new “cells as drugs” paradigm. Efficacy and critical aspects in cell therapy. Current Pharmaceutical Design. 2013;**19**(13):2459-2473

[138] Laroni A, Novi G, Kerlero de Rosbo N, Uccelli A. Towards clinical application of mesenchymal stem cells for treatment of neurological diseases of the central nervous system. Journal of Neuroimmune Pharmacology: The Official Journal of The Society on NeuroImmune Pharmacology. 2013;**8**(5):1062-1076

[139] Tang BL. The use of mesenchymal stem cells (MSCs) for amyotrophic lateral sclerosis (ALS) therapy - a perspective on cell biological mechanisms. Reviews in the Neurosciences. 2017;**28**(7):725-738

[140] Hajivalili M, Pourgholi F, Kafil HS, Jadidi-Niaragh F, Yousefi M. Mesenchymal stem cells in the treatment of amyotrophic lateral sclerosis. Current Stem Cell Research & Therapy. 2016;**11**(1):41-50

[141] Vercelli A, Mereuta OM, Garbossa D, et al. Human mesenchymal stem cell transplantation extends survival, improves motor performance and decreases neuroinflammation in mouse model of amyotrophic lateral sclerosis. Neurobiology of Disease. 2008;**31**(3):395-405

[142] Boucherie C, Schafer S. Lavand'homme P, Maloteaux JM, Hermans E. Chimerization of astroglial population in the lumbar spinal cord after mesenchymal stem cell transplantation prolongs survival in a rat model of amyotrophic lateral sclerosis. Journal of Neuroscience Research. 2009;**87**(9):2034-2046

[143] Marconi S, Bonaconsa M, Scambi I, et al. Systemic treatment with adipose-derived mesenchymal stem cells ameliorates clinical and pathological features in the amyotrophic lateral sclerosis murine model. Neuroscience. 2013;**248**:333-343

[144] Uccelli A, Milanese M, Principato MC, et al. Intravenous mesenchymal stem cells improve survival and motor function in experimental amyotrophic lateral sclerosis. Molecular Medicine. 2012;**18**:794-804

[145] Suzuki M, McHugh J, Tork C, et al. Direct muscle delivery of GDNF with human mesenchymal stem cells improves motor neuron survival and function in a rat model of familial ALS. Molecular therapy: The Journal of the American Society of Gene Therapy. 2008;**16**(12):2002-2010

[146] Krakora D, Mulcrone P, Meyer M, et al. Synergistic effects of GDNF and VEGF on lifespan and disease progression in a familial ALS rat model. Molecular therapy: The journal of the American Society of Gene Therapy. 2013

[147] Rao MS, Noble M, Mayer-Proschel MA. Tripotential glial precursor cell is present in the developing spinal cord. Proceedings of the National Academy of Sciences of the United States of America. 1998;**95**(7):3996-4001

[148] Kruminis-Kaszkiel E, Wojtkiewicz J, Maksymowicz W. Glial-restricted precursors as potential candidates for ALS cell-replacement therapy. Acta Neurobiologiae Experimentalis. 2014;**74**(3):233-241

[149] Lepore AC, Rauck B, Dejea C, et al. Focal transplantation-based astrocyte replacement is neuroprotective in a model of motor neuron disease. Nature Neuroscience. 2008;**11**(11):1294-1301

[150] Mountford JC. Human embryonic stem cells: Origins, characteristics and potential for regenerative therapy. Transfusion Medicine. 2008;**18**(1):1-12

[151] Yu J, Vodyanik MA, Smuga-Otto K, et al. Induced pluripotent stem cell lines derived from human somatic cells. Science. 2007;**318**(5858):1917-1920

[152] Kondo T, Funayama M, Tsukita K, et al. Focal transplantation of human iPSC-derived glial-rich neural progenitors improves lifespan of ALS mice. Stem Cell Reports. 2014; **3**(2):242-249

[153] Thomsen GM, Gowing G, Svendsen S, Svendsen CN. The past, present and future of stem cell clinical trials for ALS. Experimental Neurology. 2014;**262 Pt B**:127-137

[154] Atassi N, Beghi E, Blanquer M, et al. Intraspinal stem cell transplantation for amyotrophic lateral sclerosis: Ready for efficacy clinical trials? Cytotherapy. 2016;**18**(12):1471-1475

[155] Suzuki M, McHugh J, Tork C, et al. GDNF secreting human neural progenitor cells protect dying motor neurons, but not their projection to muscle, in a rat model of familial ALS. PLoS One. 2007;**2**(8):e689

[156] Mazzini L, Gelati M, Profico DC, et al. Human neural stem cell transplantation in ALS: Initial results from a phase I trial. Journal of Translational Medicine. 2015;**13**:17

[157] Glass JD, Hertzberg VS, Boulis NM, et al. Transplantation of spinal cord-derived neural stem cells for ALS: Analysis of phase 1 and 2 trials. Neurology. 2016;**87**(4):392-400

[158] Riley JP, Raore B, Taub JS, Federici T, Boulis NM. Platform and cannula design improvements for spinal cord therapeutics delivery. Neurosurgery. 2011;**69**(2 Suppl Operative):ons147-154; discussion ons55

[159] Raore B, Federici T, Taub J, et al. Cervical multilevel intraspinal stem cell therapy: Assessment of surgical risks in Gottingen minipigs. Spine. 2011;**36**(3):E164-E171

[160] Park S, Kim HT, Yun S, et al. Growth factor-expressing human neural progenitor cell grafts protect motor neurons but do not ameliorate motor performance and survival in ALS mice. Experimental & Molecular Medicine. 2009;**41**(7):487-500

[161] Hwang DH, Lee HJ, Park IH, et al. Intrathecal transplantation of human neural stem cells overexpressing VEGF provide behavioral improvement, disease onset delay and survival extension in transgenic ALS mice. Gene Therapy. 2009;**16**(10):1234-1244

[162] McGinley LM, Sims E, Lunn JS, et al. Human cortical neural stem cells expressing insulin-like growth factor-I: A novel cellular therapy for Alzheimer's disease. Stem Cells Translational Medicine. 2016;**5**(3):379-391

[163] Riley J, Glass J, Feldman EL, et al. Intraspinal stem cell transplantation in amyotrophic lateral sclerosis: A phase I trial, cervical microinjection, and final surgical safety outcomes. Neurosurgery. 2014;**74**(1):77-87

[164] Tadesse T, Gearing M, Senitzer D, et al. Analysis of graft survival in a trial of stem cell transplant in ALS. Annals of Clinical and Translational Neurology. 2014;**1**(11):900-908

[165] Mazzini L, Ferrero I, Luparello V, et al. Mesenchymal stem cell transplantation in amyotrophic lateral sclerosis: A phase I clinical trial. Experimental Neurology. 2010;**223**(1):229-237

[166] Mazzini L, Mareschi K, Ferrero I, et al. Mesenchymal stromal cell transplantation in amyotrophic lateral sclerosis: A long-term safety study. Cytotherapy. 2012;**14**(1):56-60

[167] Gothelf Y, Abramov N, Harel A, Offen D. Safety of repeated transplantations of neurotrophic factors-secreting human mesenchymal stromal stem cells. Clinical and Translational Medicine. 2014;**3**:21

[168] Petrou P, Gothelf Y, Argov Z, et al. Safety and clinical effects of mesenchymal stem cells secreting neurotrophic factor transplantation in patients with amyotrophic lateral sclerosis: Results of phase 1/2 and 2a clinical trials. JAMA Neurology. 2016;**73**(3):337-344

[169] Ki-Wook O, Chanil M, Hyun YK, et al. Phase I trial of repeated intrathecal autologous bone marrow-derived mesenchymal stromal cells in amyotrophic lateral sclerosis. Stem Cells Translational Medicine. 2015;**4**(6):590-597

Chapter 6

Astrocytes' Role in Alzheimer's Disease Neurodegeneration

Ilaria Dal Prà, Ubaldo Armato and Anna Chiarini

Additional information is available at the end of the chapter

http://dx.doi.org/10.5772/intechopen.72974

Abstract

Central nervous system (CNS) astrocytes are glial cells performing crucial tasks encompassing energy metabolism, neurotransmission, ion and water stable levels, and immune defense and control local blood flow/oxygen levels. Arising from neural stem cells, astrocytes differentiate into subtypes that vary according to animal species. Human cerebral cortex astrocytes are sturdier and cytologically and functionally more complex, control wider domains, and spread calcium signals more quickly than their rodents' counterparts. They actively partake in CNS homeostasis maintenance and functioning by teaming up with their client neurons, other glial cell types, and cerebrovascular cells. Alterations of astrocytes' activities deeply impact on age-related chronic ailments like Alzheimer's disease (AD), the commonest senile dementia; AD involves the growing accumulation of amyloid-β peptides (Aβs) and hyperphosphorylated Tau proteins the astrocytes, and neurons supply following the interaction of their calcium-sensing receptors (CaSRs) with exogenous Aβs. The activated Aβ·CaSR signaling triggers a self-propagating mechanism that spreads the neuropathology among adjacent and far away astrocytes and their neuronal clients causing neurons' death. CaSR antagonists or calcilytics suppress these noxious effects in vitro. Hence, calcilytics are potential therapeutics that could halt the spread of AD neuropathology and safeguard the patients' neuronal viability, cognition, memory, and ultimately life.

Keywords: human, astrocyte, Alzheimer's disease, amyloid-β, tau protein, calcium-sensing receptor, calcilytics

1. Introduction

Between the 16th and 18th week of intrauterine life, a pool of stem cells of the neural plate generates every neural cell type, excepting microglia, in humans. Once differentiated, the astrocytes undergo a complex maturing process through which they acquire their specific morpho-functional characteristics. When these processes achieve completion, human astrocytes account for up to 50%, if not more, of the entire CNS cell population. These cells are larger in size and endowed with more numerous branches than their much less abundant (<20% of all CNS cells) rodents' counterparts [1]. Being so plentiful, astrocytes have a relevant role in brain environment homeostasis maintenance [2, 3]. They metabolically sustain neurons, recycle neurotransmitters, affect synapse activity, control local blood flow, and partake in blood-brain barrier functional integrity (see for details [2–4] and below). Aging and CNS diseases, neurodegenerative ones included, can induce an activated or inflammatory or reactive condition in the astrocytes [5, 6].

2. Human astrocytes' varieties

As their designation indicates, astrocytes have a typical star-shaped morphology as they emit different numbers of cytoplasmic branches according to their subtype. Astrocytes of several subtypes dwell in the human CNS. Some of them display locational predilections, e.g., fibrous astrocytes for the white matter and protoplasmic astrocytes for the gray matter. More recently, it has been realized that the classical protoplasmic and fibrous astrocytes can be differentiated into several subtypes, some of which proper only of the human cerebral cortex. Such subtypes share a specific marker, the glial fibrillary acidic protein (GFAP), which is an intermediate filaments' constituent expressed by all the astrocytes cultured in vitro. However, in vivo only the fibrous astrocytes express GFAP in the white matter (see for Ref. [7]). Recent studies have singled out a novel marker expressed by both protoplasmic and fibrous astrocytes, the aldehyde dehydrogenase-1 family member L-1 (Aldh1L1) [1, 8, 9].

2.1. Radial astrocytes

Radial astrocytes are the first ones to appear in the course of embryogenesis. At that point in time, they aid neurons' migration by acting as scaffolds [10]. Later, they differentiate becoming *stellate astrocytes*. However, after birth, radial astrocytes persist as such in the cerebellum (Bergmann glia) and the retina (Müller glia).

2.2. Fibrous astrocytes

These white-matter-located astrocytes present very long and thin processes which mostly do not emit branches. The processes' terminal end-feet envelope the axonal nodes of Ranvier and also gets in touch with the walls of cerebral vessels. Most notably, fibrous astrocytes partake in the repair of injured brain tissue, especially at the spinal cord level [11].

2.3. Protoplasmic astrocytes

They are the most abundant astrocytic type. Their somata give out numerous (up to 200) long branches, which end up with leafy feet or end-feet in part touching the blood vessels' walls and in part enwrapping several thousands of synapses [1, 8]. Near the pia mater's inner surface, the astrocytes' end-feet cluster together forms the CNS *limiting peripheral membrane.*

The astrocytes' end-feet in contact with the outer wall of cerebral arteries and veins make up the *glia limitans,* a space in which the *glymphatic* drainage allows the influx and efflux of the brain interstitial fluid (lymph). Such fluxes are crucially assisted by the astrocytes' water-transporting aquaporin-4 channels. Via these paravascular pathways, nutrients reach the neurons and glial cells, while toxic metabolites and soluble amyloid-β peptides (sAβs) are removed from the CNS tissue [12]. In addition, the early connection between the endothelial cells of the brain's nascent blood vessels and the astrocytes derived from radial glia results in a tight interaction between the end-feet of mature astrocytes and the capillary endothelial cells which presides over the normal function of the blood-brain barrier (BBB) [13].

It is worth recalling here that both Golgi silver staining and GFAP immunolabeling of brain tissue sections make the astrocytes appear as star-like cells. However, the astrocytes are the possessors of a certain number of cytoplasmic branches these methods do not stain. Therefore, such methods do not reveal the astrocytes' true morphology as visible under the light and/or fluorescence microscope. Another concept of old is that during development the astrocytes' branches form an interdigitated scaffold permitting the organization of the neurons. Recently, it has become clear that independent and distinct astrocytic domains develop with no connection with similar neighboring domains within the hippocampus [14]. As abovementioned, the morpho-functional features of human protoplasmic and fibrous astrocytes differ from rodents' ones. For instance, the diameters of gray matter-located human protoplasmic astrocytes are 2.6-fold longer, and their GFAP-positive processes are 10-fold more abundant. A single protoplasmic astrocyte can control from 270,000 to 2.0 million synapses placed inside its spatial domain. Most important, the branches of a single astrocyte touch, envelop, and regulate not only a huge number of synapses but also the capillary vessels controlling the blood flow going to those same synapses. This organized structure has been interpreted as the indication of a control of synaptic activity by the astrocytes independently of neuronal activity. Although unable to transmit neural impulses, human astrocytes propagate calcium ion [Ca^{2+}] waves at speeds of up to 36 μm/s, i.e., 4–10-fold faster than rodents' astrocytes do [15–17].

2.4. Additional astrocytes' subtypes

Besides the above-described canonical kinds, several other astrocyte subtypes have been recognized. Emsley and Macklis [17] have used a combined approach consisting of S100β immunostaining, GFAP expression, and human GFAP promoter-prodded enhanced green fluorescent protein (eGFP) expression in transgenic mice, to identify within several subtypes of CNS astrocytes. The latter incorporate radial glia, protoplasmic astrocytes, fibrous astrocytes, ependymal glia, tanycytes, Bergmann glia, and velate glia. The cytoarchitectonics and functional requirements of their local placements mainly determine the morphological features, growth rates, and relative densities of these subtypes [17]. NG2 cells are an additional CNS glial cell type likely possessed of stem cell features and hence capable of giving raise to astrocytes, neurons, and oligodendrocytes (OLGs) during both intra- and extrauterine life. NG2 glial cells functionally interact with neurons at the level of synapses. Studies are under way to clarify the heterogeneity of NG2 glia [18].

2.5. Human cortex-specific astrocytic subtypes

At variance with other mammalian species, humans have developed two novel cerebral cortical astroglia subtypes: the *astrocytes with varicose projections* and the *interlaminar astrocytes.* The latter are plentiful in the cortical layer 1, whereas the former inhabit cortical layers 5 and 6. The somata of both subtypes give out prominent cytoplasmic branches. In the case of the astrocytes with varicose projections, such branches are up to 1 mm long and terminate on the cerebral vessels walls or in the neuropil. After twisting courses, the also lengthy branches of the interlaminar astrocytes end up like varicose projections in contact with vascular walls or in the neuropil. Hitherto, the specific roles of such recently identified cerebral cortical astrocytic subtypes are not understood. Anyhow, the lengthy processes of the human interlaminar astrocytes can propagate Ca^{2+} waves [15–17].

3. Astrocytes' physiology

In the past and still now, some scientists have been holding astrocytes as neuron-supporting and at the same time debris-scavenging cells protectively regulating the homeostasis of a microenvironment from which neurons derive the necessary nutrients [12, 19]. Astrocytes also control the workings of "tripartite synapses" by enveloping them with their branches, thus barring the diffusion of released neurotransmitters and preventing the firing activity of one neuron from altering that of adjacent neurons [20]. In addition, astrocytes' synaptic regulation does not influence only the tripartite synapses their branches envelop but also far away synapses via astrocytes' signals, a process named *lateral astrocyte synaptic regulation* [21]. Astrocytes can do this and also communicate with neighboring neurons, with which they form astrocyte-neuron gangs with a ratio of one "master" astrocyte and 20–30 "client" neurons [22] and adjust local blood flow by secreting various compounds called *gliotransmitters* [23]. Surges in intracellular Ca^{2+} levels drive the release of several gliotransmitters, comprising adenosine, ATP, D-serine, eicosanoids, glutamate, and TNF-α, which would adjust the activities of the astrocytes themselves, the far away synapses, and the surrounding cells [24].

Since astrocytes cannot be electrically excited, their plasma membranes do not propagate action potentials as instead neurons do. The membrane potential of astrocytes at rest has very low values, ranging from −85 to −90 mV. This is due to their intense expression of TREK-1 and TWIK-1 potassium ion [K^+] channels [25]. As recent lines of evidence show, astrocytes residing in separate brain areas express dissimilar types and levels of ion channels and hence are equipped with distinctive electrophysiological characteristics. The huge group of ion channels implicated is also differently expressed during astrocytes' developmental stages [26].

In addition, astrocytes express various kinds of metabotropic receptors, which are coupled to a number of intracellular second messenger systems. For example, astroglia are known to adjust neuronal excitability and synaptic transmission through the metabotropic glutamatergic receptor subtype 5 (mGluR5). The results of experiments using brain slices showed that in response to an assortment of neurotransmitters, comprising acetylcholine, adenosine, ATP, endocannabinoids, GABA, glutamate, norepinephrine, and prostaglandins, metabotropic receptors could raise the intracellular Ca^{2+} levels ($[Ca^{2+}]_i$) via phospholipase C (PLC)- and inositol (1,4,5)-triphosphate (IP3)-dependent activities [27].

4. Astrocytes and AD neuropathology

An aberrant reactivity of astrocytes is a telltale sign of chronic neurodegenerative ailments like AD and Parkinson's disease [1, 3, 5]. While AD advances an *astrogliosis* emerges as a sign of astrocytes' dysfunction. However, astrogliosis is a common event in all kinds of CNS injury or ailment and is marked by persistent scar-like structures made by proliferating and migrating reactive astrocytes [5, 11]. Two types of reactive astrocytes, the A1 and the A2, have been latterly identified, whose specific activities could result advantageous or detrimental according to the type of neuropathology considered. In fact, reactive astrocytes of the A2 type advance healing of ischemic injuries (e.g., stroke). Conversely, reactive astrocytes of the A1 type could either stop their physiological activities and next degenerate or become involved in detrimental activities [28]. Reportedly, astrocytes mediate Aβ neurotoxicity and Tau phosphorylation in primary cocultures with rat embryo neurons [29].

AD hits nearly 2% of the people of the Western world particularly after 60 years of age [30]. AD's clinical course can be dissected into (*a*) a quite protracted (~20–40 years) asymptomatic phase, the early diagnosis of which is hard to make because of the present lack of specific markers, (*b*) an amnestic minor cognitive impairment phase (aMCI; ~3–6 years) in which amnesia's severity progressively grows, and (*c*) a full-blown symptomatic phase (~6–8 years) typified by escalating losses of memory and cognitive abilities and ending up with patients' obit [31, 32]. Controversies still rage about the pathophysiological mechanisms promoting the opening and unforgiving progression of the sporadic or late-onset AD (SAD or LOAD) [33]. The neuropathology unhurriedly yet progressively destroys the neuronal networks. As shown by high-resolution fMRI studies, LOAD starts in the lateral entorhinal cortex of the hippocampus, the brain's memory-recording place, and next spreads along the extended projection circuits connecting the hippocampus with cognition-crucial wider and wider cognition-crucial areas of the upper cerebral cortex [34].

In the healthy brain, neurons produce and release at their synapses tiny amounts of non-toxic $A\beta_{42}$ monomers, the intra- and extracellular amounts of which remain at low (i.e., pM), physiological values owing to a set of removing mechanisms operated by several proteases, phagocytosis by microglia and astrocytes, and disposal into the blood circulation [35]. In aged brains, the ability to clear the Aβs from the CNS increasingly plummets likely because of local microcirculation problems. Consequently, as the *amyloid cascade hypothesis* posits, the accumulating $A\beta_{42}$ monomers start forming agglomerates first of toxic soluble oligomers ($A\beta_{42}$-os) and protofibrils [35] and next of insoluble, fibrils, and senile plaques, thereby driving the neuropathology progression [33, 36]. According to this *Aβs first hypothesis*, the hyperphosphorylated Tau (p-Tau) protein, the second main driver of AD, enters the stage some time later.

Conversely, as the *brainstem-Tau first hypothesis* posits, AD starts within a brainstem nucleus, the *locus coeruleus*, and its surroundings. There, presumably mutated accumulating p-Taues group into neurotoxic oligomers (p-Tau-os) which next steadily spread out across the cerebral cortex along lengthy and circuitous neural pathways that also reach the hippocampus, leaving as their aftermaths intra-neuronal neurofibrillary tangles (NFTs) [37–40]. Later, p-Tau-os can also prompt the production of $A\beta_{42}$ surpluses which too diffuse and accumulate intracerebrally [37, 39, 41]. A colocalization of Aβs and NFTs within the cytoplasm of human astrocytes can also occur [42]. Whatever is the temporal order of manifestation of the two main AD drivers [on this topic, see also below], their joined toxic activities do speed up the occurrence of synapses loss, neuroinflammation, mitochondrial damage and dysfunction, oxidative stress, astrocytes' and microglia's reactivation, senile plaques' deposition, cerebral amyloid angiopathy (CAA), NFTs, and progressive oligodendroglia and neurons death—all hallmarks of AD's neuropathology—and therefore accelerate the clinical course of AD [37, 39].

Moreover, $A\beta_{42}$-os and $A\beta_{42}$ fibrillar aggregates bind various plasma membrane receptors, comprising the calcium-sensing receptors (CaSRs) and the receptors for advanced glycation end products (RAGEs) which can activate the astrocytes (see for further details [3, 11, 43, 44]). Such multiple receptor interactions with Aβs stir up astrocytes' JAK2 and MEK1/MEK2/ERK-1/ERK-2 signaling pathways stimulate the direct binding of STAT1 and HIF-1α/HIF-1β complexes to the *BACE1* and *VEGF-A* gene promoters and activate the microglia triggering synthesis and secretion of proinflammatory cytokines like IL-1β, TNF-α and INF-γ [37, 43, 44]. Such cytokines critically advance the formation of Aβ-os and fibrils [45, 46].

5. The CaSR

A highly conserved gene, the *CASR* is a member of family C of the G-protein-coupled receptors (GPCRs). Family C GPCRs do not share any DNA sequence homology with the members of other GPCR families. However, the CaSR exhibits topological and sequence homology to the metabotropic glutamate receptors (mGluRs) [47]. The CaSR protein has seven transmembrane α-helices (TM1–TM7) linked by extra- and intracellular loops altogether making the 7TM region. The CaSR protein has a massive (612 amino acids) extracellular N-terminal domain, the so-called Venus flytrap (VFT), and a much tinier intracellular C-terminal tail, which makes up the G-protein-binding domain [22, 48]. In their membrane-bound form, CaSRs form homodimers (CaSR/CaSR) or heterodimers (e.g., CaSR/mGluR) [22, 48]. CaSR dimers are put together at the endoplasmic reticulum (ER) and next are conveyed and fitted into the plasma membrane [49]. Once there, the CaSR senses minute changes in extracellular Ca^{2+} concentration ($[Ca^{2+}]_e$). However, the CaSR is not a ligand-discriminating receptor. Rather, it may be better described without changing its acronym as a *cation-sensing receptor*. In point of fact, its ligands can be distinguished in (*a*) VFT-binding CaSR-activating orthosteric ligands, comprising Ca^2, several di- and trivalent cations, aminoglycoside antibiotics, and the polyamine spermine, and (*b*) allosteric ligands which bind different sections of the 7TM domain, including aromatic L-α-amino acids, extracellular Na^+, and pharmacological *agonists* and *antagonists* (*see below*) [22]. The activation of CaSR encompasses a complex set of interactions among amino acids, Ca^{2+} and conceivably anions like PO_4^{3-} ions. Recently, Geng et al. [50] demonstrated that the CaSR can display an inactive state both in the absence and in the presence of Ca^{2+} ions and adopts the active state only when one L-amino acid, and one or more Ca^{2+} ions are bound to it. L-amino acids like L-Trp and Ca^{2+} ions are co-agonists of the CaSR, operating together to elicit the receptor's activation. Finally, it should be mentioned that in human adult astrocytes, CaSR expression increases in proliferatively quiescent cells with respect to actively growing ones, but is not affected by high or low levels of $[Ca^{2+}]_e$ [51].

Notably, being positively charged, both soluble or fibrillar Aβs specifically form complexes with the plasma membrane CaSRs. Subsequently, the Aβs·CaSR complexes coalesce into patches which are rapidly endocytosed and can be detected within EEA1-positive early endosomes in the cytoplasm (**Figure 1**) [54, 55]. However, it has not been ascertained whether Aβs' binding site[s] is [are] of the orthosteric or allosteric kind or both [22, 44].

Various species of G-proteins mediate CaSR's intracellular signaling by (*a*) activating a set of enzymes such as protein kinases (e.g., AKT, JNK, PKCs, and MAPKs like MEK/ERK) and lipid kinases (e.g., phospholipase A2, C, D), (*b*) triggering gene expression through transcription factors, (*c*) inhibiting adenylyl cyclase, and (*d*) inducing Ca^{2+} influx via TCPC6-encoded channels [56]. The relevant consequences are modifications to enzyme activities (e.g., proteases), cell proliferation, cell secretion, and/or cell death. In addition, CaSR-expressing neurons and all types of glial cells expressing the CaSR are liable to be harmed by the cytotoxic effects of CaSR-binding and CaSR-activating soluble Aβ oligomers [sAβ-os] and/or insoluble fibrillar Aβ (fAβ) aggregates [22, 44].

CaSR's expression occurs in every portion of the rat and human brain. By using the in situ hybridization method, Yano et al. [57] demonstrated that the CaSR is intensely expressed in several areas of the adult rat CNS. In relation to AD, we recall here that CaSR's expression abounds in the hippocampus especially at the level of the somata and axon terminals of the pyramidal neurons, suggesting the functional modulation of such cells by CaSR's signaling [47, 58]. Notably, the N-methyl-D-aspartate receptor (NMDAR) brain location is superimposable on the CaSR's. Both NMDARs and CaSRs play crucial roles in the induction of

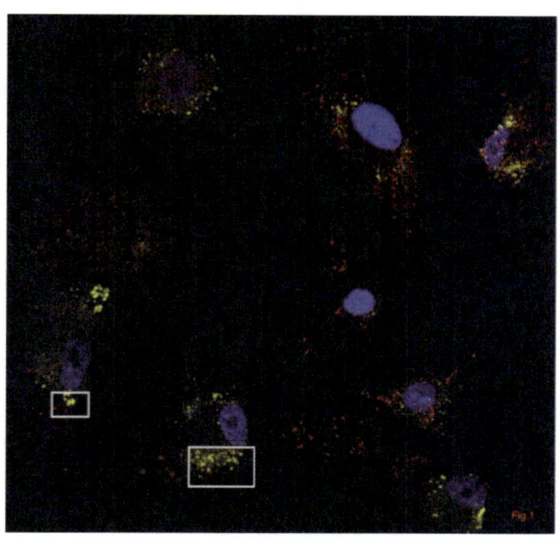

Figure 1. Cultured untransformed adult human astrocytes CaSRs bind $A\beta_{25-35}$ and internalize the $A\beta_{25-35}$·CaSR complexes within in EEA1-positive cytoplasmic early endosomes. Cells were incubated for 15 min at 37°C with $A\beta_{25-35}$ [5.0 μM] and next fixed and permeabilized using the in situ proximity ligation assay (PLA) (see for details [52, 53]), it is possible to specifically reveal the $A\beta_{25-35}$·CaSR complexes as *red dots*. Using an antibody against the EEA1 antigen marker, early endosomes [54] can be seen as *green dots*. The yellow fluorescence reveals the discrete colocalization of the $A\beta_{25-35}$·CaSR complexes with the EEA1-positive early endosomes. *Top panel* magnification, 600×. The other two panels are zoomed from the middle (middle panel) and left (bottom panel) rectangles in the top panels.

long-term potentiation (LTP) [59]. Typically, CaSR's expression occurs not only in neurons but also in human primary astrocytes, astrocytoma cell lines, oligodendroglia, and microglial cells [57]. Interestingly, total CaSR protein levels increase significantly though transiently in Aβ-exposed NAHAs [44]. Furthermore, the intensity of CaSR's immunoreactivity significantly increases with age in the hippocampus of 3xTg AD-model mice [60], particularly where Aβs and p-Taues also accumulate, a clear indication of the involvement of this receptor in AD pathophysiology in vivo (see also below).

The intracellular Ca^{2+} concentration ($[Ca^{2+}]_i$) can vary widely under both normal and pathological conditions. The Ca^{2+} influx into cultured astrocytes is linear and normally increases only up to 1.8 mM, suggesting that CaSR signaling controls it [61, 62]. In the past, aberrations of cell surface and intracellular Ca^{2+}-controlling mechanisms were posited to happen in various neurodegenerative ailments, AD included [61–65]. Reportedly, exogenous $A\beta_{42}$ and its well-established proxy, $A\beta_{25-35}$, trigger $[Ca^{2+}]_i$ surges and oscillations which persist for hours in the neurons and astrocytes too and concur with the loss of the inner mitochondrial membrane potential. This in turn promotes the release of reactive oxygen species (ROS) and oxidative stress in both neurons and astrocytes. Coculturing such reactive astrocytes with neurons caused the neurons' death within 24 h unless the Aβ-elicited $[Ca^{2+}]_i$ surges were forestalled [61].

Recent findings from our laboratory lend credence to the view that the CaSR, one of the receptors astrocytes express, drives the pathogenic mechanisms of AD [48, 66–69].

6. Human cortical astrocytes, CaSRs, and AD promotion

It is time for us to zoom in on our preclinical model of cortical untransformed phenotypically stable, i.e., *normal* adult human astrocytes (NAHAs) obtained from temporal cortex surgical leftovers of motorbike accident victims with perforating skull trauma. After culturing and expanding the numbers of the NAHAs in vitro and next inducing them into proliferative quiescence, we have been investigating their metabolic responses to added exogenous Aβ-os or Aβ fibrils either in the presence or absence of a microglial cytokine mixture (i.e. IL-1β, TNF-α, and INF-γ) [44, 55, 70, 71].

As we recalled above, CaSR's expression takes place with dissimilar intensities, in every CNS cell type, astrocytes included [44, 57]. Recent studies have brought to light some of the physiological roles the CaSR plays in the human CNS, like modulation of neurons' dendrites and axons growth and of OLGs development [57, 72]. Using the NAHAs as our experimental system, we first demonstrated that exogenous $A\beta_{25-35}$—instigated CaSR signaling elicits the concurrent expression of nitric oxide synthase-2 (NOS-2) and of GTP cyclohydrolase-1 (GCH-1). GCH-1 makes the BH4 [tetrahydrobiopterin] cofactor that dimerizes and activates the NOS-2 moieties, thus allowing the synthesis of nitric oxide (NO) to occur [44, 73, 74]. Exogenous fibrillar Aβs also induce via direct CaSR signaling activation the cytoplasmic stabilization and nuclear translocation of the hypoxia-inducible HIF-1α•HIF-1β transcription complex in NAHAs. This elicits the vascular endothelial growth factor-A (*VEGF-A*) gene expression and the de novo synthesis of three splice protein variants (i.e., $VEGF\text{-}A_{121}$, $VEGF\text{-}A_{165}$, and $VEGF\text{-}A_{189}$) and the secretion mainly of the VEGF-A_{165} variant [55, 70]. A typical feature of AD is an overproduction and release of VEGF-A from neurons, glial cells, and cerebrovascular endothelium. Such VEGF-A surpluses are toxic for neurons, astrocytes, and endothelial cells, the constituents of the neurovascular units, and result in BBB's functional impairment (see for Refs. [75–78]). In vivo, an Aβ·CaSR-mediated VEGF-A_{165} oversecretion from the human astrocytes' end-feet of their blood-vessel contacting processes could drive local surges of the blood flow in the hippocampus of aMCI stage patients [79, 80]. This event could be revealed as unexpected intensified blood oxygen level-dependent (BOLD) signals by means of high-resolution functional magnetic resonance imaging [fMRI] analysis [81, 82]. Hence, such BOLD signal is not due, as would be wrongly expected, to a presumptive hyperactivity of overtasked neurons in shrunken dentate gyrus/CA3 Aβ-damaged hippocampal areas of aMCI patients [80–82]. The increased VEGF-A release elicits a greater local vascular density via neoangiogenesis which augments blood oxygen delivery and BOLD signal intensity of these hippocampal areas once they are functionally activated. Yet, the progression of AD neuropathology destroys the overgrown local vessels, thus reducing the blood flow to the point that the fMRI-intensified BOLD signal vanishes. At any rate, this boosted BOLD signal at the hippocampal level of aMCI subjects is a harbinger of the impending symptomatic stage of AD [79].

However, the most exciting discoveries were subsequently made possible by the advent of very sensitive ELISA kits assaying Aβs. In untreated NAHAs, the metabolic processing of amyloid precursor holoprotein (APP) takes place along the nonamyloidogenic pathway [NAP] being mediated by the activity of the α-secretases (mainly ADAM10) and extracellularly sheds all the soluble sAPPα it produces. Notably, sAPPα is a neurotrophic and neuroprotective compound positively affecting neurons' functions and viability. Moreover, sAPPα synthesis precludes any $A\beta_{40/42}$ production from APP as it is cut from the middle amino acid sequence of $A\beta_{40/42}$. Therefore, NAP largely prevails over APP's amyloidogenic processing [AP] in the untreated astrocytes, which secrete only very low basal $A\beta_{40/42}$ amounts [71]. Conversely, adding fibrillar $A\beta_{25-35}$ by itself and hence stirring off $A\beta_{25-35}$·CaSR signaling remarkably reduces sAPPα's extracellular shedding while driving an overproduction and oversecretion of neurotoxic $A\beta_{42}$/$A\beta_{42}$-os owing to concurrent raises in the sequential activities of BACE-1 and γ-secretase. The further addition of a microglial cytokine mixture only accelerates but not increases the total amount of $A\beta_{42}$/$A\beta_{42}$-os secretion by the NAHAs despite a concurring APP overexpression [44, 71]. Thus, these events could start of self-sustaining vicious cycle of $A\beta_{42}$/$A\beta_{42}$-os spreading within the brain [37, 44]. The same Aβ·CaSR-induced signaling mechanism stimulates the secretion of neurotoxic $A\beta_{42}$/$A\beta_{42}$-os from human cortical postnatal HCN-1A neurons [44]. Thereafter, the neurons start dying slowly like they do in vivo [44]. Most important, we also gained preliminary evidence indicating that Tau and hyperphosphorylated (p)-Tau are both expressed by untreated NAHAs in culture and that their exposure to the usual $A\beta_{42}$ proxy, $A\beta_{25-35}$, significantly increases via Aβ·CaSR-induced signaling the activity of GSK-3β [83], the main Tau protein kinase [84, 85]. The upshot is an increased production of p-Tau/p-Tau-os which both accumulate inside the cells and are extracellularly released inside exosomes [83]. Novel lines of evidence suggest that extracellular vesicles, which comprise exosomes, play important physiological and pathological roles in the CNS [86]. The above mechanism could promote the concurrent diffusion of both p-Tau/p-Tau-os and $A\beta_{42}$-os, the two main AD drivers, within the brain, though the tauopathy's noxious effects will take longer to manifest [37, 83].

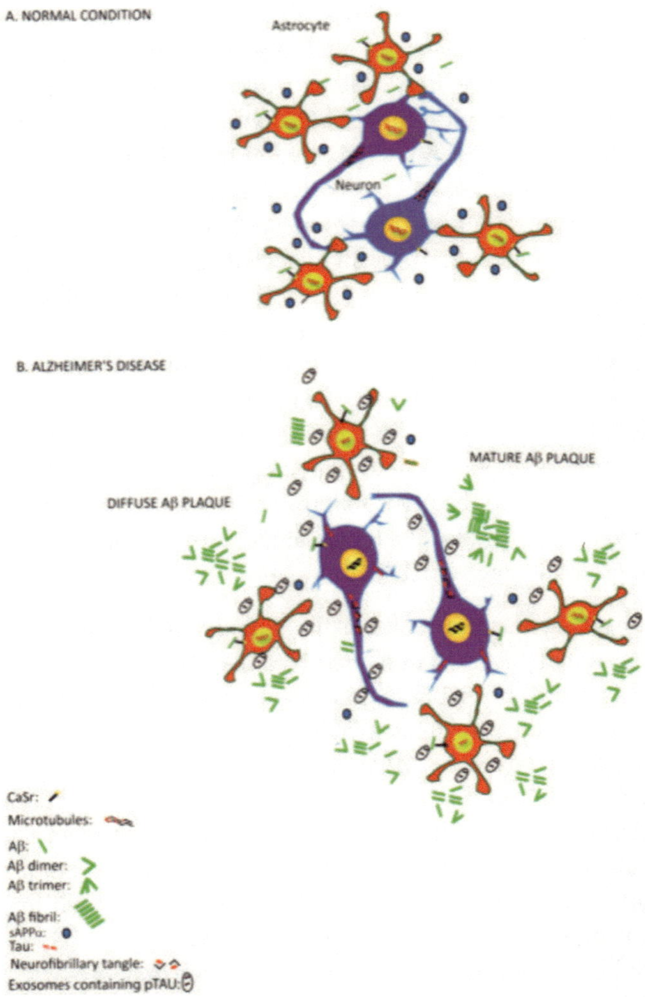

Figure 2. Cartoon depicting the calcilytic-suppressible differences between healthy and AD brain tissue brought about by Aβ-os·CaSR signaling. (A) Under healthy conditions, human astrocytes and neurons of the astrocyte-neuron gangs mutually interact to upkeep the environment's homeostasis. Via the prevailing nonamyloidogenic processing of APP the astrocytes release the neurotrophic and neuroprotective sAPPα, the synthesis of which obliterates any excess production and release of toxic Aβ-os and hence of Aβ fibrillar polymers. In parallel, multiple fully working clearance systems help keep the nontoxic but trophic $A\beta_{42}$ monomers at very low levels (not shown). The astrocytes release exosomes which enclose minimal amounts of p-Tau (not shown). No accumulation of Aβ-os or p-Tau-os occurs within the neurons and astrocytes. (B) Ongoing AD neuropathology involves several changes brought about by Aβ-os·CaSR signaling in the activated human astrocytes and neurons. The now prevailing amyloidogenic processing of APP leads to the overproduction of $A\beta_{42}$-os in both cell types at the expense of the NAP which severely curtails the extracellular shedding and beneficial activities of sAPPα. Thus $A\beta_{42}$-os both accumulate inside the cells and are oversecreted: this allows $A\beta_{42}$-os diffusion and interaction with the CaSRs of adjacent and far off neurons and astrocytes. This mechanism spreads the neuropathology promoting the progression of AD. Fibrillar polymers of oversecreted $A\beta_{42}$ also accumulate extracellularly giving raise to either diffuse or mature Aβ plaques, which can also release Aβ-os. Moreover, Aβ-os·CaSR signaling increases Tau protein phosphorylation by GSK-3β and the accumulation of p-Tau inside the astrocytes (and likely neurons). In the neurons, toxic p-Tau accumulates as NFTs, which cause severe dysfunctions. Moreover, the astrocytes release significantly increased amounts of p-Tau enclosed within membrane-bound exosomes, an activity which can aid a later emergence of the tauopathy. The Aβ-os·CaSR signaling also increases the production and release of NO and VEGF-A surpluses from the astrocytes [not shown]. Remarkably, administering a calcilytic-like NPS 2143 upkeeps the physiological condition shown in (A), thus disclosing its anti-AD therapeutic potential.

Given the relevance of the roles that the several upshots of the Aβ·CaSR-elicited signaling could have on the promotion of AD, we were enticed to test whether an allosteric highly specific CaSR antagonist [short-termed as *calcilytic*] could have any anti-AD therapeutic potential. Thus, we demonstrated that calcilytic NPS 2143 [87, 88] can persistently downregulate CaSR protein expression thus not only antagonizing but also curbing Aβ·CaSR signaling [44]. And the calcilytic enhances the proteolysis of endogenously amassing $A\beta_{42}$ by enhancing the 20S chymotrypsin-like activity of the proteasome. Moreover, NPS 2143 keeps down the Golgi/trans-Golgi network transport of endogenous $A\beta_{42}$/$A\beta_{42}$-os and, consequently, fully suppresses any oversecretion of the latter driven by the Aβ·CaSR signaling both in the case of NAHAs and of cortical human neurons [37, 44]. In addition, calcilytic NPS 2143 also wholly curbs the concurrent Aβ·CaSR signaling-elicited surplus production and secretion of NO and $VEGF\text{-}A_{165}$ from the NAHAs [37, 44, 55]. Conversely, the CaSR allosteric *agonist* or *calcimimetic* NPS R-568 enhances the surplus release of $A\beta_{42}$/$A\beta_{42}$-os, NO, and VEGF-A from the NAHAs confirming the positive involvement of the CaSR in these metabolic changes [44]. Also, NPS 2143 promotes APP and ADAM10 α-secretase translocation to the NAHAs plasma membrane, thereby restoring the extracellular shedding of neurotrophic and neuroprotective sAPPα to nearly normal (i.e., untreated) levels. Yet, NPS 2143 does not change the concurrent APP's increased expression suggesting its promotion via mechanisms involving Aβs and other receptors but not the Aβ·CaSR signaling [76]. Notably, NPS 2143 remains beneficially effective even when a mixture of microglial proinflammatory cytokines is added to the Aβs treatment, indicating that a calcilytic could keep its beneficial effects even under AD-typical neuroinflammatory conditions [71]. Most important, NPS 2143 also fully suppresses the Aβ·CaSR-induced concurrent increase in GSK-3β activity and, consequently, the surges in both intracellular p-Tau/p-Tau-os levels and exosomal p-Tau/p-Tau-os release [83]. Extracellular vesicles, including exosomes, are likely to play both physiological and pathological roles in the CNS [86]. And, last but not least, adding NPS 2143 keeps the human cortical neurons *alive* and kicking notwithstanding the simultaneous presence of otherwise toxic levels of exogenous Aβs [44].

We wish to stress that these results could be gained by using untransformed human cortical adult astrocytes and postnatal neurons, *arguably the preclinical experimental models which at present are the closest one to human AD patients*. Our findings show that calcilytics terminate both stimulatory effects of pathological Aβ·CaSR signaling on $A\beta_{42}$ and p-Tau, the two AD's main drivers, surplus production and extracellular diffusion. On these grounds, we posit that such highly selective CaSR antagonists could effectively halt AD's progressive spread and preserve patients' cognition and life quality even when a neuroinflammation has already been ignited (**Figure 2**).

7. Conclusions and future perspectives

Mounting lines of evidence lend credence to the view that the human astrocytes—the characteristics of which remarkably differ from those of their rodent counterparts—play manifold roles in the molecular mechanisms associated with AD's pathophysiology. A growing accumulation of Aβs, p-Taues, NO, and VEGF-A hinges upon the signaling of Aβs·CaSR complexes. This initiates a self-spreading cascade of events which culminate in neuronal synaptic disconnection, dysfunction, and death coupled with the oligodendrocyte dysfunction, axonal myelin sheaths damage and death, the activation of the microglia, the alteration of BBB permeability, and the expression of all the other neuropathological hallmarks of AD. The upshot is a concurrent degeneration of the gray and white matters. Thus, the CNS will keep shrinking; AD clinical symptoms will emerge and increase in intensity until the patients having lost their memories and cognitive abilities die. It is obvious that given their mounting numbers, the care of LOAD patients does heavily impact on their relatives and, for the huge costs of their assistance, on their National Health Services. In this disheartening scenario, the repurposing of highly specific CaSR antagonists or calcilytics as anti-AD therapeutics has the potential for shining a ray of hope.

Abbreviations

Aβs	amyloid-β peptides
AD	Alzheimer's disease
aMCI	amnestic minor cognitive impairment
APP	Aβ precursor protein
BBB	blood-brain barrier
BOLD	blood oxygen level-dependent
CaSR	calcium-sensing receptor
CNS	central nervous system
fMRI	functional magnetic resonance imaging
GPCRs	G-protein-coupled receptors
GSK-3β	glycogen synthase kinase-3β
LOAD	late-onset AD
NAHAs	normal (untransformed) adult human astrocytes
NFTs	neurofibrillary tangles
NO	nitric oxide
OLGs	oligodendrocytes
-os	oligomers
p-Tau	hyperphosphorylated Tau protein
VEGF	vascular endothelial growth factor

Author details

Ilaria Dal Prà*, Ubaldo Armato and Anna Chiarini

*Address all correspondence to: ilaria.dalpra@univr.it

Histology and Embryology Unit, University of Verona Medical School, Verona, Italy

References

[1] Khakh BS, Sofroniew MW. Diversity of astrocyte functions and phenotypes in neural circuits. Nature Neuroscience. 2015;**18**:942-552. DOI: 10.1038/nn.4043

[2] Avila-Muñoz E, Arias C. When astrocytes become harmful: Functional and inflammatory responses that contribute to Alzheimer's disease. Ageing Research Reviews. 2014;**18**: 29-40. DOI: 10.1016/j.arr.2014.07.004

[3] Filous AR, Silver J. Targeting astrocytes in CNS injury and disease: A translational research approach. Progress in Neurobiology. 2016;**144**:173-187. DOI: 10.1016/j.pneurobio.2016.03.009

[4] Eroglu C, Barres BA. Regulation of synaptic connectivity by glia. Nature. 2010;**468** (**7321**):223-231. DOI: 10.1038/nature09612

[5] Pekny M, Wilhelmsson U, Pekna M. The dual role of astrocyte activation and reactive gliosis. Neuroscience Letters. 2014;**565**:30-38. DOI: 10.1016/j.neulet.2013.12.071

[6] Ferrer I. Diversity of astroglial responses across human neurodegenerative disorders and brain aging. Brain Pathology. 2017;**27**:645-674. DOI: 10.1111/bpa.12538

[7] Middeldorp J, Hol EM. GFAP in health and disease. Progress in Neurobiology. 2011;**93**: 421-443. DOI: 10.1016/j.pneurobio.2011.01.005

[8] Bushong EA, Martone ME, Jones YZ, Ellisman MH. Protoplasmic astrocytes in CA1 stratum radiatum occupy separate anatomical domains. The Journal of Neuroscience. 2002; **22**:183-192

[9] Boesmans W, Rocha NP, Reis HJ, Holt M, Vanden Berghe P. The astrocyte marker Aldh1L1 does not reliably label enteric glial cells. Neuroscience Letters. 2014;**566**:102-105. DOI: 10.1016/j.neulet.2014.02.042

[10] Ge WP, Jia GM. Local production of astrocytes in the cerebral cortex. Neuroscience. 2016;**323**:3-9. DOI: 10.1016/j.neuroscience.2015.08.057.

[11] Hamby ME, Sofroniew MV. Reactive astrocytes as therapeutic targets for CNS disorders. Neurotherapeutics. 2010;**7**:494-506. DOI: 10.1016/j.nurt.2010.07.003

[12] Lliff JJ, Wang M, Liao Y, Plogg BA, Peng W, Gundersen GA, Benveniste H, Vates GE, Deane R,Goldman SA, Nagelhus EA, Nedergaard M. A paravascular pathway facilitates

CSF flow through the brain parenchyma and the clearance of interstitial solutes, including amyloid β. Science Translational Medicine. 2012;**4**:147ra111. DOI: 10.1126/scitranslmed.3003748

[13] Cheslow L, Alvarez JI. Glial-endothelial crosstalk regulates blood-brain barrier function. Current Opinion in Pharmacology. 2015;**26**:39-46. DOI: 10.1016/j.coph.2015.09.010.

[14] Xu G, Wang W, Zhou M. Spatial organization of NG2 glial cells and astrocytes in rat hippocampal CA1 region. Hippocampus. 2014;**24**:383-395. DOI: 10.1002/hipo.22232

[15] Oberheim NA, Takano T, Han X, He W, Lin JH, Wang F, Xu Q, Wyatt JD, Pilcher W, Ojemann JG, Ransom BR, Goldman SA, Nedergaard M. Uniquely hominid features of adult human astrocytes, The Journal of Neuroscience 2009;**29**.3276-3287. DOI: 10.1523/JNEUROSCI.4707-08.2009.

[16] Oberheim NA, Wang GS, Nedergaard M. Astrocytic complexity distinguishes the human brain. Trends in Neurosciences. 2006;**29**:547-553

[17] Emsley JG, Macklis JD. Astroglial heterogeneity closely reflects the neuronal-defined anatomy of the adult murine CNS. Neuron Glia Biology. 2006;**2**:175-186

[18] Viganò F, Dimou L. The heterogeneous nature of NG2-glia. Brain Research. 2016;**1638** ([PtB]):129-137. DOI: 10.1016/j.brainres.2015.09.012

[19] Zhang H, YJ S, Zhou WW, Wang SW, PX X, XL Y, Liu RT. Activated scavenger receptor a promotes glial internalization of Aβ. PLoS One. 2014;**9**:e94197. DOI: 10.1371/journal.pone.0094197

[20] Pérez-Alvarez A, Araque A. Astrocyte-neuron interaction at tripartite synapses. Current Drug Targets. 2013;**14**:1220-1224

[21] Covelo A, Araque A. Lateral regulation of synaptic transmission by astrocytes. Neuroscience. 2016;**323**:62-66. DOI: 10.1016/j.neuroscience.2015. 02.036

[22] Dal Prà I, Chiarini A, Pacchiana R, Gardenal E, Chakravarthy B, Whitfield JF, Armato U. Calcium-sensing receptors of human astrocyte-neuron teams: Amyloid-β-driven mediators and therapeutic targets of Alzheimer's disease. Current Neuropharmacology. 2014; **12**:353-364. DOI: 10.2174/ 1570159X12666140828214701

[23] Harada K, Kamiya T, Tsuboi T. Gliotransmitter release from astrocytes: Functional, developmental, and pathological implications in the brain. Frontiers in Neuroscience. 2016;**9**:499. DOI: 10.3389/fnins.2015.00499. eCollection 2015.

[24] Newman EA. Glial cell regulation of neuronal activity and blood flow in the retina by release of gliotransmitters. Philosophical Transactions of the Royal Society of London. Series B, Biological Sciences. 2015;**370**[1672]:pii:20140195. DOI: 10.1098/rstb.2014.0195.

[25] Zhou M, Xu G, Xie M, Zhang X, Schools GP, Ma L, Kimelberg HK, Chen H. TWIK-1 and TREK-1 are potassium channels contributing significantly to astrocyte passive conductance in rat hippocampal slices. The Journal of Neuroscience. 2009;**29**:8551-8564. DOI: 10.1523/JNEUROSCI.5784-08.2009

[26] Olsen ML, Khakh BS, Skatchkov SN, Zhou M, Lee CJ, Rouach N. New insights on astrocyte ion channels: Critical for homeostasis and neuron-glia Signaling. The Journal of Neuroscience. 2015;**35**:13827-13835. DOI: 10.1523/JNEUROSCI.2603-15.2015

[27] Panatier A, Robitaille R. Astrocytic mGluR5 and the tripartite synapse. Neuroscience. 2016;**323**:29-34. DOI: 10.1016/j.neuroscience.2015.03.063

[28] Zamanian JL, Xu L, Foo LC, Nouri N, Zhou L, Giffard RG, Barres BA. Genomic analysis of reactive astrogliosis. The Journal of Neuroscience. 2012;**32**:6391-6410. DOI: 10.1523/JNEUROSCI.6221-11.2012

[29] Garwood CJ, Pooler AM, Atherton J, Hanger DP, Noble W. Astrocytes are important mediators of Aβ-induced neurotoxicity and tau phosphorylation in primary culture. Cell Death & Disease. 2011;**2**:e167. DOI: 10.1038/cddis.2011.50

[30] Alzheimer's Association. Alzheimer's disease facts and figures. Alzheimer's & Dementia. 2008;**4**:110-133

[31] Querfurth HW, LaFerla FM. Alzheimer's disease. The New England Journal of Medicine. 2010;**362**:329-344

[32] Gallagher M, Koh MT. Episodic memory on the path to Alzheimer's disease. Current Opinion in Neurobiology. 2011;**21**:929-934. DOI: 10.1016/j.conb.2011.10.021

[33] Armato U, Chakravarthy B, Pacchiana R, Whitfield JF. Alzheimer's disease: An update of the roles of receptors, astrocytes and primary cilia. International Journal of Molecular Medicine. 2013;**31**:3-10. DOI: 10.3892/ijmm.2012.1162

[34] Khan UA, Liu L, Provenzano FA, Berman DE, Profaci CP, Sloan R, Mayeux R, Duff KE, Small SA. Molecular drivers and cortical spread of lateral entorhinal cortex dysfunction in preclinical Alzheimer's disease. Nature Neuroscience. 2014;**17**:304-311. DOI: 10.1038/nn.3606

[35] Sehlin D, Englund H, Simu B, Karlsson M, Ingelsson M, Nikolajeff F, Lannfelt L, Pettersson FE. Large aggregates are the major soluble Aβ species in AD brain fractionated with density gradient ultracentrifugation. PLoS One. 2012;**7**:e32014. DOI: 10.1371/journal.pone.0032014

[36] Selkoe DJ. Soluble oligomers of the amyloid beta-protein impair synaptic plasticity and behavior. Behavioural Brain Research. 2008;**192**:106-113. DOI: 10.1016/j.bbr.2008.02.016

[37] Dal Prà I, Chiarini A, Gui L, Chakravarthy B, Pacchiana R, Gardenal E, Whitfield JF, Armato U. Do astrocytes collaborate with neurons in spreading the "infectious" aβ and tau drivers of Alzheimer's disease? The Neuroscientist. 2015;**21**:9-29. DOI: 10.1177/1073858414529828

[38] Braak H, Thal DR, Ghebremedhin E, Del Tredici K. Stages of the pathologic process in Alzheimer disease: Age categories from 1 to 100 years. Journal of Neuropathology and Experimental Neurology. 2011;**70**:960-969. DOI: 10.1097/NEN.0b013e318232a379

[39] Braak H, Del Tredici K. The preclinical phase of the pathological process underlying sporadic Alzheimer's disease. Brain. 2015;**138**(Pt 10):2814-2833. DOI: 10.1093/brain/awv236

[40] Gerson JE, Kayed R. Formation and propagation of tau oligomeric seeds. Frontiers in Neurology. 2013;**4**:93. DOI: 10.3389/fneur.2013.00093. eCollection 2013

[41] Jin M, Shepardson N, Yang T, Chen G, Walsh D, Selkoe DJ. Soluble amyloid beta-protein dimers isolated from Alzheimer cortex directly induce tau hyperphosphorylation and neuritic degeneration. Proceedings of the National Academy of Sciences of the United States of America. 2011;**108**:5819-5824. DOI: 10.1073/pnas.1017033108

[42] Wakabayashi K, Mori F, Hasegawa M, Kusumi T, Yoshimura I, Takahashi H, Kaneko S. Co-localization of beta-peptide and phosphorylated tau in astrocytes in a patient with corticobasal degeneration. Neuropathology. 2006;**26**:66-71

[43] Chiarini A, Armato U, Liu D, Dal Prà I. Calcium-sensing receptors of human neural cells play crucial roles in Alzheimer's disease. Frontiers in Physiology. 2016;**7**:134. DOI: 10.3389/fphys.2016.00134. eCollection 2016

[44] Armato U, Chiarini A, Chakravarthy B, Chioffi F, Pacchiana R, Colarusso E, Whitfield JF, Dal Prà I. Calcium-sensing receptor antagonist [calcilytic] NPS 2143 specifically block the increased secretion of endogenous Ab42 prompted by exogenous fibrillary or soluble Ab25-35 in human cortical astrocytes and neurons—Therapeutic relevance to Alzheimer's disease. Biochimica et Biophysica Acta (BBA): Molecular Basis of Disease. 2013;**1832**:1634-1652. DOI: 10.1016/j.bbadis.2013.04.020

[45] Gold M, El Khoury J. β-amyloid, microglia, and the inflammasome in Alzheimer's disease. Seminars in Immunopathology. 2015;**37**:607-611. DOI: 10.1007/s00281-015-0518-0

[46] Blasko I, Veerhuis R, Stampfer-Kountchev M, Saurwein-Teissl M, Eikelenboom P, Grubeck-Loebenstein B. Costimulatory effects of interferon-gamma and interleukin-1beta or tumor necrosis factor alpha on the synthesis of Abeta1-40 and Abeta1-42 by human astrocytes. Neurobiology of Disease. 2000;**7**[6PtB]:682-689.

[47] Brown EM, Gamba G, Riccardi D, Lombardi M, Butters R, Kifor O, Sun A, Hediger MA, Lytton J, Hebert SC. Cloning and characterization of an extracellular Ca^{2+}-sensing receptor from bovine parathyroid. Nature. 1993;**366**(6455):575-580

[48] Armato U, Bonafini C, Chakravarthy B, Pacchiana R, Chiarini A, Withfiled JF, Dal Prà I. The calcium-sensing receptor: A novel Alzheimer's disease crucial target? Journal of the Neurological Sciences. 2012;**322**:137-140

[49] Pidasheva S, Grant M, Canaff L, Ercan O, Kumar U, Hendy GN. Calcium-sensing receptor dimerizes in the endoplasmic reticulum: Biochemical and biophysical characterization of CASR mutants retained intracellularly. Human Molecular Genetics. 2006;**15**:2200-2209

[50] Geng Y, Mosyak L, Kurinov I, Zuo H, Sturchler E, Cheng TC, Subramanyam P, Brown AP, Brennan SC, Mun HC, Bush M, Chen Y, Nguyen TX, Cao B, Chang DD, Quick M, Conigrave AD, Colecraft HM, McDonald P, Fan QR. Structural mechanism of ligand activation in human calcium-sensing receptor. Elife. 2016;**5**:pii: e13662. DOI: 10.7554/eLife.13662

[51] Dal Prà I, Chiarini A, Nemeth EF, Armato U, Whitfield JF. Roles of Ca^{2+} and the Ca^{2+}-sensing receptor [CASR] in the expression of inducible NOS [nitric oxide synthase]-2

and its BH4 [tetrahydrobiopterin]-dependent activation in cytokine-stimulated adult human astrocytes. Journal of Cellular Biochemistry. 2005;**96**:428-438

[52] Pacchiana R, Abbate M, Armato U, Dal Prà I, Chiarini A. Combining immunofluorescence with in situ proximity ligation assay: A novel imaging approach to monitor protein-protein interactions in relation to subcellular localization. Histochemistry and Cell Biology. 2014;**142**:593-600. DOI: 10.1007/s00418-014-1244-8

[53] Söderberg O, Gullberg M, Jarvius M, Ridderstråle K, Leuchowius KJ, Jarvius J, Wester K, Hydbring P, Bahram F, Larsson LG, Landegren U. Direct observation of individual endogenous protein complexes in situ by proximity ligation. Nature Methods. 2006;**3**:995-1000

[54] Voltan AR, Sardi Jde C, Soares CP, Pelajo Machado M, Fusco Almeida AM, Mendes-Giannini MJ. Early endosome antigen 1 [EEA1] decreases in macrophages infected with *Paracoccidioides brasiliensis*. Medical Mycology. 2013;**51**:759-764. DOI: 10.3109/13693786.2013.777859

[55] Dal Prà I, Armato U, Chioffi F, Pacchiana R, Whitfield JF, Chakravarthy B, Gui L, Chiarini A. The Aβ peptides-activated calcium-sensing receptor stimulates the production and secretion of vascular endothelial growth factor-A by normoxic adult human cortical astrocytes. Neuromolecular Medicine. 2014;**16**:645-657. DOI: 10.1007/s12017-014-8315-9

[56] Chakravarty B, Chattopadhyay N, Brown EM. Signaling through the extracellular calcium-sensing receptor [CaSR]. Advances in Experimental Medicine and Biology. 2012;**740**:103-142. DOI: 10.1007/978-94-007-2888-2_5

[57] Yano S, Brown EM, Chattopadhyay N. Calcium-sensing receptor in the brain. Cell Calcium. 2004;**35**:257-264. DOI: 10.1016/j.ceca.2003.10.008

[58] Chen W, Bergsman JB, Wang X, Gilkey G, Pierpoint CR, Daniel EA, Awumey EM, Dauban P, Dodd RH, Ruat M, Smith SM. Presynaptic external calcium signaling involves the calcium-sensing receptor in neocortical nerve terminals. PLoS One. 2010;**5**:e8563. DOI: 10.1371/journal.pone.0008563

[59] Chattopadhyay N, Legradi G, Bai M, Kifor O, Ye C, Vassilev PM, Brown EM, Lechan RM. Calcium-sensing receptor in the rat hippocampus: A developmental study. Brain Research. Developmental Brain Research. 1997;**100**:13-21

[60] Gardenal E, Chiarini A, Armato U, Dal Prà I, Verkhratsky A, Rodríguez JJ. Increased calcium-sensing receptor immunoreactivity in the hippocampus of a triple transgenic mouse model of Alzheimer's disease. Frontiers in Neuroscience. 2017;**11**:81. DOI: 10.3389/fnins.2017.00081. eCollection 2017

[61] Mattson MP, Cheng B, Davis D, Bryant K, Lieberburg I, Rydel RE. beta-Amyloid peptides destabilize calcium homeostasis and render human cortical neurons vulnerable to excitotoxicity. The Journal of Neuroscience. 1992;**12**:376-389

[62] Mattson MP. Calcium and neurodegeneration. Aging Cell. 2007;**6**:337-350

[63] Khakh BS, McCarthy KD. Astrocyte calcium signaling: From observations to functions and the challenges therein. Cold Spring Harbor Perspectives in Biology. 2015;**7**:a020404. DOI: 10.1101/cshperspect.a020404

[64] Fairless R, Williams SK, Diem R. Dysfunction of neuronal calcium signalling in neuroinflammation and neurodegeneration. Cell and Tissue Research. 2014;**357**:455-462

[65] Berridge MJ. Calcium regulation of neural rhythms, memory and Alzheimer's disease. The Journal of Physiology. 2014;**592**:281-293. DOI: 10.1113/jphysiol.2013.257527

[66] Chiarini A, Dal Prà I, Marconi M, Chakravarthy B, Whitfield JF, Armato U. Calcium-sensing receptor [CaSR] in human brain's pathophysiology: Roles in late-onset Alzheimer's disease [LOAD]. Current Pharmaceutical Biotechnology. 2009;**10**:317-326

[67] Ye C, Ho-Pao CL, Kanazirska M, Quinn S, Rogers K, Seidman CE, Seidman JG, Brown EM, Vassilev PM. Amyloid-beta proteins activate Ca^{2+}-permeable channels through calcium-sensing receptors. Journal of Neuroscience Research. 1997;**47**:547-554

[68] Dal Prà I, Chiarini A, Armato U. Antagonizing amyloid-β/calcium-sensing receptor signaling in human astrocytes and neurons: A key to halt Alzheimer's disease progression? Neural Regeneration Research. 2015;**10**:213-218. DOI: 10.4103/1673-5374.152373

[69] Conley YP, Mukherjee A, Kammerer C, DeKosky ST, Kamboh MI, Finegold DN, Ferrell RE. Evidence supporting a role for the calcium-sensing receptor in Alzheimer disease. American Journal of Medical Genetics. Part B, Neuropsychiatric Genetics. 2009;**150B**:703-709. DOI: 10.1002/ajmg.b.30896

[70] Chiarini A, Whitfield J, Bonafini C, Chakravarthy B, Armato U, Dal Prà I. Amyloid-β[25-35], an amyloid-β[1-42] surrogate, and proinflammatory cytokines stimulate VEGF-A secretion by cultured, early passage, normoxic adult human cerebral astrocytes. Journal of Alzheimer's Disease. 2010;**21**:915-926. DOI: 10.3233/JAD-2010-100471

[71] Chiarini A, Armato U, Liu D, Dal Prà I. Calcium-sensing receptor antagonist NPS 2143 restores amyloid precursor protein physiological non-Amyloidogenic processing in Aβ-exposed adult human astrocytes. Scientific Reports. 2017;**7**:1277. DOI: 10.1038/s41598-017-01215-3

[72] Ferry S, Traiffort E, Stinnakre J, Ruat M. Developmental and adult expression of rat calcium-sensing receptor transcripts in neurons and oligodendrocytes. The European Journal of Neuroscience. 2000;**12**:872-884

[73] Chiarini A, Dal Prà I, Gottardo R, Bortolotti F, Whitfield JF, Armato U. BH[4] [tetrahydrobiopterin]-dependent activation, but not the expression, of inducible NOS [nitric oxide synthase]-2 in proinflammatory cytokine-stimulated, cultured normal human astrocytes is mediated by MEK-ERK kinases. Journal of Cellular Biochemistry. 2005;**94**:731-743

[74] Chiarini A, Armato U, Pacchiana R, Dal Pra I. Proteomic analysis of GTP cyclohydrolase 1 multiprotein complexes in cultured normal adult human astrocytes under both basal and cytokine-activated conditions. Proteomics. 2009;**9**:1850-1860. DOI: 10.1002/pmic.200800561

[75] Sanchez A, Tripathy D, Luo J, Yin X, Martinez J, Grammas P. Neurovascular unit and the effects of dosage in VEGF toxicity: Role for oxidative stress and thrombin. Journal of Alzheimer's Disease. 2013;**34**:281-291. DOI: 10.3233/JAD-121636

[76] Ruhrberg C, Bautch VL. Neurovascular development and links to disease. Cellular and Molecular Life Sciences. 2013;**70**:1675-1684. DOI: 10.1007/s00018-013-1277-5

[77] Carmeliet P, Ruiz de Almodovar CVEGF. Ligands and receptors: Implications in neurodevelopment and neurodegeneration. Cellular and Molecular Life Sciences. 2013;**70**:1763-1778. DOI: 10.1007/s00018-013-1283-7. Erratum in: Cell Mol Life Sci. 2013;**70**:2221. Carmen, Ruiz de Almodovar [corrected to Ruiz de Almodovar, Carmen].

[78] Tang H, Mao X, Xie L, Greenberg DA, Jin K. Expression level of vascular endothelial growth factor in hippocampus is associated with cognitive impairment in patients with Alzheimer's disease. Neurobiology of Aging. 2013;**34**:1412-1415. DOI: 10.1016/j.neurobiolaging.2012.10.029

[79] Chiarini A, Armato U, Whitfield JF, Dal Prà I. Targeting human astrocytes' calcium-sensing receptors for treatment of Alzheimer's disease. Current Pharmaceutical Design. 2017 Jul 10. DOI: 10.2174/1381612823666170710162509

[80] Dickerson BC, Salat DH, Greve DN, Chua EF, Rand-Giovannetti E, Rentz DM, Bertram L, Mullin K, Tanzi RE, Blacker D, Albert MS, Sperling RA. Increased hippocampal activation in mild cognitive impairment compared to normal aging and AD. Neurology. 2005;**65**:404-411

[81] Yassa MA, Stark SM, Bakker A, Albert MS, Gallagher M, Stark CE. High-resolution structural and functional MRI of hippocampal CA3 and dentate gyrus in patients with amnestic mild cognitive impairment. NeuroImage. 2010;**51**:1242-1252. DOI: 10.1016/j.neuroimage.2010.03.040

[82] Yassa MA. Ground zero in Alzheimer's disease. Nature Neuroscience. 2014;**17**:146-147. DOI: 10.1038/nn.3631

[83] Chiarini A, Armato U, Gardenal E, Gui L, Dal Prà I. Amyloid β-exposed human astrocytes overproduce phospho-tau and overrelease it within exosomes, effects suppressed by calcilytic NPS 2143-further implications for Alzheimer's therapy. Frontiers in Neuroscience. 2017;**11**:217. DOI: 10.3389/fnins.2017.00217. eCollection 2017

[84] Buée L, Bussière T, Buée-Scherrer V, Delacourte A, Hof PR. Tau protein isoforms, phosphorylation and role in neurodegenerative disorders. Brain Research. Brain Research Reviews. 2000;**33**:95-130

[85] Schraen-Maschke S, Sergeant N, Dhaenens CM, Bombois S, Deramecourt V, Caillet-Boudin ML, Pasquier F, Maurage CA, Sablonnière B, Vanmechelen E, Buée L. Tau as a biomarker of neurodegenerative diseases. Biomarkers in Medicine. 2008;**2**:363-384. DOI: 10.2217/17520363.2.4.363

[86] Rajendran L, Bali J, Barr MM, Court FA, Krämer-Albers EM, Picou F, Raposo G, van der Vos KE, van Niel G, Wang J, Breakefield XO. Emerging roles of extracellular vesicles in the nervous system. The Journal of Neuroscience. 2014;**34**:15482-11549. DOI: 10.1523/JNEUROSCI.3258-14.2014

[87] Nemeth EF. Pharmacological regulation of parathyroid hormone secretion. Current Pharmaceutical Design. 2002;**8**:2077-2087

[88] Nemeth EF. The search for calcium receptor antagonists [calcilytics]. Journal of Molecular Endocrinology. 2002;**29**:15-21

Chapter 7

Mitochondrial Function in Alzheimer's Disease: Focus on Astrocytes

Riikka Lampinen, Irina Belaya, Isabella Boccuni,
Tarja Malm and Katja M. Kanninen

Additional information is available at the end of the chapter

http://dx.doi.org/10.5772/intechopen.71825

Abstract

The brain is one of the most energy-requiring organs in the human body. Mitochondria not only generate this energy, but are centrally involved critical cellular functions including maintenance of calcium homeostasis, synthesis of biomolecules, and cell signaling. Even though neurons and astrocytes preferentially use different energy substrates and metabolic pathways, these two cell types are intricately linked in their energy metabolism. Recently it has become clear that astrocytes have a key role in the regulation and support of the neuronal mitochondrial quality control, yet several questions remain unanswered to fully understand the mechanisms of mitochondrial function, transport, turnover and degradation in astrocytes. Alzheimer's disease is the most common neurodegenerative disorder, the exact mechanisms of which remain incompletely understood. The fact that astrocytic mitochondrial dysfunction is an early event in the pathogenesis of Alzheimer's disease suggests that more research on mitochondrial function and impairment is required in the hopes of disease alleviation in the future.

Keywords: mitophagy, energy metabolism, brain, neurodegeneration, mitochondrial quality control

1. Introduction

This chapter summarizes the importance of proper mitochondrial functioning in the central nervous system, with a special focus on astrocytic mitochondria and their quality control. Mitochondrial function is next discussed in the context of Alzheimer's disease (AD), before finally casting a look at potential future therapeutic approaches to modulate these events in astrocytes.

2. Energy metabolism in the brain

The brain is one of the most energy-requiring organs in the human body, yet it contains relatively few energy reserves. The daily energy consumption of the brain is 20 times higher than that of skeletal muscle [1]. Related to its mass, the brain utilizes a large proportion of all the oxygen and glucose available in the body. Despite the fact that the mass of the human brain corresponds only to 2% of the total body weight, the brain utilizes around 20% of the all energy received from glucose [2]. In mammals, glucose is considered to be the main energy source for the brain and especially for the neuronal cells with a high-energy demand, it is converted to adenosine triphosphate (ATP) in the cell's mitochondria [2]. In neurons, the requirement for energy is highest in the synaptic regions where the signal transmission between two neurons takes place [3].

The brain is fuelled mainly by blood-derived glucose, but during some conditions, such as starvation or physical activity, ketone and lactate from blood flow are also used for energy [4, 5]. Glucose and lactate enter the brain through specific glucose transporters (GLUTs) and monocarboxylate transporter (MCTs) for further metabolic processing. There are three main glucose metabolic pathways: aerobic and anaerobic glycolysis (generates pyruvate and lactate, respectively), pentose phosphate pathway (generates NADPH and pentose), and glycogenesis (generates glycogen) [6, 7].

Neurons are highly energy demanding in comparison to other brain cell types [8]. Even though neurons and astrocytes preferentially use different energy substrates and metabolic pathways, these two cell types are intricately linked in their energy metabolism. Astrocytes are responsible for energy production, storage and delivery in the brain, and are considered as the main energy supplier for neurons [7]. For example, astrocyte-derived lactate has been shown to play a crucial role in long-term memory formation and neuronal activity control [6, 9]. Astrocytes are critical for brain energy cooperation and in addition to carrying out metabolic pathways such as aerobic glycolysis and glycogenesis, they release lactate and regulate glutamate homeostasis [7, 8].

Astrocytes uptake glucose from capillaries through GLUT1 transporters. Through glycolysis glucose is converted to pyruvate and then to lactate, which is released into the extracellular space [10]. Astrocytes are the main cellular reservoir of lactate, which is mainly produced from glycogen [9, 11, 12]. Through the so-called astrocyte–neuron lactate shuttle, lactate enters neuronal cells from the extracellular space through MCTs to be used in the tricarboxylic acid (TCA) cycle for generation of ATP – the major player in intracellular energy transfer [10]. Despite the fact that astrocytes and neurons both consume glucose and lactate, these two types of cells have very different metabolic profiles. Under normal physiological conditions astrocytes take up more than 80% of glucose, whereas neurons utilize limited amounts of glucose [7]. Astrocytes also have a higher glycolysis rate than neurons [6]. The specific activity of 6-phosphofructo-1-kinase (PFK1), a master regulator of glycolysis, is fourfold higher in astrocytes than in neurons [13].

Glutamate, most well known for being the main excitatory neurotransmitter in the brain, is also a key player in energy metabolism. Astrocytes take up glutamate from the synaptic cleft via glutamate transporters, and either transform it into glutamine, or utilize it in the TCA cycle [10]. Interestingly, glutamate uptake also increases glucose utilization and promotes astrocytic lactate production to provide energy sources for neurons [5, 14, 15].

3. Mitochondrial function in the brain

In the human body the fatty acids and carbohydrates acquired from the diet form a base material for a chain of oxidative reactions where the energy is stored in small energy rich molecules such as ATP. Mitochondria are called the small powerhouses of the cell, which in oxidative conditions take the major responsibility for ATP production. Based on an endosymbiosis theory, the mitochondria originate from an aerobic proteobacteria engulfed by a prokaryotic cell. Nowadays they are important organelles of the eukaryotic cell, with various tasks critical for cellular health and well-being [16].

In addition to being the key organelles for energy production, mitochondria also take care of other critical cellular functions including maintenance of calcium homeostasis, synthesis of biomolecules, and cell signaling [17]. Related to calcium homeostasis, the mitochondria function as Ca^{2+} storage reservoirs in cells. Calcium is an important signaling molecule, the release of which from the mitochondria to the cytosol is tightly controlled [18]. Depolarization of the mitochondrial membrane potential releases Ca^{2+} to the cytosol, which can induce cell apoptosis [19]. Induction of apoptosis leads to cytochrome c release, which activates pro-apoptotic caspases when released to cell cytoplasm from the inner membrane of the mitochondria.

In comparison to astrocytes, neurons express or have less active enzymes for protection against oxidative stress [20]. Because of this, neurons are dependent on the nearby astrocytes in their strategies to cope with reactive oxygen species (ROS). The ROS have in tightly controlled amounts an important function as signaling molecules in the cell. However, in situations of uncontrolled high concentrations of ROS, the cell may face a harmful cascade leading to disruption of cell structures, apoptosis and senescence. In the brain the ROS can originate from either exogenous or endogenous sources. Exogenous sources for ROS include for example ultraviolet (UV) radiation and toxins, chemicals or drugs that produce ROS as their by-products in the body [21]. Importantly, mitochondria are considered as a significant endogenous source for ROS [22, 23]. It has also been reported that exogenous ROS may also induce the release of endogenous ROS from the mitochondria [24]. In summary, mitochondrial ROS are important signaling molecules, controlling the balance of which is important to limit the harmful effects of ROS overload in the brain.

In addition to their various important roles, mitochondria have also been reported to affect cognitive function and memory in the brain. Recently it was observed that the amount and morphology of the presynaptic mitochondria in specific brain regions affects memory and synaptic health in non-human primates [25]. The study shows that estrogen treatment, which has been considered to enhance working memory, prevents working memory impairment in aged ovariectomized monkeys. The monkeys treated with cyclic estradiol had a higher number in total and less morphologically malformed donut-shaped mitochondria in their presynaptic regions compared to controls. This observation sets as of yet unanswered questions of even wider functions of mitochondria in the mammalian brain.

4. Mitochondrial function in astrocytes

According to recent calculations, the human brain is estimated to contain glial cells and neurons in a ratio of 1:1 [26]. The major glial cells are classified as oligodendrocytes, microglia and astrocytes. The astrocytes play a central role in maintaining of CNS homeostasis, expression of neurotransmitters and neuroprotection [27]. The astrocytes co-operate closely with the neurons, being critical components of important processes such as synapse formation, maintenance of synaptic plasticity, maintenance of blood brain barrier integrity and removal of excessive neurotransmitters from the synaptic cleft [28]. The morphology of astrocytes is ideal for their various functions. Each astrocyte has its own territory in the brain, with minimal overlapping with other cells [29]. The astrocytes can communicate with neurons and reach the synaptic regions with their fine shaped processes, and reach the brain vasculature with larger protrusions (endfeet). Notably, the astrocytic endfeet is potent at regulating the cerebral blood flow [30].

Mitochondrial dynamics of astrocytes is less studied than that of neurons. Enzymes metabolizing glycogen are highly expressed in astrocytes and thus astrocytes in the human brain are usually considered more glycolytic in their energy metabolism compared to highly oxygen dependent neurons. However, besides glycolytic metabolism, there is also evidence of a strong aerobic metabolism in astrocytes [31]. Glycolysis in astrocytes is directly linked to the energy metabolism in neurons via the astrocyte–neuron lactate shuttle. There the lactate, produced in astrocytes, can be transferred to neurons as a supplement for their TCA cycle in mitochondria [32]. Therefore, neurons and astrocytes are intricately linked in their energy metabolism, and in mitochondrial function.

Following signal transmission between two neurons, astrocytes surrounding the synapse clear the neurotransmitter glutamate from the synaptic cleft via specific glutamate transporters expressed in their cell membrane. The glutamate taken up by astrocytes is then converted either to glutamine and released back to neurons, or used as fuel in the TCA cycle in the mitochondria in the form of α-ketoglutarate. The enzymes required for this glutamate metabolism are expressed in astrocytes at high levels [31]. The neuronal activity and following glutamate uptake by astrocytes has also been reported to affect mitochondrial movement inside the astrocytes. The astrocytes are endowed with the ability to pause or move mitochondria in cell compartments with highest activity [33, 34].

5. Mitochondrial quality control

Due to the significance of mitochondria to the well-being of cells, the mitochondrial quality is hierarchically regulated and controlled, aiming to maintain a healthy population of mitochondria. The quality control system regulates mitochondrial biogenesis, dynamics, and degradation, and through influencing mitochondrial health, has major potential to improve health and lifespan [17]. In order to maintain this population of fully functional and morphologically optimally shaped mitochondria, the mitochondria constantly take part in a cycle of fusion and fission events [35]. However, the cell also requires another strategy to degrade severely damaged or surplus mitochondria. Due to the fact that compromised mitochondria release potentially harmful substances such as cytochrome c and calcium [36], it is very important that defective mitochondria are eliminated quickly and efficiently. Efficient degradation of damaged mitochondria is particularly important for neurons because their survival and activity depends on mitochondrial homeostasis [37, 38]. In general, macroautophagy is a process through which organelles and cytosolic components are engulfed in membrane-bound vesicles and degraded upon fusion with lysosomes. It serves housekeeping function essential for homeostasis and survival of the cells. The specific process through which severely damaged or surplus mitochondria are degraded through an autophagic process is called mitophagy [39, 40]. Mitophagy is a crucial mechanism for mitochondrial quality control [41]. The fact that the majority of mature lysosomes are concentrated close to the cell soma [42] brings yet another challenge for neuronal mitophagy: axonal transport of damaged mitochondria to the soma takes time although rapid degradation is required to prevent the release of toxic substances.

Until very recently, it was presumed that each cell in the central nervous system degrades its own cell organelles. This notion was revoked by a study showing that the majority of neuronal mitochondria in axons are internalized and degraded by adjacent astrocytes with high phagocytic activity under normal physiological conditions in vivo [43]. This process of transcellular mitochondrial degradation is known as transmitophagy (TM). Using a tandem fluorophore protein reporter of acidified mitochondria, the study showed that acidified axonal mitochondria are associated with astrocytic lysosomes in the optic nerve head. After this phenomenon was found there have emerged also other studies stating that the transfer of mitochondria between neurons and astrocytes occurs the other way around as well. For example, astrocytic mitochondria transferred in extracellular particles have been shown to be functional in neurons. The transfer of mitochondria is suggested to be mediated via CD38 signaling, an important enzyme for calcium signaling in the cell [44]. However, it should be noted that the results presented by Hayakawa et al. [44] have also received commentaries about proof of the actual internalization and functionality of the astrocytic mitochondria in neurons [45].

Previous studies show that the fine astrocytic processes contacting the synaptic regions contain plenty of mitochondria [31]. In addition, the mitochondria in astrocytic fine processes are smaller in size and less elongated than those located in the major branches around the cell soma [46]. These results awake further interest of whether TM or the transfer of mitochondria between brain cells are universal phenomena critical for the proper functioning of mitochondria in the healthy and diseased brain.

6. Astrocytes in Alzheimer's disease

AD causes an enormous socio-economic burden on societies as it impacts millions of people. It is the most common chronic neurodegenerative disorder that is associated with cognitive decline and progressive memory loss [47]. AD pathology is characterized by accumulation of misfolded amyloid beta (Aβ) proteins in extracellular amyloid plaques, deposition of modified tau proteins in intraneural neurofibrillary tangles, and sustained neuroinflammation and oxidative stress [48]. There are two types of AD: familial (FAD) and sporadic. Familial AD affects a small minority of patients and is associated with mutations in genes encoding amyloid precursor protein (APP) or the presenilins (PSEN1 and PSEN2) [49, 50]. Approximately 95% cases of AD are sporadic and are associated with age-related increase in free-radical production, oxidative stress, impaired mitochondrial energy metabolism and mitochondrial dysfunction [51]. There is a great deal of research that has contributed to our understanding of the etiological and pathological features of AD, but the cause and underlying mechanisms of this disease remains incompletely understood. Because of this, there is no effective cure for AD.

To study AD mechanisms and test new therapeutic approaches preclinically, a large number of animal models have been developed. For example, in the non-transgenic AD model, Aβ or tau proteins are injected into the rodent brain. In transgenic AD animals, single or multiple mutations in genes associated with AD (such as APP, PSEN1/2, tau) are introduced to model familial AD. Transgenic AD models can be divided into two different groups depending on plaque deposition – early plaque AD models such as APPswePS1dE9, 3xTG-AD, 5xFAD, and late plaque AD models such as TG2576, PDAPP-J20 [52]. In addition to rodent models, recent advances in stem cell technologies have promoted the use of human-based cell models for AD research. For example, it is now possible to model AD in vitro by using induced pluripotent stem cells (iPSCs) and cells derived from these by differentiation [53–55].

A full understanding of the importance of astrocytes in AD has become evident only recently. For a long time it has been known that astrocytes have numerous functions that act at maintaining of CNS homeostasis and the blood brain barrier, expression of neurotransmitters and neuroprotection, supplying neurons with energy and antioxidants [27, 28]. Even though Alois Alzheimer first observed pathological astrocyte modifications in the AD brain over a century ago [56], it is only now becoming clear that the dysfunction of astrocytes is an essential and even early component of many neurodegenerative diseases, including AD [27, 57].

Researchers have utilized several AD animal models for studying astrocyte alterations associated with AD. For example, in the 5xFAD mouse model, expressing five FAD mutations in genes encoding APP and PSEN1 [58], impairment in energy metabolism and activation status in neonatal astrocytes of transgenic mice was very recently discovered [59]. In addition, an impairment in Aβ uptake and neuronal support was demonstrated in old 5xFAD astrocytes [60]. In another mouse model of AD, the 3xTG-AD mice (with three FAD mutations in genes encoding APP, PSEN1 and tau) atrophy of astrocytes was described to start early, at the age of 3 months [61, 62]. The double transgenic APPswePS1dE9 AD mouse model has revealed a decline in normal functioning of old astrocytes leading to diminution of neuronal support [63]. At the same time, astrocytic pathology associated with AD is also found in late plaque AD models. In [64] authors shown the involvement of astrocytes in the degradation of amyloid plaques and autophagic processes in PDAPP-J20 mouse model of AD. In contrast, results in the TG2576 mouse model demonstrated that reactive astrocytes become Aβ producers through expression of BACE1, which catalyzes the first step in the formation of the Aβ peptide from APP [65].

It is important to note that rodent astrocytes are different from human astrocytes. For example, human astrocytes are larger and more complex in morphology and they have faster calcium responses and more robust responses to glutamate [66]. Very recently, AD-associated astrocyte dysfunction has also been described in human iPSC-derived cell models. Using this model, atrophy of astrocytes and abnormal expression of astrocytic markers were demonstrated in iPSC-derived astrocytes from patients with familial and sporadic forms of AD [54]. We have also shown that iPSC-derived AD astrocytes are compromised in neuronal supportive function, and display increased β-amyloid production and oxidative stress, altered cytokine release, and dysregulated $Ca2+$ homeostasis [67]. In addition to cellular models, human post-mortem brain from AD patients also can be used for the study astrocytic pathology at the disease end stage. In recent studies, astrocytic atrophy also was found in FAD human post-mortem brain [57].

Recently it has become realized that there are two types of reactive astrocytes: A1 astrocytes, which are harmful and induced by neuroinflammation, and A2 astrocytes, which are helpful and induced by acute brain injury [68, 69]. The A2 astrocytes have a protective role and promoting neuronal survival, whereas A1 astrocytes are destructive for neurons and have neurotoxic properties [70]. In human AD, harmful A1 astrocytes constitute the majority of all astrocytes in CNS and can play a crucial role in induction and progression of AD [70].

Astrocyte dysfunction, so called "reactive astrogliosis," is associated with all neurodegenerative diseases including AD, and characterized with various complex molecular and functional changes in the cells [71]. Both in the human and in rodent AD brain, reactive astrocytes are characterized by hypertrophy and overexpression of intermediate filaments like glial fibrillary acidic protein (GFAP) [69, 72]. Alterations in astrocytes lead to changes in synaptic activity and neuronal survival [73]. It is interesting to note that in the CA1 subfields of the hippocampus, reactive astrocytes, proximal to Aβ plaques, have significantly higher GFAP expression than astrocytes distal to amyloid plaques [62, 71]. Moreover, these distal astrocytes display atrophy [62], which is thought to occur before plaque formation, suggesting that astrocytes may be associated with early changes occurring during the development of AD [32].

AD astrocytes are also characterized by a number of molecular alterations. Dysregulation in the release of chemical neurotransmitters including glutamate, D-serine, GABA, as well as calcium in astrocytes leads to a disturbance in the normal communication between neurons and astrocytes and eventually impairs synaptic plasticity [32, 71]. Moreover, the majority of hippocampal astrocytes (86%) in the AD brain express heme oxygenase (HO-1), while normal astrocytes almost do not express HO-1 at all (6–7%). This is indicative of oxidative stress occurring in the astrocytes during AD [74].

In the AD brain, reactive astrogliosis is associated with a reduction of normal astrocyte glycolytic activity in response to Aβ [75]. As mentioned above, astrocytic glycolysis has a central role in supplying neurons with lactate, which is crucial for long-term memory formation [6, 9, 76]. Reduction of lactate released from astrocytes has been demonstrated in arctic Aβ mice [77]. Moreover, correlation of memory impairment with reduced level of hippocampal lactate has been reported to occur in response to Aβ in rats [78].

7. Impaired mitochondrial function in Alzheimer's disease: focus on astrocytes

In the last years, research on neurodegenerative diseases has begun to change its focus from neurons to the neighboring supportive cells. For example, it is now known that astrocytes have a key role in the regulation and support of the neuronal mitochondrial quality control [79, 80]. Furthermore, recent studies in the AD field have shifted attention from the "amyloid hypothesis" to the "neuroenergetic hypothesis" [81], thereby focusing on the importance of the cellular bioenergetic interplay in disease conditions. In this part of the chapter we summarize what is thus far known about the impairment of astrocytic mitochondria in AD.

Impairments in mitochondria of brain cells lead to cerebral hypometabolism - specifically neurons are very sensitive to alterations in basal energy levels since they need a fine energetic homeostasis to employee their function (**Figure 1**). As the mitochondria are the principal source of ATP as well as of ROS, they retain a critical role at the centre of a complex web of processes leading to cellular and organismal aging and neurodegeneration [82]. Studies on mitochondrial function specifically in astrocytes have shed some light on the pathological features of AD. Already almoust 10 years ago Kaminsky and Kosenko [83] investigated the effects of Aβ peptides on mitochondrial and non-mitochondrial sources of ROS and antioxidant enzymes in rat brain in vivo: the authors demonstrated that the continuous infusion of Aβ for up to 14 days stimulated the generation of hydrogen peroxide in isolated neocortical mitochondria through an alteration of the antioxidant enzymes activity. Abramov et al. [84] demonstrated that Aβ peptides induce a loss of mitochondrial potential ($\Delta\psi m$) in astrocytes but not in neurons, with a remarkable augmentation of intracellular calcium concentrations [85]. Calcium overload is considered the main biochemical feature of Aβ excitotoxic stress and it causes free radical accumulation in neurons and the formation of the mitochondrial permeability transition pore (mPTP) [86]. The formation of the

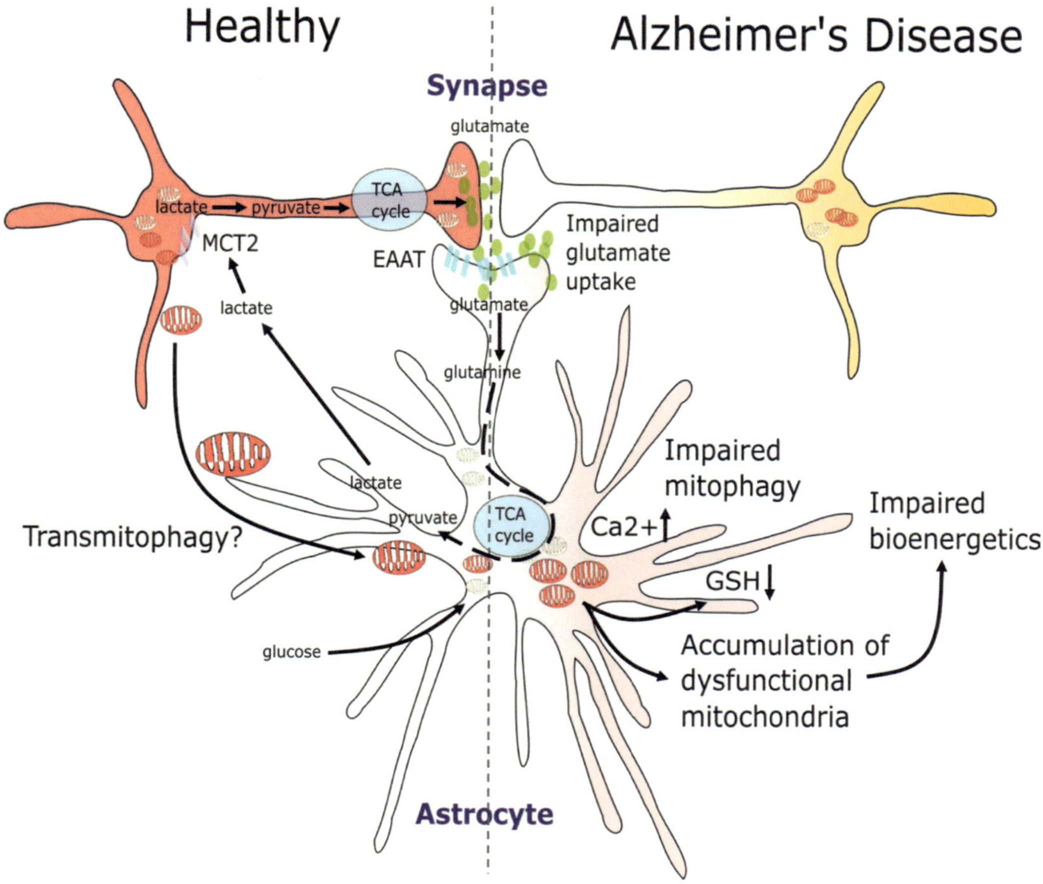

Figure 1. Alzheimer's disease pathology alters astrocytic neurosupportive functions.

mPTP leads to a phenomenon known as mitochondrial swelling, which occurs along with several mitochondrial perturbations described in "the mitochondrial cascade hypothesis in AD" [87]. Mitochondrial impairment precedes AD-associated synaptic damage, neuronal cell death and deficits in learning and memory [88]. Importantly, mitochondrial dysfunction is a key cellular feature of both sporadic and genetic AD and observed also in apolipoprotein E-4 (ApoE4) carriers [89]. This suggests that mitochondrial dysfunction is a key pathological feature of AD [90].

The central nervous system presents a high rate of production of oxidative molecules and relative low levels of antioxidant agents. It is particularly sensitive to oxidative damage because of the high consumption of oxygen, the presence of membrane polyunsaturated fatty acids susceptible to free radical attack, and the low ratio between ROS and antioxidant enzymes [91]. Astrocytes support neurons in the fight against oxidative damage by production of glutathione (GSH), the main antioxidant of the brain. Already some 25 years ago it was reported that impairment of astrocytic antioxidant systems causes neuronal death: Sagara et al. [92] demonstrated that there is a relationship between the GSH decline in neurons exposed to Aβ1-42 neurotoxic peptide and the concomitant decrease of GSH levels and the increase of intracellular calcium influx in astrocytes. The reduction of GSH and the increase of oxidation of proteins related to energy metabolism could be a consequence of the altered regulation of the transcription factors controlling nuclear and mitochondrial oxidative phosphorylation (OXPHOS) genes in brain cells. Reduced levels of nuclear respiratory factor 2 (NRF2), peroxisome proliferator-activated receptor γ coactivator-1α (PGC-1α) and mitochondrial transcription factor A (TFAM) are reported in hippocampal tissues from AD brain [93]. These transcription factors regulate the mitochondrial quality control system through mitochondrial biogenesis, the fission-fusion cycle of mitochondria and mitophagy.

A defective mitochondrial dynamic induces a structural change of the organelles. Baloyannis [94] described morphological alterations of the mitochondrial cristae, accumulation of osmiophilic material, and decrease of mitochondrial size to be associated with AD. The quantification of mitochondrial DNA (mtDNA) revealed low levels in AD subjects in the cortical and hippocampal areas [95, 96], which may reflect a diminished number and mass of mitochondria in AD. However, a complex picture was presented by [97], where the authors demonstrated that by measuring the mtDNA present in phagosomes together with the mtDNA in healthy mitochondria the quantification resulted in higher levels in AD subjects than in controls. The observation of an augmented number of unhealthy mitochondria in AD is corroborated by a study showing an increased number of fragmented mitochondria in Aβ stimulated astrocytes [98]. In addition to having effects on mitochondrial fragmentation, Aβ results in increased glycolysis, augmented ATP levels and the maintenance of the mitochondrial potential ($\Delta\psi$m) in exposed astrocytes [99].

Mitochondrial trafficking through the astrocytes and the localization of these organelles along the fine processes (<600 nm of diameter) of reactive astrocytes may be disrupted due to loss of genes implicated in neurodegenerative diseases. For example, PARK-2 mutations may alter the Parkin-mediated turnover of Mitochondrial Rho GTPase 1 (Miro1), a key regulator of mitochondrial trafficking. Miro1 is required to tether kinesin motor protein complexes to the outer mitochondrial membrane (OMM) and modulate the fission-fusion ratio, mitophagy and mitochondria-endoplasmic reticulum interaction [100]. Alterations to the trafficking of astrocyte mitochondria could disrupt the supportive functions of astrocytes. For example, it is well-known that astrocytes deplete the glutamate present in the synaptic left through glutamate transporters, and this is fundamental for the functionality of neurotransmission [101]. Loss of astrocyte mitochondrial function is related to the inability of astrocytes to convert glutamate to glutamine and is known to precede neuronal glutamate excitotoxicity [102]. Genda et al. [103] demonstrated the co-localization of the glutamate transporter GLT-1 with the sites of high neuronal transmission activity in hippocampal sections: furthermore, the authors observed the co-compartmentalization of mitochondria in the areas of higher concentration of glutamate transporter GLT-1. Mitochondria are not-uniformly distributed along the astrocytes but they are an important source of energy in the contact areas with neurons to contribute to neuroprotective function against toxic insults. The mitochondria of astrocytes thereby play a direct role in glutamate-mediated synapsis homeostasis and in the hippocampal neuronal transmission: the organelles provide the ATP for the glutamate-glutamine shuttle to supply the energy demand in situ.

Very recently it was shown that human AD astrocytes have an altered display of mitochondrial encoding genes when compared to healthy controls [104]. The authors performed total RNA sequencing of the astrocytes to shed light on the molecular differences caused by the disease. PITRM1/PREP/MP1, localized in mitochondrial matrix and encoding an enzyme that degrades the Aβ peptide, was shown to be downregulated in AD. NDUFA4L2, encoding a protein that inhibits Complex I activity, was upregulated in AD astrocytes. In addition, MTND1P22, most likely a long non-coding RNA involved in the regulation of NADH dehydrogenase 1, was also altered in the AD astrocytes. This evidence pointing to the importance of mitochondria specifically in AD astrocytes is supported by further studies on the effect of Aβ on the functions of astrocyte mitochondria. Aβ induces ATP synthase uncoupling in astrocytes [105], increased β-amyloid/APP lead to reduced expression of superoxide dismutase and results in increased age-related oxidative stress in astrocytes [106], and Aβ/APP localizes on the mitochondrial inner membrane of astrocytes and disrupts Complex IV (COX) activity and APP processing by β-secretase [107]. Taken together, these studies support the evidence that exogenous Aβ treatment is sufficient to induce mitochondria-mediated apoptosis and that a dysfunction in astrocytic mitochondrial quality control is a key part of the pathophysiology associated with AD.

Astrocytes are an essential source of energy for neurons by providing the neurons lactate. Astrocytes also participate in the clearance of glutamate from the synaptic cleft, take up neuronal mitochondria and are an important source of antioxidant enzymes, such as GSH. In AD, these normal astrocytic functions are altered leading to increases in astrocytic intracellular calcium, reductions in the levels of GSH and mitochondrial dysfunction. The normal intracellular degradation pathway for non-functional mitochondria, mitophagy, is impaired, leading to accumulation of non-functional mitochondria. In summary, these events lead to impaired astrocytic bioenergetics and impaired glutamate uptake from the synaptic cleft, greatly influencing neuronal health and contributing to the pathology progression.

8. Therapeutic approaches targeted to modulation of mitochondrial function in Alzheimer's disease

There are a huge number of therapeutic approaches that have been trialed in AD, yet the only approved treatments only delay the inevitable and no cure for this devastating disorder exists. A critical difficulty in neurodegenerative disorders such as AD is the relative late onset of the symptoms united to a progressive degeneration, and late disease diagnosis.

At the time of diagnosis, neuronal impairment is often too far for effective intervention. Furthermore, the anatomical site affected in these disorders is often difficult to access by potential therapies.

Pharmaceutical companies have invested heavily in a variety of potential therapies to modulate AD: the well-known memantine, reducing the glutamate excitotoxicity, is considered one of the best available therapeutics for AD but still the possible long-term side effects are unknown [108]. In order for new approaches for a future therapeutic to be effective it is believed that early and better diagnosis methods are needed in order to prevent AD progression [109]. Mitochondria-targeting therapies are a novel approach that have potential to be used in the early onset of cognitive impairment. Mitochondrial oxidative damage is considered an early event of the disease process, which becomes more pronounced as AD progresses [110]. Mitochondrial dysfunction precedes Aβ plaque deposition [111] and is accompanied by a progressive reduction of the cerebral metabolic rates of glucose. Thus, several new therapeutic approaches have tested the efficacy of mitochondria-targeted molecules in delaying AD progression. For example, around ten clinical trials demonstrate that modulation of mitochondrial function rescue neuronal death and synaptic toxicity caused by Aβ exposure [112].

Mitochondrial medicine includes both life style intervention and pharmacological approaches. The Mediterranean diet [113], exercise [114] and caloric restriction [115, 116] have been shown to modulate AD risk factors including the mitochondrial healthy homeostasis. In combination with these, several preventive approaches have been studied in AD patients, for example the antioxidant N-acetyl cysteine (NAC) [117], α-lipoic acid (LA) [118] and curcumin [119] have been tested. Some clinical studies in particular demonstrate that NAC reduces brain oxidative stress through increasing GSH-mediated protective activity against Aβ deposits and lipid peroxidation, and decreasing acetylcholine levels and choline acetyltransferase (ChAT) activity [120]. In addition, several clinical trials used well-known molecules to limit oxidative damage: vitamin E (α-tocopherol) rescues cognitive impairment and oxidative stress in early phase of AD in pre-clinical studies [121] even though there are controversial results in clinical trials in human AD subjects [122]; Donepezil enhances the mitochondrial resistance by inhibiting the mitochondrial permeability transition pore (mPTP) in a mouse model of AD [123]. Other pre-clinical studies demonstrating potent mitochondrial effects have not yet been assessed in clinical trials but show great promise. For example, conjugated Coenzyme Q with a lipophilic triphenylphosphonium (TPP^+) form MitoQ that protect primary cortical neurons from Aβ toxicity, loss of mitochondrial membrane potential and ROS production [124]; Szeto-Shiller antioxidant peptides allow the localization of antioxidant molecules in the mitochondrial matrix, the major source of ROS, and in particular SS31 shows a neuroprotective effect [125, 126]. Furthermore, endogenous compounds such as peroxiredoxine (Prdx) [127] and the natural molecules such as alkaloid caffeine [128], polyphenol resveratrol [129] and gypenoside XVII (GP-17) [130] have been used to modulate the bioenergetic homeostasis at different levels in AD mouse models. The antioxidant approach may have wide applications; however, it could also present some controversial effects on mitochondrial adaptation. For example, mitohormesis, an adaptive response that improves overall oxidative stress resistance induced by caloric restriction and exercise, may be inhibited by antioxidants [131].

The hypothesis that impaired mitophagy in both neurons and astrocytes may lead to AD neurodegeneration and the potential of the mitophagy process as a therapeutic target needs further clarification. Pre-clinical studies introduce novel therapeutic molecules such as p62-mediated mitophagy inducer (PMI) and Mitochondrial division inhibitor 1 (Midvi-1) for this purpose. PMI is a recently described compound developed to upregulate p62 via stabilization of the transcription factor Nrf2 and to promote mitophagy [132]. This molecule has not yet been tested against neurodegeneration. Midvi-1 is a small molecule non-competitive inhibitor of dynamin-related protein 1 (Drp1) GTPase activity, which attenuates Drp1 mediated mitochondrial-fission and enhances the mitochondrial rescue through inactivation of PINK1 [133]. Recently, Manczak et al. [134] proposed a Drp1 based therapy in the context of AD: the authors demonstrated that the interaction of Drp1 with Aβ increases as AD progresses and that a partial reduction of Drp1 reduces Aβ deposition, reduces mitochondrial dysfunction and enhances mitochondrial biogenesis.

It is noteworthy that most of the therapies for AD applied target neurons as the main cell type involved in neurodegeneration. Given that several therapeutic approaches have been attempted that do not completely rescue AD progression suggests that we should once more consider the cellular target against which we focus. A step towards the right direction has been taken by the scientific community in beginning to consider microglia as a therapeutic target for neurodegeneration because of their involvement in neuroinflammation. For example, the synthetic compound Midvi-1 attenuates mitochondrial-induced apoptosis in primary microglial cells in an Aβ-induced model of AD, thereby counteracting the neuroinflammation [135], and the endogenous compound melatonin has a protective role against cognitive decline and restores mitochondrial respiratory rate in microglial cells of the APPsw mouse model of AD [136].

The increasingly evident key role of astrocytes in supporting neurons against neurodegeneration suggests that probing the unexplored field of mitochondrial-targeted therapies in astrocytes is needed. Currently, there is no relevant literature about astrocyte-targeted therapies, possibly because they are thought to be more involved in the late phases of AD progression. However, modulating early changes in these cells might prove to be more beneficial than targeting downstream pathways.

9. Future aspects

Several questions remain unanswered to fully understand the mechanisms of mitochondrial function, transport, turnover and degradation in astrocytes. Given the complexity of astrocyte sub-populations and region-specific phenotypes [137] several experimental approaches and models are needed to study mitochondrial function and possible impairment in these cells.

It is important to note that very little literature exists about AD-associated mitochondrial dysfunction specifically in astrocytes, although recent reports have highlighted the importance of this cell type in neurodegeneration. In the future, it will be critically important to carry out more studies that focus on alterations of astrocytic mitochondria in AD because of the arising role of these cells in the early onset of this disease. Furthermore, the utilization of human models in AD research is expected to provide valuable tools and detailed mechanistic insight into the role of astrocytes that is central in understanding the features of this devastating human disease.

As research steers towards an in depth understanding of the molecular basis of mitochondria and the mitochondrial quality control system it is possible that this might in the future provide both a diagnostic and a therapeutic tool for neurodegeneration.

Acknowledgements

We gratefully acknowledge the financial support from the Academy of Finland and The Sigrid Juselius Foundation.

Author details

Riikka Lampinen, Irina Belaya, Isabella Boccuni, Tarja Malm and Katja M. Kanninen*

*Address all correspondence to: katja.kanninen@uef.fi

A. I. Virtanen Institute for Molecular Sciences, University of Eastern Finland, Kuopio, Finland

References

[1] Wang Z, Ying Z, Bosy-Westphal A, et al. Specific metabolic rates of major organs and tissues across adulthood: Evaluation by mechanistic model of resting energy expenditure. The American Journal of Clinical Nutrition. 2010;**92**(6):1369-1377

[2] Mergenthaler P, Lindauer U, Dienel GA, et al. Sugar for the brain: The role of glucose in physiological and pathological brain function. Trends in Neurosciences. 2013;**36**(10): 587-597

[3] Howarth C, Gleeson P, Attwell D. Updated energy budgets for neural computation in the neocortex and cerebellum. Journal of Cerebral Blood Flow & Metabolism. 2012;**32**(7): 1222-1232

[4] van Hall G, Stømstad M, Rasmussen P, et al. Blood lactate is an important energy source for the human brain. Journal of Cerebral Blood Flow & Metabolism. 2009;**29**(6): 1121-1129

[5] Magistretti PJ. Role of glutamate in neuron-glia metabolic coupling. The American Journal of Clinical Nutrition. 2009;**90**(3):875-880

[6] Bélanger M, Allaman I, Magistretti P. Brain energy metabolism: Focus on astrocyte-neuron metabolic cooperation. Cell Metabolism. 2011;**14**(6):724-738

[7] Fu W, Jhamandas JH. Role of astrocytic glycolytic metabolism in Alzheimer's disease pathogenesis. Biogerontology. 2014;**15**(6):579-586

[8] Bolaños JP, Almeida A, Moncada S. Glycolysis: A bioenergetic or a survival pathway? Trends in Biochemical Sciences. 2010;**35**(3):145-149

[9] Suzuki A, Stern S, Bozdagi O, et al. Astrocyte-neuron lactate transport is required for long-term memory formation. Cell. 2011;**144**(5):810-823

[10] Rose J, Brian C, Woods J, et al. Mitochondrial dysfunction in glial cells: Implications for neuronal homeostasis and survival. Toxicology. 2017;**391**:109-115

[11] Walls AB, Heimbürger CM, Bouman SD, et al. Robust glycogen shunt activity in astrocytes: Effects of glutamatergic and adrenergic agents. Neuroscience. 2009;**158**(1):284-292

[12] Obel LF, Müller MS, Walls AB, et al. Brain glycogen-new perspectives on its metabolic function and regulation at the subcellular level. Frontiers in Neuroenergetics. 2012;**4**: 1-15

[13] Almeida A, Moncada S, Bolaños JP. Nitric oxide switches on glycolysis through the AMP protein kinase and 6-phosphofructo-2-kinase pathway. Nature Cell Biology. 2004;**6**(1): 45-51

[14] Voutsinos-Porche B, Bonvento G, Tanaka K, et al. Glial glutamate transporters mediate a functional metabolic crosstalk between neurons and astrocytes in the mouse developing cortex. Neuron. 2003;**37**(2):275-286

[15] Pellerin L, Magistretti PJ. Glutamate uptake into astrocytes stimulates aerobic glycolysis: A mechanism coupling neuronal activity to glucose utilization. Proceedings of the National Academy of Sciences of the United States of America. 1994;**91**(22): 10625-10629

[16] Sagan L. On the origin of mitosing cells. Journal of Theoretical Biology. 1967;**14**(3):255-274

[17] Held NM, Houtkooper RH. Mitochondrial quality control pathways as determinants of metabolic health. BioEssays. 2015;**37**(8):867-876

[18] Duchen MR. Mitochondria and calcium: From cell signalling to cell death. The Journal of Physiology. 2000;**529**:57-68

[19] Giorgi C, Baldassari F, Bononi A, et al. Mitochondrial Ca(2+) and apoptosis. Cell Calcium. 2012;**52**(1):36-43

[20] Raps SP, Lai JC, Hertz L, et al. Glutathione is present in high concentrations in cultured astrocytes but not in cultured neurons. Brain Research. 1989;**493**(2):398-401

[21] Ziech D, Franco R, Georgakilas AG, et al. The role of reactive oxygen species and oxidative stress in environmental carcinogenesis and biomarker development. Chemico-Biological Interactions. 2010;**188**(2):334-339

[22] Starkov AA. The role of mitochondria in reactive oxygen species metabolism and signaling. Annals of the New York Academy of Sciences. 2008;**1147**:37-52

[23] Boveris A, Chance B. The mitochondrial generation of hydrogen peroxide. General properties and effect of hyperbaric oxygen. The Biochemical Journal. 1973;**134**(3):707-716

[24] Zorov DB, Filburn CR, Klotz LO, et al. Reactive oxygen species (ROS)-induced ROS release: A new phenomenon accompanying induction of the mitochondrial permeability transition in cardiac myocytes. The Journal of Experimental Medicine. 2000;**192**(7): 1001-1014

[25] Hara Y, Yuk F, Puri R, et al. Presynaptic mitochondrial morphology in monkey prefrontal cortex correlates with working memory and is improved with estrogen treatment. Proceedings of the National Academy of Sciences of the United States of America. 2014;**111**(1):486-491

[26] von Bartheld CS, Bahney J, Herculano-Houzel S. The search for true numbers of neurons and glial cells in the human brain: A review of 150 years of cell counting. The Journal of Comparative Neurology. 2016;**524**(18):3865-3895

[27] Verkhratsky A, Olabarria M, Noristani HN, et al. Astrocytes in Alzheimer's disease. Neurotherapeutics. 2010;**7**(4):399-412

[28] Sofroniew MV, Vinters HV. Astrocytes: Biology and pathology. Acta Neuropathologica. 2010;**119**(1):7-35

[29] Ogata K, Kosaka T. Structural and quantitative analysis of astrocytes in the mouse hippocampus. Neuroscience. 2002;**113**(1):221-233

[30] Nedergaard M, Ransom B, Goldman SA. New roles for astrocytes: Redefining the functional architecture of the brain. Trends in Neurosciences. 2003;**26**(10):523-530

[31] Lovatt D, Sonnewald U, Waagepetersen HS, et al. The transcriptome and metabolic gene signature of protoplasmic astrocytes in the adult murine cortex. The Journal of Neuroscience. 2007;**27**(45):12255-12266

[32] Acosta C, Anderson HD, Anderson C. Astrocyte dysfunction in Alzheimer disease. Journal of Neuroscience Research. 2017;**95**(12):2430-2447

[33] Jackson JG, Robinson MB. Reciprocal regulation of mitochondrial dynamics and calcium signaling in astrocyte processes. The Journal of Neuroscience. 2015;**35**(45):15199-15213

[34] Jackson JG, O'Donnell JC, Takano H, et al. Neuronal activity and glutamate uptake decrease mitochondrial mobility in astrocytes and position mitochondria near glutamate transporters. The Journal of Neuroscience. 2014;**34**(5):1613-1624

[35] Cagalinec M, Safiulina D, Liiv M, et al. Principles of the mitochondrial fusion and fission cycle in neurons. Journal of Cell Science. 2013;**126**(10):2187-2197

[36] Jeong SY, Seol DW. The role of mitochondria in apoptosis. BMB Reports. 2008;**41**(1):11-22

[37] Lionaki E, Markaki M, Palikaras K, et al. Mitochondria, autophagy and age-associated neurodegenerative diseases: New insights into a complex interplay. Biochimica et Biophysica Acta. 2015;**1847**(11):1412-1423

[38] Amadoro G, Corsetti V, Florenzano F, et al. Morphological and bioenergetic demands underlying the mitophagy in post-mitotic neurons: The pink-parkin pathway. Frontiers in Aging Neuroscience. 2014;**6**:18

[39] Lemasters JJ. Selective mitochondrial autophagy, or mitophagy, as a targeted defense against oxidative stress, mitochondrial dysfunction, and aging. Rejuvenation Research. 2005;**8**(1):3-5

[40] Kissova I, Deffieu M, Manon S, et al. Uth1p is involved in the autophagic degradation of mitochondria. The Journal of Biological Chemistry. 2004;**279**(37):39068-39074

[41] Narendra DP, Youle RJ. Targeting mitochondrial dysfunction: Role for PINK1 and Parkin in mitochondrial quality control. Antioxidants & Redox Signaling. 2011;**14**(10): 1929-1938

[42] Cai Q, Lu L, Tian JH, et al. Snapin-regulated late endosomal transport is critical for efficient autophagy-lysosomal function in neurons. Neuron. 2010;**68**(1):73-86

[43] Davis CH, Kim KY, Bushong EA, et al. Transcellular degradation of axonal mitochondria. Proceedings of the National Academy of Sciences of the United States of America. 2014;**111**(26):9633-9638

[44] Hayakawa K, Esposito E, Wang X, et al. Transfer of mitochondria from astrocytes to neurons after stroke. Nature. 2016;**535**(7613):551-555

[45] Berridge MV, Schneider RT, McConnell MJ. Mitochondrial transfer from astrocytes to neurons following ischemic insult: Guilt by association? Cell Metabolism. 2016;**24**(3): 376-378

[46] Derouiche A, Haseleu J, Korf HW. Fine astrocyte processes contain very small mitochondria: Glial oxidative capability may fuel transmitter metabolism. Neurochemical Research. 2015;**40**(12):2402-2413

[47] Mayeux R. Early Alzheimer's disease. The New England Journal of Medicine. 2010;**362**(23): 2194-2201

[48] Nelson P, Braak H, Markesbery W. Neuropathology and cognitive impairment in Alzheimer disease: A complex but coherent relationship. Journal of Neuropathology and Experimental Neurology. 2009;**68**(1):1-14

[49] Karch CM, Goate AM. Alzheimer's disease risk genes and mechanisms of disease pathogenesis. Biological Psychiatry. 2015;**77**(1):43-51

[50] Tanzi RE. The genetics of Alzheimer disease. Cold Spring Harbor Perspectives in Medicine. 2012;**2**(10):1-10

[51] Demetrius LA, Driver J. Alzheimer's as a metabolic disease. Biogerontology. 2013;**14**(6): 641

[52] Lee J, Han P. An update of animal models of Alzheimer disease with a reevaluation of plaque depositions. Experimental Neurobiology. 2013;**22**(2):84-95

[53] Arber C, Lovejoy C, Wray S. Stem cell models of Alzheimers disease: Progress and challenges. Alzheimer's Research & Therapy. 2017;**9**(1):42

[54] Jones VC, Atkinson-dell R, Verkhratsky A, et al. Aberrant iPSC-derived human astrocytes in Alzheimer's disease. Cell Death and Disease. 2017;**8**(3):e2696

[55] Liao M, Muratore CR, Gierahn TM, et al. Single-cell detection of secreted Aβ and sAPPα from human IPSC-derived neurons and astrocytes. The Journal of Neuroscience. 2016;**36**(5):1730-1746

[56] Alzheimer A. Contribution about the knowledge of the pathologic neuroglia, and its relationships with the course of the decomposition of the nervous system. Histologic and Histopathologic Studies on Cerebral Cortex. 1910:401-562

[57] Rodríguez-Arellano JJ, Parpura V, Zorec R, et al. Astrocytes in physiological aging and Alzheimer's disease. Neuroscience. 2016;**323**:170-182

[58] Oakley H, Cole SL, Logan S, et al. Intraneuronal beta-amyloid aggregates, neurodegeneration, and neuron loss in transgenic mice with five familial Alzheimer's disease mutations: Potential factors in amyloid plaque formation. Journal of Neuroscience. 2006;**26**(40):10129-10140

[59] van Gijsel-Bonnello M, Baranger K, Benech P, et al. Metabolic changes and inflammation in cultured astrocytes from the 5xFAD mouse model of Alzheimer's disease: Alleviation by pantethine. PLoS One. 2017;**12**(4):1-22

[60] Iram T, Trudler D, Kain D, et al. Astrocytes from old Alzheimer's disease mice are impaired in Aβ uptake and in neuroprotection. Neurobiology of Disease. 2016;**96**:84-94

[61] Kulijewicz-Nawrot M, Verkhratsky A, Chvátal A, et al. Astrocytic cytoskeletal atrophy in the medial prefrontal cortex of a triple transgenic mouse model of Alzheimer's disease. Journal of Anatomy. 2012;**221**(3):252-262

[62] Olabarria M, Noristani HN, Verkhratsky A, et al. Concomitant astroglial atrophy and astrogliosis in a triple transgenic animal model of Alzheimer's disease. Glia. 2010;**58**(7): 831-838

[63] Orre M, Kamphuis W, Osborn LM, et al. Isolation of glia from Alzheimer's mice reveals inflammation and dysfunction. Neurobiology of Aging. 2014;**35**(12):2746-2760

[64] Pomilio C, Pavia P, Gorojod RM, et al. Glial alterations from early to late stages in a model of Alzheimer's disease: Evidence of autophagy involvement in Aβ internalization. Hippocampus. 2016;**26**(2):194-210

[65] Hartlage-Rübsamen M, Zeitschel U, Apelt J, et al. Astrocytic expression of the Alzheimer's disease β-secretase (BACE1) is stimulus-dependent. Glia. 2003;**41**(2):169-179

[66] Oberheim NA, Takano T, Han X, et al. Uniquely hominid features of adult human astrocytes. Journal of Neuroscience. 2009;**29**(10):3276-3287

[67] Oksanen M, Petersen AJ, Naumenko N, et al. PSEN1 mutant iPSC-derived model reveals severe astrocyte pathology in alzheimer's disease. Stem Cell Reports. 2017. pii: S2213-6711(17)30471-X [Epub ahead of print]

[68] Pekny M, Wilhelmsson U, Pekna M. The dual role of astrocyte activation and reactive gliosis. Neuroscience Letters. 2014;**565**:30

[69] Zamanian JL, Xu L, Foo LC, et al. Genomic analysis of reactive astrogliosis. The Journal of Neuroscience. 2012;**32**(18):6391-6410

[70] Liddelow SA, Guttenplan KA, Clarke LE, et al. Neurotoxic reactive astrocytes are induced by activated microglia. Nature. 2017;**541**(7638):481-487

[71] Osborn LM, Kamphuis W, Wadman WJ, et al. Astrogliosis: An integral player in the pathogenesis of Alzheimer's disease. Progress in Neurobiology. 2016;**144**:121-141

[72] Dossi E, Vasile F, Rouach N. Human astrocytes in the diseased brain. Brain Research Bulletin. 2017. pii: S0361-9230(17)30082-5 [Epub ahead of print]

[73] Cotrina ML, Nedergaard M. Astrocytes in the aging brain. Journal of Neuroscience Research. 2002;**67**(1):1-10

[74] Schipper H, Gupta A, Szarek W. Suppression of glial HO-1 activitiy as a potential neurotherapeutic intervention in AD. Current Alzheimer Research. 2009;**6**(5):424-430

[75] Schubert D, Soucek T, Blouw B. The induction of HIF-1 reduces astrocyte activation by amyloid beta peptide. The European Journal of Neuroscience. 2009;**29**(7):1323-1334

[76] Cai Z, Cheng-Qun W, Zhou L. Astrocyte and Alzheimer's disease. Journal of Neurology. 2017;**264**(10):2068-2074

[77] Merlini M, Meyer E, Ulmann-Schuler A, et al. Vascular β-amyloid and early astrocyte alterations impair cerebrovascular function and cerebral metabolism in transgenic arcAβ mice. Acta Neuropathologica. 2011;**122**(3):293-311

[78] Lu W, Huang J, Sun S, et al. Changes in lactate content and monocarboxylate transporter 2 expression in Aβ_{25-35}-treated rat model of Alzheimer's disease. Neurological Sciences. 2015;**36**(6):871

[79] Kubik LL, Philbert MA. The role of astrocyte mitochondria in differential regional susceptibility to environmental neurotoxicants: Tools for understanding neurodegeneration. Toxicological Sciences. 2015;**144**(1):7-16

[80] Stephen T, Gupta-Agarwal S, Kittler JT. Mitochondrial dynamics in astrocytes. Biochemical Society Transactions. 2014;**42**(5):1302-1310

[81] Demetrius LA, Simon DK. The inverse association of cancer and Alzheimer's: A bioenergetic mechanism. Journal of the Royal Society Interface. 2013;**10**(82):20130006

[82] Slemmer JE, Shacka JJ, Sweeney MI, et al. Antioxidants and free radical scavengers for the treatment of stroke, traumatic brain injury and aging. Current Medicinal Chemistry. 2008;**15**(4):404-414

[83] Kaminsky YG, Kosenko EA. Effects of amyloid-beta peptides on hydrogen peroxide-metabolizing enzymes in rat brain in vivo. Free Radical Research. 2008;**42**(6):564-573

[84] Abramov AY, Canevari L, Duchen MR. Beta-amyloid peptides induce mitochondrial dysfunction and oxidative stress in astrocytes and death of neurons through activation of NADPH oxidase. The Journal of Neuroscience. 2004;**24**(2):565-575

[85] Kuchibhotla KV, Lattarulo CR, Hyman BT, et al. Synchronous hyperactivity and intercellular calcium waves in astrocytes in Alzheimer mice. Science. 2009;**323**(5918):1211-1215

[86] Begley JG, Duan W, Chan S, et al. Altered calcium homeostasis and mitochondrial dysfunction in cortical synaptic compartments of presenilin-1 mutant mice. Journal of Neurochemistry. 1999;**72**(3):1030-1039

[87] Swerdlow RH, Burns JM, Khan SM. The Alzheimer's disease mitochondrial cascade hypothesis: Progress and perspectives. BBA - Molecular Basis of Disease. 2014;**1842**(8): 1219-1231

[88] Pagani L, Eckert A. Amyloid-Beta interaction with mitochondria. International Journal of Alzheimer's Disease. 2011;**2011**:925050

[89] Anandatheerthavarada HK, Biswas G, Robin M, et al. Mitochondrial targeting and a novel transmembrane arrest of Alzheimer's amyloid precursor protein impairs mitochondrial function in neuronal cells. The Journal of Cell Biology. 2003;**161**(1):41-54

[90] Swerdlow RH. The neurodegenerative mitochondriopathies. Journal of Alzheimer's Disease. 2009;**17**(4):737-751

[91] Halliwell B. Reactive oxygen species and the central nervous system. Journal of Neurochemistry. 1992;**59**(5):1609-1623

[92] Sagara JI, Miura K, Bannai S. Maintenance of neuronal glutathione by glial cells. Journal of Neurochemistry. 1993;**61**(5):1672-1676

[93] Sheng B, Wang X, Su B, et al. Impaired mitochondrial biogenesis contributes to mitochondrial dysfunction in Alzheimer's disease. Journal of Neurochemistry. 2012;**120**(3): 419-429

[94] Baloyannis SJ. Mitochondrial alterations in Alzheimer's disease. Journal of Alzheimers Disease. 2006;**9**(9):119-126

[95] Rice AC, Keeney PM, Algarzae NK, et al. Mitochondrial DNA copy numbers in pyramidal neurons are decreased and mitochondrial biogenesis transcriptome signaling is disrupted in Alzheimer's disease hippocampi. Journal of Alzheimer's Disease. 2014;**40**(2): 319-330

[96] Brown AM, Sheu RK, Mohs R, et al. Correlation of the clinical severity of alzheimer's disease with an aberration in mitochondrial DNA (mtDNA). Journal of Molecular Neuroscience. 2001;**16**(1):41-48

[97] Hirai K, Aliev G, Nunomura A, et al. Mitochondrial abnormalities in Alzheimer's disease. Journal of Neuroscience. 2001;**21**(9):3017-3023

[98] Fukui H, Moraes CT. The mitochondrial impairment, oxidative stress and neurodegeneration connection: Reality or just an attractive hypothesis? Trends in Neurosciences. 2008;**31**(5):251-256

[99] Fu W, Shi D, Westaway D, et al. Bioenergetic mechanisms in astrocytes may contribute to amyloid plaque deposition and toxicity. The Journal of Biological Chemistry. 2015;**290**(20):12504-12513

[100] Misko A, Jiang S, Wegorzewska I, et al. Mitofusin 2 is necessary for transport of axonal mitochondria and interacts with the Miro/Milton complex. Journal of Neuroscience. 2010;**30**(12):4232-4240

[101] Bak LK, Schousboe A, Waagepetersen HS. The glutamate/GABA-glutamine cycle: Aspects of transport, neurotransmitter homeostasis and ammonia transfer. Journal of Neurochemistry. 2006;**98**(3):641-653

[102] Voloboueva LA, Suh SW, Swanson RA, et al. Inhibition of mitochondrial function in astrocytes: Implications for neuroprotection. Journal of Neurochemistry. 2007;**102**(4): 1383-1394

[103] Genda EN, Jackson JG, Sheldon AL, et al. Co-compartmentalization of the astroglial glutamate transporter, GLT-1, with glycolytic enzymes and mitochondria. The Journal of Neuroscience. 2011;**31**(50):18275-18288

[104] Sekar S, McDonald J, Cuyugan L, et al. Alzheimer's disease is associated with altered expression of genes involved in immune response and mitochondrial processes in astrocytes. Neurobiology of Aging. 2015;**36**(2):583-591

[105] Sarkar P, Zaja I, Bienengraeber M, et al. Epoxyeicosatrienoic acids pretreatment improves amyloid -induced mitochondrial dysfunction in cultured rat hippocampal astrocytes. AJP - Heart and Circulatory Physiology. 2014;**306**(4):475-484

[106] Lee H, Pancholi N, Esposito L, et al. Early induction of oxidative stress in mouse model of Alzheimer disease with reduced mitochondrial superoxide dismutase activity. PLoS One. 2012;**7**(1):e28033

[107] Tamagno E, Guglielmotto M, Aragno M, et al. Oxidative stress activates a positive feedback between the γ- and β-secretase cleavages of the β-amyloid precursor protein. Journal of Neurochemistry. 2008;**104**(3):683-695

[108] Matsunaga S, Kishi T, Iwata N. Memantine monotherapy for Alzheimer's disease: A systematic review and meta-analysis. PLoS One. 2015;**10**(4):e0123289

[109] Amanatkar HR, Papagiannopoulos B, Grossberg GT. Analysis of recent failures of disease modifying therapies in Alzheimer's disease suggesting a new methodology for future studies. Expert Review of Neurotherapeutics. 2017;**17**(1):7-16

[110] Reddy AP, Reddy PH. Mitochondria-targeted molecules as potential drugs to treat patients with Alzheimer's disease. Progress in Molecular Biology and Translational Science. 2017;**146**:173-201

[111] Yao J, Irwin RW, Zhao L, et al. Mitochondrial bioenergetic deficit precedes Alzheimer's pathology in female mouse model of Alzheimer's disease. Proceedings of the National Academy of Sciences of the United States of America. 2009;**106**(34):14670-14675

[112] Wilkins HM, Morris HM. New therapeutics to modulate mitochondrial function in neurodegenerative disorders. Current Pharmaceutical Design. 2017;**23**(5):731-752

[113] Morris MC, Tangney CC, Wang Y, et al. MIND diet associated with reduced incidence of Alzheimer's disease. Alzheimer's & Dementia. 2015;**11**(9):1007-1014

[114] Chirles TJ, Reiter K, Weiss LR, et al. Exercise training and functional connectivity changes in mild cognitive impairment and healthy elders. Journal of Alzheimer's Disease. 2017; **57**:845-856

[115] Van Cauwenberghe C, Vandendriessche C, Libert C, et al. Caloric restriction: Beneficial effects on brain aging and Alzheimer's disease. Mammalian Genome. 2016;**27**(7):300-319

[116] Martin B, Mattson MP, Maudsley S. Caloric restriction and intermittent fasting: Two potential diets for successful brain aging. Ageing Research Reviews. 2006;**5**(3):332-353

[117] Bavarsad Shahripour R, Harrigan MR, Alexandrov AV. N-acetylcysteine (NAC) in neurological disorders: Mechanisms of action and therapeutic opportunities. Brain and Behavior. 2014;**4**(2):108-122

[118] Maczurek A, Hager K, Kenklies M, et al. Lipoic acid as an anti-inflammatory and neuroprotective treatment for Alzheimer's disease. Advanced Drug Delivery Reviews. 2008;**60**(13):1463-1470

[119] Baum L, Lam CWK, Cheung SK, et al. Six-month randomized, placebo-controlled, double-blind, pilot clinical trial of curcumin in patients with Alzheimer disease. Journal of Clinical Psychopharmacology. 2008;**28**(1):110-113

[120] Pocernich CB, Butterfield DA. Elevation of glutathione as a therapeutic strategy in Alzheimer disease. BBA - Molecular Basis of Disease. 2012;**1822**(5):625-630

[121] Sung S, Yao Y, Uryu K, et al. Early vitamin E supplementation in young but not aged mice reduces Abeta levels and amyloid deposition in a transgenic model of Alzheimer's disease. FASEB Journal. 2004;**18**(2):323-325

[122] Usoro OB, Mousa SA. Vitamin E forms in Alzheimer's disease: A review of controversial and clinical experiences. Critical Reviews in Food Science and Nutrition. 2010;**50**(5):414-419

[123] Ye CY, Lei Y, Tang XC, et al. Donepezil attenuates Aβ-associated mitochondrial dysfunction and reduces mitochondrial Aβ accumulation in vivo and in vitro. Neuropharmacology. 2015;**95**:29-36

[124] Ng LF, Gruber J, Cheah IK, et al. The mitochondria-targeted antioxidant MitoQ extends lifespan and improves healthspan of a transgenic *Caenorhabditis elegans* model of Alzheimer disease. Free Radical Biology & Medicine. 2014;**71**:390-401

[125] Reddy PH, Manczak M, Kandimalla R. Mitochondria-targeted small molecule SS31, a potential candidate for the treatment of Alzheimer's disease. Human Molecular Genetics. 2017;**26**(8):1483-1496

[126] Szeto H. Mitochondria-targeted peptide antioxidants: Novel neuroprotective agents. The AAPS Journal. 2006;**8**(3):521-531

[127] Kim IK, Lee KJ, Rhee S, et al. Protective effects of Peroxiredoxin 6 overexpression on amyloid β-induced apoptosis in PC12 cells. Free Radical Research. 2013;**47**(10): 836-846

[128] Dragicevic N, Delic V, Cao C, et al. Caffeine increases mitochondrial function and blocks melatonin signaling to mitochondria in Alzheimer's mice and cells. Neuropharmacology. 2012;**63**(8):1368-1379

[129] Rege SD, Geetha T, Griffin GD, et al. Neuroprotective effects of resveratrol in Alzheimer disease pathology. Frontiers in Aging Neuroscience. 2014;**6**:218

[130] Meng X, Wang M, Sun G, et al. Attenuation of Aβ25-35-induced parallel autophagic and apoptotic cell death by gypenoside XVII through the estrogen receptor-dependent activation of Nrf2/ARE pathways. Toxicology and Applied Pharmacology. 2014;**279**(1): 63-75

[131] Onyango IG, Dennis J, Khan SM. Mitochondrial dysfunction in Alzheimer's disease and the rationale for bioenergetics based therapies. Aging and Disease. 2016;**7**(2):201-214

[132] East DA, Fagiani F, Crosby J, et al. PMI: A ΔΨm independent pharmacological regulator of mitophagy. Chemistry & Biology. 2014;**21**(11):1585-1596

[133] Cui M, Tang X, Christian WV, et al. Perturbations in mitochondrial dynamics induced by human mutant PINK1 can be rescued by the mitochondrial division inhibitor mdivi-1. The Journal of Biological Chemistry. 2010;**285**(15):11740-11752

[134] Manczak M, Kandimalla R, Fry D, et al. Protective effects of reduced dynamin-related protein 1 against amyloid beta-induced mitochondrial dysfunction and synaptic damage in Alzheimer's disease. Human Molecular Genetics. 2016;**25**(23):5148-5166

[135] Xie N, Wang C, Lian Y, et al. Inhibition of mitochondrial fission attenuates Aβ-induced microglia apoptosis. Neuroscience. 2014;**256**:36-42

[136] Jang M, Jung S, Lee M, et al. Melatonin attenuates amyloid beta25-35-induced apoptosis in mouse microglial BV2 cells. Neuroscience Letters. 2005;**380**(1-2):26-31

[137] Schitine C, Nogaroli L, Costa MR, et al. Astrocyte heterogeneity in the brain: From development to disease. Frontiers in Cellular Neuroscience. 2015;**9**:76

Chapter 8

The Role of Astrocytes in Tumor Growth and Progression

Emily Gronseth, Ling Wang, David R. Harder and Ramani Ramchandran

Additional information is available at the end of the chapter

http://dx.doi.org/10.5772/intechopen.72720

Abstract

Current research is continually implicating the importance of astrocytes as active participants in neurological injury, disease, and tumor progression. This chapter will discuss some of these emerging concepts, especially as they relate to tumor biology. Astrocytes themselves can become tumorigenic, such as the case in gliomas, which often have aberrant signaling in key regulating genes of astrocyte development. Astrocytes secrete factors that maintain the tight junctions of the blood brain barrier (BBB), which in turn regulates the success or failure of metastatic cells extravasating into the brain. This astrocytic association with the brain vasculature also promotes brain tumor stem cell characteristics, which are known to be necessary for tumor initiation. Tumor cells within the brain make direct contacts with astrocytes through gap junctions, which subsequently lead to increased chemoresistance of the tumor cells. Astrocytes have also been shown to effect tumors cells via secretion of degradative enzymes, cytokines, chemokines, and growth factors, all of which have been shown to promote tumor cell proliferation, survival, and invasion. Thus, research in astrocyte biology and the role of astrocytes in the tumor microenvironment has and will likely continue to reveal novel targets for cancer intervention.

Keywords: astrocytes, metastasis, blood-brain barrier, reactive astrogliosis, cancer

1. Introduction

The tumor microenvironment plays a critical role in tumor progression. Tumors within the central nervous system (CNS) include primary brain tumors originating from a CNS resident cell, or secondary tumors that came from extraneural origins. The brain microenvironment consists of multiple cell types including the most abundant glial cell, astrocytes. Astrocytes have very diverse and microenvironment-dependent morphologies; for a long time, this structural contribution was considered their main purpose. Present in gray matter, protoplasmic astrocytes are the most common types of astrocytes and are stellate in nature with branching processes or "endfeet" [1]. These endfeet make important contacts with neurons and other cells within the brain microenvironment. Importantly for this chapter, one of these interfaces, which we will discuss further, is the astrocyte endfeet connections made with endothelial cells and pericytes, commonly referred to as the blood brain barrier (BBB). This barrier allows for select metabolites to enter and toxic waste to exit the brain.

Homeostasis in the brain is of utmost importance to maintain neural function and prevent potentially detrimental immune responses from occurring. An invading tumor cell normally encounters enormous barriers before it can colonize the brain. On entering the brain, it will need to overcome brain defense mechanisms, which are partly mediated by astrocytes and brain macrophage cells called microglia. These and other mechanisms are in place to thwart tumor cell entrance, however, in some cases these mechanisms are either not adequate to prevent tumor cell invasion, or exploited to aid in tumor cell extravasation into the brain. In addition to regulating brain metastases, astrocytes, which develop from neural stem cells (NSCs), can become transformed and undergo developmental dysregulation due to aberrant gene activation, resulting in various types of brain tumors, including gliomas.

In this chapter, we will further discuss autocrine, paracrine, and juxtacrine mechanisms in which astrocytes influence surrounding cells in the brain microenvironment and tumor progression within the CNS. We will discuss the underlying mechanisms that regulate these processes, and provide examples of possible interventions that could eventually be translated into successful clinical treatment for patients.

2. Primary tumors of astrocytic origin

We begin this chapter by understanding how astrocytes themselves may become transformed and discuss the key features of these types of tumors. The cellular origin of many brain tumors can be traced back to multipotent NSCs, which are able to self-renew and differentiate into all subtypes of mature neurons and glial cells. However, many tumors with more distinct cellular origins exist along the glial cell differentiation axis, and are traced back to more restricted and differentiated astrocyte progeny [2]. During development of mature astrocytes, NSCs first partially differentiate into neuronal precursor cells where, in the presence of specific growth factors and their cognate receptors, they differentiate into various cellular lineages [3]. Early astrocyte precursors are characterized by their expression of fibroblast growth factor receptor (FGFR), nestin, and epidermal growth factor receptor (EGFR), while mature astrocytes express markers such as glutamate aspartate transporter (GLAST), FGFR3, S100β and glial fibrillary acidic protein (GFAP) [4–7]. These astrocyte precursor cells are perhaps most vulnerable to transformation, and depending on the stage of these cells, fatal adult primary brain tumors (gliomas) may arise. Because mature astrocytes maintain their ability to proliferate throughout adulthood (an uncommon characteristic of many CNS cells), it is hypothesized that this is a contributing reason for why astrocytic tumors are so common overall and most common in adults [8, 9].

The term "glial cells" describes a broader group of cells including astrocytes, ependymal cells and oligodendrocytes, not all gliomas are specifically astrocytic in nature. Gliomas which are thought to originate or histologically resemble astrocytes include astrocytomas, mixed gliomas or oligoastrocytomas, diffuse intrinsic pontine gliomas [10], and high grade astrocytomas called glioblastoma multiforme (GBM). There are also several types of mixed neuronal-glial tumors. These tumors are extremely heterogeneous, differing in histology, location in the brain, molecular biology, karyotype, age of onset, and survival prognosis of the patient. Gliomas share many characteristics with astrocytes, particularly activated astrocytes, which will be discussed in a later section of this chapter. Some of these include migration capabilities, growth factor expression pattern, stem cell-like characteristics, and the ability for anchorage-independent growth which is correlated with invasiveness of a tumor [11–13].

In general, cellular origins of the previously mentioned gliomas are astrocyte precursor cells. However, the diversity in the distinct molecular/genetic alterations of the tumors suggests that different stages or types of precursor cells have different sensitivities to specific genetic mutations. One of the most notable genetic signatures of GBM is EGFR amplification and overexpression which, as previously mentioned, is also involved in regulating astrocyte differentiation [14–17]. There have been several mechanisms associating EGFR overexpression with astrocyte tumor malignancy. Several known ligands of EGFR, including EGF and transforming growth factor-α (TGF-α), promote proliferation of astrocytes and astrocyte precursor cells, thus contributing to the malignancy of the tumors [14, 18, 19]. Additionally, cell cycle regulators such as Rb, p53 and CDKN2A are commonly mutated and inactivated in low grade gliomas and GBM, [15, 20–23]. Mutations in isocitrate dehydrogenase (IDH)-1 and -2 are also extremely common, but only in certain gliomas; they are present in 70% of grade II and III astrocytomas and oligodendrogliomas, as well as secondary GBMs, but are rare in primary GBMs [15, 24].

3. The role of astrocytes in tumor growth and progression

As will be discussed in more detail throughout this chapter, astrocytes are very heterogeneous in regards to function and influence on tumors within the CNS. This fact, combined with the heterogeneity that encompasses the transformation of cells results in unique tumor genotypes and phenotypes, plus many other contextual factors, equates to interactions that are both tumor promoting and tumor suppressive (**Figure 1**). Arguably, there is more evidence suggesting how astrocytes can be tumor promoting, which will be covered in this section. Some functions of astrocytes that are known within the literature to be tumor promoting to both primary and metastatic brain tumors are summarized and illustrated (**Figure 2**).

3.1. Metastatic tumors: Interactions with astrocytes at the blood-brain barrier

One of the critical steps in the life time of tumor progression is tumor metastasis, especially brain metastasis. This step results in catastrophic consequences from a patient perspective. The metastases from extraneural tumors in the brain are actually the most common sources of tumors in the CNS, as shown in **Table 1** [25, 26].

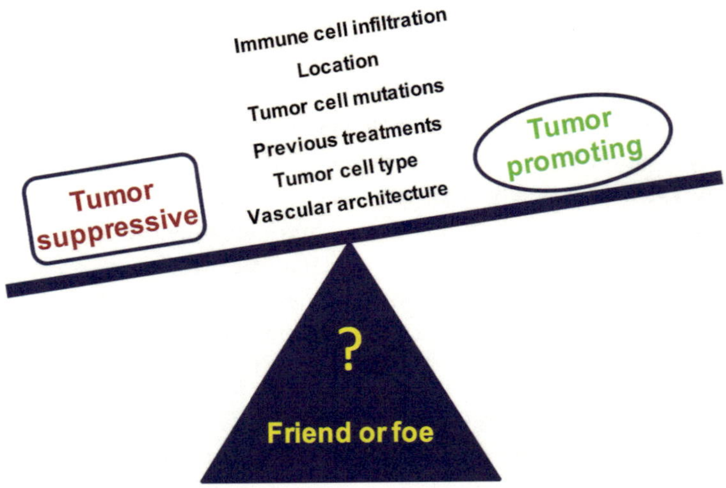

Figure 1. Research shows astrocytes have functions that result in tumor supporting and tumor suppressing mechanisms, and sometimes both. Like many physiological responses, this demonstrates the context dependent balancing act that occurs when homeostasis is breached, and the many factors that play a role in tipping the balance one way or another.

The process of metastasis, in brief, involves invasion of a tumor cell away from the tumor to a blood vessel, entry into and survival in the blood circulation, extravasation from the blood vessel into the secondary organ, and survival, engraftment, and proliferation into a secondary tumor. Extravasating into the brain provides an added challenge: that of getting past the BBB. The most functionally important component of the BBB are the tight junctions held between brain microvascular endothelial cells. Thus, substances that get into the brain parenchyma are tightly controlled. Both para-cellular and trans-cellular diffusion are low; most solutes that get in and out through the BBB, such as glucose and other nutrients, do so through transporters expressed on endothelial cells [27–29]. Despite this added barrier, many extraneural tumors have a strong tendency to metastasize to the brain. To note, there are regions within the brain that lack BBB, and could also be a potential avenue of metastasis [30]. The recent discovery of brain lymphatics is also suggestive of an alternative route given the already known function of lymphatics to carry tumor cells [31].

Breast cancer, melanoma, and lung cancer are three tumor types that show proclivity to go to the brain. The most common type of brain metastases originate from lung cancer, accounting for up to 56% of brain metastases, followed by breast cancer metastases at 13–30% [32, 33]. Interestingly, specific subtypes of these tumors have a much higher frequency of brain metastases, including non-small cell lung cancer (NSLC), triple negative breast cancer cells that are estrogenic receptor (ER), progesterone receptor (PR) and epidermal growth factor receptor-2 (HER2) (ER^-, PR^-, $HER2^-$), and HER2-enriched ($HER2^+$) breast cancer cells [32–35]. One theory behind a specific tumors' proclivity to the brain is explained by Paget's seed and soil hypothesis, which suggests that for a seed (tumor cell) to take up in a soil (brain), it must adapt itself and make changes that will favor the soil [26, 36]. In support of this idea, genes associated with breast cancer metastasis to brain have been discovered and efforts continue to identify new targets for lung cancer cell metastasis to the brain and for other cancers as well [37–40]. However, the question raised by the

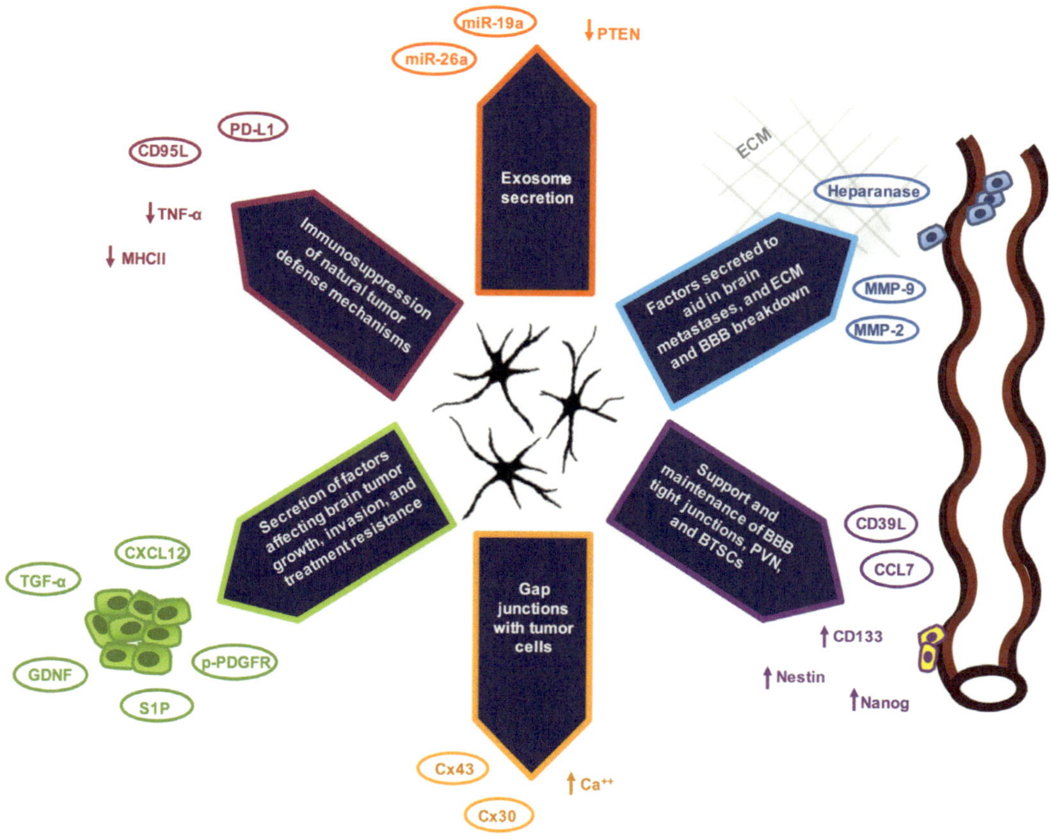

Figure 2. Many signaling mechanisms have been identified that implicate astrocytes in tumor progression. Some of these functions include secretion of factors that have been shown to increase invasiveness and malignancy of established brain tumors, in addition to factors that enable brain metastasizing cells to enter the brain. Astrocytes have also been shown to maintain the vascular niche in the brain which can promote stem-like characteristics in BTSCs. Astrocytes directly interact with tumor cells and communicate via gap junctions, leading to increased intracellular calcium and resistance to treatments. Indirect or paracrine communication with surrounding cells often occurs via secretion of exosomes known to carry miRNAs to target key tumor suppressor genes in tumor cells and surrounding microenvironment. Lastly, astrocytes have been shown to regulate CNS immune suppression, weakening the innate tumor killing response of the body.

seed-soil hypothesis is whether the soil influences the seed, and if so, how it is accomplished. One could argue that in the first place, the soil is influenced by the seed. Therefore, in this "circular logic," both seed and soil appear to contribute together, ultimately, for the growth of the tumor cell.

Astrocytes are vital to the development and maintenance of the BBB, therefore understanding their role in this process is necessary to understand how they also may influence brain metastatic tumor cells attempting to breach the BBB. The tight junctions between the endothelial cells of the BBB are comprised of many junctional proteins, notably claudin-5 and occludin [41, 42]. Vascular endothelial (VE)-cadherin is also of importance within adherens junctions which associate with tight junctions, as well as cytoplasmic scaffolding proteins such as zonula occludens (ZO)-1 and -2 [27, 43–45]. In normal conditions, the BBB homeostasis and junctional complexes are partially supported at the structural and physiological functional levels by astrocytes. Astrocytes contact

CNS tumor type	Incidence rate (per 100,000 persons) (all ages)	References
All brain metastases	8.3/11.1/14.3	[195–197]
Lung cancer brain metastases	~ 3.2–8(estimation based on 39–56% of all brain metastases)	[32]
Breast cancer brain metastases	~ 1.1–4.3 (estimation based on 13–30% of all brain metastases)	[32]
Melanoma brain metastases	~ 0.5–1.6 (estimation based on 6–11% of all brain metastases)	[32]
Primary malignant CNS tumors	7.2	[198]
GBM	3.2	[198]
Nerve sheath tumors	1.82	[198]
Other astrocytomas	1.2	[198]
CNS lymphoma	0.43	[198]
Embryonal tumors (medulloblastoma, ATRT, and PNET)	0.62 (*ages 0–19 only*)	[198]

Table 1. Primary and metastatic CNS tumors with their respective incidence rates per 100,000 persons. All tumors are accounting for all ages, except embryonal tumors which only includes persons' age 0–19 in the population study.

brain endothelial cells via their end feet processes. This contact was shown to maintain BBB permeability characteristics. However, it was later found that secreted factors alone in astrocyte-conditioned media also upheld the tight junction characteristics in endothelial cells, demonstrating the importance of both astrocyte contact and paracrine actions in BBB function [46–48]. For example, Sonic hedgehog (Shh), an important developmental signaling protein, is known to be secreted by astrocytes and bind its cognate receptor, Patched-1, expressed at the cell membrane of brain endothelial cells. This induces a signaling cascade mediated by β-catenin that bolsters tight junctions by increasing expression of occludin [49, 50]. Other proteins secreted by astrocytes that regulate and maintain tight junctions of brain ECs (most often by increased gene expression of junctional proteins) include angiotensin-1, FGF, TGF-β, glia derived neurotropic factor (GDNF), and retinoic acid (RA) [51–55].

Just as astrocytes are important for maintaining the BBB in homeostatic conditions, astrocytes also play key roles when the BBB is disrupted, which can occur during extravasation of tumor cells metastasizing to the brain. Several groups utilized mouse models of melanoma, lung, and breast cancer combined with histological and fluorescent imaging modalities to visualize very early interactions with tumor cells and the BBB. This work demonstrates that tumor cells first arrest in the brain capillaries, often at branch points [56, 57]. Lorger et al. (2010) show that very early on, astrocytes become activated and associate around vasculature in the brain where breast tumor cells are present, but in some cases have not yet extravasated or visibly altered the BBB [56]. This suggests that signals secreted by tumor cells are reaching astrocytes either directly or indirectly through the endothelial cells; a topic that requires further investigation. This association of tumor cells with reactive astrocytes persists throughout metastases formation, characterized by increased astrocyte expression of GFAP, nestin, and matrix metalloproteinase 9 (MMP-9), all of which aid in tumor extravasation mechanisms that will be discussed in later sections.

3.2. Astrocytes' direct cell-cell interactions with tumor cells

Astrocytes have multiple primary and branching endfeet which expand and contract, allowing them to dynamically contact both synapses and the microvasculature. Also, astrocytes regulate communication between neuronal networks and glial-vascular coupling by forming independent contact network [58–61]. Therefore, it has been widely accepted that astrocytes directly contact and communicate with neurons to regulate neuronal function at the synaptic and network levels, which provides a significant impact on physiological and pathological state of the CNS. Subsequently, direct interactions with astrocytes and tumor cells, often in the form of gap junctions, has also been discovered to be significant for tumor progression and resistance to therapy.

As discussed, gliomas are the most lethal primary intracranial tumors. The proliferative dysfunction and invasion of gliomas are associated with changes in gap junction communication [62, 63]. In metastatic brain tumors, reactive astrocytes protect melanoma cells from chemotherapy induced cell death by sequestering intracellular calcium through gap junctions [64]. In the brain, metastases from breast and lung cancer show upregulation of many survival genes which is dependent on the direct contact through gap junctions between the astrocytes and tumor cells, which was found to be causal for developing resistance [65]. These data suggest that reactive astrocytes participate in tumor progression and chemo-resistance by their direct physical contacts and gap junctional communication with tumor cells in the brain.

Gap junctions are efficient tools for intercellular communication. In astrocytes, they are composed of connexins 30 and 43 (Cx30, Cx43) [66]. Cx43 is widely expressed in adult astrocytes and exhibits increased expression in reactive astrocytes induced by various brain pathologies and intercellular calcium signaling [67–73]. Also, Cx43-mediated intercellular communication between astrocytes plays an important role in the invasion of glioma cells in the brain [63]. A recent study has also revealed that breast and lung cancer cells express proto-cadherin 7 (PCDH7) to promote tumor-astrocyte gap junction formation by recruiting Cx43, which allows the transfer of cGAMP from tumor cells to astrocytes to trigger the secretion of inflammatory cytokines, which further promote tumor growth and chemo-resistance [74].

3.3. Astrocytes' secretome and paracrine signaling mechanisms that influence tumor cells

3.3.1. Cytokines and growth factors

Astrocytes can synthesize a host of biologically interesting growth factors and cytokines. Previous studies have shown that sphingosine-1-phosphate (S1P), which shows the highest expression in the brain and is only expressed by astrocytes, induces cell motility in GBM cell lines that express S1P receptor-1 and S1P receptor-3 [75, 76]. Other neurotrophic factors secreted by astrocytes, such as TGF-α, C-X-C motif chemokine 12 (CXCL12), and GDNF, have also revealed the potential to increase the invasive capacity of GBM cells [77, 78]. In brain metastatic tumors, an early study found that metastatic MDA-MB-435 breast cancer cells, when cultured with astrocyte conditioned media, exhibit better growth in response to the conditioned medium. However, the growth-stimulatory effect was partially reversed by anti-IL-6, anti-TGF-β, and anti-insulin like growth factor-1 (IGF-I) antibodies [79]. Another study showed that reactive astrocytes expressed phosphorylated platelet-derived growth factor receptor β at tyrosine 751 (p751-PDGFRβ). Pazopanib, an inhibitor of PDGFRs, inhibited the activation of p-PDGFR expressing astrocytes, and thus prevented brain metastasis formation in the HER2-transfected MDA-MB-231 breast cancer cells [80]. Taken together, this work demonstrates that paracrine signaling by astrocyte secreted cytokines and growth factors facilitates tumor metastasis formation in the brain.

3.3.2. Extracellular matrix (ECM) proteins and degradative enzymes

ECM proteins are important participants in the tumorigenic process, as they are involved in not only the physical adhesion and migration of tumors cells, but also the regulation of intracellular signaling. The brain parenchyma is high in proteoglycans, glycoproteins, and matricellular proteins, all of which astrocytes express and secrete [4]. Specifically, some astrocyte secreted matricellular proteins have been studied in regulation of various brain tumors, including secreted protein acidic and rich in cysteine (SPARC) and CYR61/CTGF/NOV (CCN). Both SPARC and CCN2 have been shown to be secreted by activated astrocytes proximal to brain tumors or injuries [81, 82]. While increases in CCN2 secretion have been correlated with negative glioblastoma outcomes, expression of SPARC and its effect on tumor cells is tumor dependent. In gliomas and astrocytomas, tumor secretion of SPARC promotes invasion, angiogenesis, and a negative prognosis [83, 84]; however medulloblastoma tumor cells have increased loss of SPARC, which when rescued induces cell cycle arrest, neuronal differentiation, and limits radioresistant DNA damage response [85–87].

Previously, we discussed MMP-related mechanisms in which astrocytes assist tumor cells in extravasating the BBB. The secretion of these matrix degrading enzymes also supports brain tumor progression by breaking down the barriers induced by the ECM. Heparanase degrades the glycosaminoglycan side chains of heparan sulfate proteoglycans, which are essential and ubiquitous macromolecules associated with the cell surface [88–90]. Reactive astrocytes have been frequently found in areas surrounding melanoma-related lesions and produce nerve growth factor (NGF), the prototypic neurotrophin [91]. Neurotrophins can stimulate heparanase production in astrocytes and thus contribute to the brain colonization of melanoma cells [88].

MMP-2 and -9 have been observed in secretory vesicles in astrocytes [92]. Stimulation of astrocytes with lipopolysaccharide, IL1-α, IL1-β, or TNF-α induces MMP-2 and -9 secretion [93]. MMP-9 also promotes the growth of primary brain tumors by releasing vascular endothelial growth factor (VEGF) sequestered in the surrounding matrix [94]. The expression of MMP-9 was up-regulated in reactive astrocytes, which was involved in the brain metastases of MDA-MB-435 cells [56]. Moreover, both MMP-2 and -9 secreted by astrocytes contribute to breast cancer MDA-MB-231 cell invasion and brain metastases [95]. In addition to secreting MMPs themselves, astrocytes can also induce tumor cells to secrete MMPs, as shown by Mendes et al. (2007), where they found breast cancer cells to secrete significantly more MMP-2 in the presence of astrocyte conditioned media, aiding metastasis to the brain [96].

3.3.3. Exosomes

The topic of exosomes, which are endosome-derived microvesicles between 50 and 100 nm in size that carry specific protein and RNA cargo, has become a subject of intense interest in tumor biology. Exosomes are released from cells by fusion of multi-vesicular structures with the plasma membrane through the process of exocytosis [97]. Exosomes are a general mode of intercellular communication and can interact with neighboring cells, thus mediating signals between astrocytes and other cells in the brain microenvironment [98, 99].

Among RNA cargo, microRNA (miRNA) transcripts, specifically miR-26a, is highly expressed in astrocytes and is present in astrocyte-derived exosomes [100, 101]. MiR-26a targets mRNAs that impact neuronal function and morphology, and was first implicated in many neuronal disorders [102–104]. Moreover, miR-26a can be sorted to exosomes and transported by these vesicles in the plasma, serum, whole blood, urine, or secreted *in vitro* by human umbilical vein endothelial cells [105–109]. In addition, miR-26a autonomously regulates primary gliomas by increasing *de novo* tumor formation and radiosensitivity through targeting of suppressor phosphatase and tensin homolog (PTEN) and ataxia-telangiectasia mutated (ATM), respectively [110, 111]. Therefore, it is plausible that miR-26a in astrocyte-derived exosomes may function to regulate the surrounding tumor environment. A recent study found that primary breast tumor cells express tumor suppressor PTEN, however this expression of *PTEN* was lost reversibly after tumor cells metastasized into the brain [112]. Astrocyte-derived exosomal miR-19a reversibly mediated the downregulation of *PTEN* expression in cancer cells, thus providing one mechanism for loss of PTEN in tumor cells that enter the brain. Further, miR-19a also increased C-C motif chemokine ligand 2 (CCL2) secretion and recruitment of myeloid cells, thus facilitating changes in the brain microenvironment to promote metastasis [112].

4. The role of astrocytes in brain tumor stem cell biology

An important attribute of brain tumor biology regarding tumor initiation and propagation is the existence of brain tumor stem cells (BTSCs). These cells have been found to, in many ways, resemble adult NSCs that exist in distinct regions of the brain, including the subventricular zone (SVZ) and the subgranular zone (SGZ) [113, 114]. Many groups identified CD133, Nestin, and sex determining region Y-box 2 (SOX2) as markers to isolate NSCs which maintain the essential properties of stem cells (self-renewal and ability to differentiate into multiple progeny) [115–118]. Using the NSC neurosphere culturing method, CD133 and/or CD15 have also been found to be expressed on BTSCs from GBM, medulloblastoma, ependymoma, and astrocytoma tumors [118–120]. Interestingly, Singh et al. (2003) found $CD133^{+}$ cells to be tumor initiating, whereas $CD133^{-}$ cells could not initiate a tumor or self-renew in a mouse xenograft model [118, 121]. The levels of $CD133^{+}$ BTSCs has since been correlated to negative prognoses in gliomas, and have been found to be particularly enriched in recurrent tumors after radiation and chemotherapy [122–124]. These findings highlight the importance of stem cells in the overall initiation, malignancy, and recurrence of brain tumors.

4.1. Astrocytes' direct influence on cancer stem cells

It is clear that BTSCs play an important role in the progression of all brain tumors. Therefore, cells in the microenvironment that influence BTSCs are of interest from a clinical therapy perspective. Interestingly, astrocytes seem to affect normal NSCs and BTSCs quite differently.

While astrocyte secreted factors have been shown to promote neurogenesis of normal adult NSCs, astrocytes within the microenvironment of brain tumors have also been shown to promote stem-like characteristics in BTSCs and enrich the stem cell population, thus worsening the malignancy of such brain tumors [125–128]. GBM $CD133^+$ stem cells co-cultured both directly and indirectly with astrocytes show gene expression signatures known to be involved in GBM invasion and metastasis, such as a disintegrin and metalloproteinase domain-containing protein 10 (*ADAM10*), hyaluronan synthase 2 (*HAS2*), and vascular cell adhesion molecule-1 (*VCAM1*). Interestingly, although there were many overlapping genes in conditions where astrocytes and tumor cells were and were not in direct contact, even the distinct gene expression changes in each condition were still related to tumor cell invasion. This emphasizes the role of astrocytes in GBM invasion, which is one of the most challenging traits of GBM [127]. Indeed, $CD133^+$ GBM cells were found to be more invasive, whereas $CD133^-$ GBM cells did not have the same gene expression and invasion changes [127]. Later, it was shown that indirect co-culture with $CD133^+$ GBM cells and astrocytes resulted in cytokine release from astrocytes that reduced radiosensitivity of the GBM cells; again, this same phenotype and crosstalk with astrocytes was absent in $CD133^-$ GBM cells [128]. Some of the astrocyte secreted cytokines that induced radioresistance include CXCL1, IL-4, IL-6, and CCL7 [128]. These differences suggest that cancer stem (or stem-like) cells signal differently with astrocytes compared to tumor cells lacking stem characteristics. The reverse effect, which is tumor stem cells influencing astrocytes has also been observed in GBM. GBM stem cells provide signals that block the expression of p53 in surrounding astrocytes [129]. P53 is a tumor suppressor often found mutated in many tumors [130], and is classically known for its function in DNA damage response. However, recently p53 has been shown to have non-autonomous cellular functions, particularly in the tumor microenvironment, by influencing secretion of proteins, including ECM proteins [129, 131, 132]. Thus, the interaction between astrocytes and BTSCs are bi-directional and influence each other's development.

In addition to primary brain tumors, cancer stem cells of brain metastatic tumors are also influenced by astrocytes. It has been shown that cyclooxygenase 2 (COX2) is highly expressed in breast cancer brain metastatic cells, which autonomously induces expression of MMP-1 and prostaglandins [133]. While MMP-1 allows for BBB tight junction and basement membrane degradation to aid brain metastasis, prostaglandins are able to activate astrocytes and subsequently increase astrocyte expression of CCL7, which was shown to significantly increase self-renewal and survival of breast cancer stem cells through increased expression of Nanog, a key stem cell regulator [133, 134]. This study provides evidence that astrocytes enrich breast cancer stem cells in brain metastases and aid in their ability to extravasate the BBB.

4.2. Astrocytes as a part of the perivascular niche

Normal NSCs in the SVZ and SGZ are maintained by specialized vascular regions called the perivascular niche (PVN) [135]. The PVN consists of the endothelial cells lining the vasculature, as well as astrocytes, pericytes, macrophages, microglia, fibroblasts, and vascular smooth muscle cells. These cells function and signal together to maintain structure and provide signals to NSCs. Evidence exists which demonstrates the vital role endothelial cells play in maintaining and regulating NSC/BTSCs' survival and differentiation status [136–139]. Astrocytes also play a vital role within the PVN. First and foremost, they play an indirect but obvious role in the structural and chemical maintenance of endothelial cell-BBB phenotypes, as discussed earlier. Studies have shown that BTSCs maintain close proximity to angiogenic regions of the tumor microenvironment, providing evidence that these regions phenocopy the PVN within the SVZ/SGZ to provide enrichment signals to BTSCs [140].

5. Astrocytes as an immune regulator in the tumor microenvironment

The immune system within the CNS is tightly controlled. In addition to the BBB, there are other barriers that maintain the CNS as an immune-privileged system, including the blood-meningeal barriers and the blood-cerebrospinal fluid (CSF) barriers [141, 142]. During homeostasis, these barriers do not allow entry of pathogens or blood-borne immune cells. Only upon CNS injury do some of these cellular barriers become fenestrated to allow for immune cell entrance. Although microglia are thought to be the main regulator of immune responses within the brain, astrocytes (and other cells) also play key roles in this function [143]. A vast amount of work investigating the astrocyte function in either normal or activated state is often related to the regulation of the immune environment in the CNS, as shown in functional studies and astrocyte secretome studies, summarized well by Sofroniew et al. [144–147]. As suggested by Yang et al. (2013), the presence of classical immunological surface molecules, such as major histocompatibility (MHC) antigen and intercellular adhesion molecule-1 (ICAM-1) on astrocytes underlines their importance in CNS immune function [11, 148, 149]. We will discuss next how astrocytes control immune responses to invading tumor cells, and the immune-related concepts associated with this process.

5.1. Immune responses to tumor cell presence

As mentioned in the discussion of astrocytes and tumor cell interactions at the BBB, there have been a few key studies observing the cellular events that take place when metastatic cells extravasate into the brain parenchyma [56, 57]. From these studies, it is known that astrocytes are the first to respond to extravasating metastatic tumor cells entering the brain, followed by microglia [56]. Regardless of whether a CNS tumor is primary or metastatic, microglia and astrocytes control the immune response; therefore, it is upon their activation that other immune cells, such as macrophages or lymphocytes, may infiltrate [144–146, 150]. Activated astrocytes secrete pro-inflammatory molecules such as CXCL12, CCI2, Il15, CCL8, and CXCL1, all of which are known to regulate recruitment, activation and proliferation of T-cells, B-cells, or natural killer (NK) cells [144–146].

As it is often seen with any local or systemic inflammation, CNS immune responses can often persist or be dysregulated by tumor cells to become pathogenic. Many of these signaling responses are mediated by astrocytes. For example, Valiente et al. [151] reported that astrocytes produce FasL and plasmin ligands as defense mechanisms to kill brain-invading tumor cells. In response, tumor cells secrete serpins, which thwart the lethal action of plasmin [151]. Thus, Fas-mediated tumor cell apoptosis is blocked, leading to tumor survival. Other cells, such as endothelial cells, in the brain microenvironment are also co-opted, which is facilitated by up-regulation of L1 cell adhesion molecules (L1CAM). All these mechanisms work together to initiate brain metastasis [151].

Astrocytes are also known to function in immunosuppression. This is accomplished by downregulating the pro-inflammatory cytokine TNF-α in surrounding microglia, and suppressing the antigen presenting abilities of various immune cells by downregulating their expression of MHCII and CD80 [152, 153]. Additionally, activated astrocytes can co-localize and induce apoptosis in T-cells attempting to infiltrate the brain parenchyma by expression of the "death ligand," CD95L, which binds the receptor on T-cells [152, 154].

5.2. Reactive Astrogliosis

Arguably, the most important feature of astrocytes in relation to their immune function is their ability to activate, a process called reactive astrogliosis. What determines whether an astrocyte is "activated" or not has not been clearly defined, however Sofroniew summarized the existing research into four key features. First, reactive astrogliosis is a spectrum of molecular, cellular, and functional changes among astrocytes in response to CNS injury of many kinds [147]. Second, the changes can vary in severity and the response can be sequential and/or progressive. Third, the changes are regulated by intra- and inter-cellular signals and lastly, signaling events can be both gain and loss of function in nature, resulting in both beneficial and detrimental outcomes [147, 155]. In other words, reactive astrogliosis is spectral in nature; the triggers can vary and therefore the "activation" or response can vary and is context dependent, which is also true in regards to how reactive astrocytes affect tumor progression and/or tumor death.

The activation responses can be as small as a transient upregulation of GFAP, to permanent structural changes in the brain from a process called glial scar formation. Scar formation occurs when astrocytes proliferate and overlap to a point that causes dense, compact barriers around necrotic tissue [147, 156]. In between these two extremes, other phenotypic changes that occur include hypertrophy of the cell body and processes, a vast array of gene expression changes, and varying degrees of proliferation up to the point of scar formation. Some of the chemical activators of astrocytes known to be secreted by or induced by tumor cells include EGF (glioblastoma and medulloblastoma), TGF-α (medulloblastoma), receptor activator of nuclear factor kappa-B (NFκB) ligand (RANKL) (glioma), macrophage migration inhibitory factor (MIF), interleukin-8 (IL-8), and plasminogen activator inhibitor-1 (PAI-1) (lung cancer metastases) [11, 157–160].

In addition to chemical activation, astrocytes can also be activated by tumor cells mechanically. Although extremely abundant, astrocytes hold a highly regulated, non-overlapping distribution that plays an important role in morphology and contact-dependent inhibition of proliferation [11, 61]. This distribution and homeostasis is mediated by contact inhibition and adherens junctions. Therefore, mechanical disruption occurs when processes such as migration and/or proliferation of surrounding cells is initiated. Such mechanical signals could come potentially emerge from tumor cells, subsequently triggering astrocyte activation via disruption of these cell surface complexes such as cadherins and β-catenin [161, 162]. The genes activated by β-catenin signaling are regulatory and often lead to proliferation and migration [11, 163]. Interestingly, Yang et al. (2012) found this contact initiated activation of astrocytes to parallel what occurs in the transformation of astrocytomas, further coupling the process of astrocyte activation and tumor progression [162].

6. Therapeutic opportunities for cancer emerging from astrocyte-tumor cross talk

As stated previously, homeostasis in brain environment is key for the functionality of the brain, and therefore key checkpoints, such as the BBB, are responsible for maintaining homeostasis [30]. The BBB also prevents access of key drugs into the brain for targeting tumor cells. Any surgical intervention in the brain clearly has quality of life considerations, and does not offer complete disease-free state. Therefore, it is of importance to prevent tumor cells from entering the brain or block the target routes and underlying mechanisms used by tumors to circumvent checkpoints. It is worth noting that the regions of the brain which are free from the protections of the junctional characteristics of the BBB, such as the stroma of the choroid plexus and area postrema have increased vascular permeability which can be problematic, and therefore must be considered when trying to block tumor cell entrance into the brain [30].

As we know, astrocytes are capable of signaling to trigger tumor cell (breast, lung, skin, and brain) migration, invasion and metastasis *in vivo* [88, 95, 127, 160]. There are many targets in the brain microenvironment that provide effective intervention strategies for metastasis, and is reviewed elsewhere [164]. Here, we will discuss targets and mechanisms at the signaling interface of tumor cells and astrocytes that offer fresh perspective on intervention strategies.

6.1. Enzyme targets

As discussed earlier, we and others have identified astrocyte secreted MMP-2, MMP-9, and MMP-1 to promote tumor progression, and blocking them with broad spectrum MMP inhibitors does influence tumor metastasis in pre-clinical models [95, 96, 165–167]. Interestingly, MMP-1 was one of 21 MMPs that showed clinical significance in regards to breast cancer brain metastasis, and expression analysis of brain-seeking triple negative breast cancer clonal cells confirm MMP-1 and MMP-9 as potential targets [133, 168]. Therefore, these studies suggest either MMPs or the underlying pathways that regulate their expression as pharmaceutical targets. Given that targeting MMPs in the past using first generation MMP inhibitors resulted in disappointing results in the clinic, we also suggest that next generation, highly-specific MMP inhibitors, applied locally, could be effective new strategies to consider in preventing further growth and movement of tumor cells to a second location in the brain [169].

6.2. Gap junction protein targets

Astrocytes are co-opted to up-regulate survival genes in tumor cells and induce protection from chemotherapy [65]. Downregulation of the astrocyte-initiated survival gene expression in tumor cells will render tumor cells sensitive to chemotherapy [65]. This chemoprevention role, however, appears to be contact dependent, utilizing gap junctions to mediate the changes in tumor cells. Previously, gap junction proteins Cx43 and Cx26 were utilized by breast cancer and melanoma cells to initiate brain metastatic lesion formation in cohort with the vasculature [170]. Indeed, patient data analysis revealed increased cancer recurrence and metastasis with increased expression of Cx26 and Cx43 in primary melanoma and breast tumor cells. The recent work done by Chen et al. shows that brain metastatic breast and lung cancer cells initiate contact with astrocytes through gap junctions, which produces a signaling response (discussed in detail earlier in the chapter) resulting in chemoresistance [74]. Bio-available modulators of gap junctions, meclofenamate and tonabersat, could influence this paracrine signaling loop, and thus could be proposed for treatment of established brain metastases [74].

6.3. PTEN, exosomes and miRNA targeting

Breast cancer metastases often show common alterations in the EGFR and HER2 driven pathways, both of which are regulated by *PTEN* gene [171]. PTEN is mutated in human brain, breast and prostate cancer, and loss of PTEN was found in a substantial portion of breast cancer brain metastases samples significantly associated with triple negative breast cancer [172, 173]. Interestingly, PTEN loss promotes a feedback loop between tumor cells and glial cells, which contributes to disease progression. We already know one mechanism in which *PTEN* expression is lost; through the targeting and degradation of transcript by miR-26a and miR-19a from astrocyte secreted exosomes [110–112].

Blocking the astrocytes from secreting the PTEN-targeting microRNA rescues the PTEN loss and importantly suppresses brain metastasis *in vivo* [112, 174]. Similarly, miR-200 containing extracellular vesicles, which regulates the mesenchymal to epithelial transition, can be transferred from metastatic cells to non-metastatic cells leading to promotion of metastasis [175]. Therefore, collectively, approaches that promote PTEN expression or prevent loss of PTEN expression has the potential to influence metastatic outcome in the clinic for select cancers such as breast, brain and prostate cancer.

6.4. Adaptations (environment)

The finding that breast cancer cells take up a neuronal phenotype when they are in the brain suggests co-evolution adaptive mechanisms associated with metastatic cells and their microenvironment. The variable PTEN expression in metastatic tumor cells in response to different organ environments suggests a genetic component that drives co-evolution adaptive behavior between metastatic cells and their microenvironment [176]. Brain homing MDA-MB-231 cells secrete bone morphogenic protein-2 (BMP-2), which mediates the differentiation of NSCs into astrocytes; subsequently, downregulation of BMP-2 in the brain homing tumor cells diminished their engraftment and colonization abilities [176]. Further, when co-cultured with NSCs, primary (non-brain homing) MDA-MB-231 cells fail to proliferate over 15 days, but brain homing MDA-MB-231 cells escaped this growth inhibition, and proliferation occurred in parallel with NSCs' differentiation into astrocytes [176]. This suggests that both the brain homing MDA-MB-231 cells' adaptive phenotype and the NSCs' differentiation into astrocytes are codependent, meaning the brain homing MDA-MB-231 cells require astrocytic signals to survive. This group extended these observations further and demonstrated that human breast cancer cells found in the brain and not in the primary tumor, upregulated γ-aminobutyric acid (GABA) pathway genes, and displayed GABAergic phenotypes that are similar to neuronal cells [177]. This phenotype offers a proliferative advantage to tumor cells because GABA is catabolized into succinate which generates NADH, a critical metabolite necessary for tumor cell sustenance. It is noteworthy that GABA is abundant in the brain, and perhaps tumor cells have adapted to this environment that gives them a proliferative advantage. Of the different cells in the brain, neurons, because of their function, require the majority of ATP [178]. As such, astrocytes expend less energy, and secrete lactate that is generated by glycolysis [179]. This evolutionary adaptation feature of tumors and their reliance on astrocytic signals open up avenues for targeting; several inhibitors of metabolites such as GABA are available and could be repurposed for brain metastases treatment. Of course, more research and context-specific treatment of such modalities will be needed.

6.5. CNS tumor immunotherapies and astrocytes

The emergence and success of immunotherapy techniques in many blood, lymph, and some solid tumors is bringing groundbreaking and exciting work in the cancer research field [180]. Currently, researchers are now looking for ways to modulate this therapy so it can be applied to more tumors, including tumors in the CNS [141]. Importantly, the effectiveness of strategies such as vaccine and immune checkpoint therapies rely on a strong response and presence of tumor infiltrating immune cells for antigen presentation, which is low in most brain tumors due to the limited presence of resident immune cells within the brain [141, 181]. Some strategies to stimulate the immune response, such as adjuvants or tetanus and diphtheria boosters with vaccine administration have increased effectiveness [141, 182, 183]. As discussed earlier, astrocytes play an important role in immunosuppression in the brain tumor microenvironment, however this function has not yet been targeted. Therefore, one could postulate investigation of a combination therapy targeting an immunosuppressive factor(s) produced by astrocytes as an additional option worthy of research.

Much excitement in the immune therapy world surrounds the programmed death ligand-1 (PD-L1), an immune checkpoint signal that is immunosuppressive by binding its cognate receptor, programmed death-1 (PD-1) receptor, expressed on T-cells to induce apoptosis [184]. Targeting and blocking PD-L1 or PD-1 with antibody therapies has been an effective treatment for several cancers [185, 186]. It has been shown that GBM tumors highly express PD-L1, in addition to infiltrating microglia [187, 188]. Normal astrocytes have also been found to highly express PD-L1, however astrocyte expression of PD-L1 in a tumor setting has not yet been investigated [189]. Future work investigating astrocyte (normal and reactive) expression of PD-L1 is needed and will provide mechanistic hypothesis to current clinical trial that utilizes nivolumab, a PD-1 antibody, in combination with temozolomide for treatment GBM. PD-L1 has also been investigated in metastatic brain tumors, however expression and correlation to outcomes appear to be tumor dependent, leading to conflicting reports on whether PD-L1 expression correlates to a positive or negative prognosis, therefore more research is needed [190–192].

7. Conclusions

Until recently, the complexities of astrocyte signaling and influence on human pathologies were not fully appreciated in the literature, especially in regards to astrocytes' influence on tumor biology. Cancer researchers began recognizing that tumor cells themselves may not be the sole perpetrators in tumor initiation and progression, and the resulting research has made it increasingly clear that tumor cells and the host environment they reside in are constantly communicating to facilitate growth, sustenance and metastasis [193, 194]. To facilitate tumor progression, the host environment is either co-opted by tumor cells or defense mechanisms of host cells are overcome by the tumor cells. Whether astrocytes are "friends" or "foes" of tumor cells is a matter of context, as evidence exists for both scenarios. **Figure 1** depicts the balancing act of these functions, in addition to the outside factors which dictate them, eventually determining the fate of the respective tumor cells and tumor as a whole. There are many known (and unknown) factors that must be considered in understanding CNS tumors and their relation to astrocytes. We summarize some of the tumor promoting mechanisms of astrocytes, which have been highlighted in this chapter (**Figure 2**), effecting both primary brain tumors and secondary brain metastases. The diversity of astrocyte mechanism modalities will hopefully bring about unique and novel intervention strategies, some of which were also discussed in this chapter. In conclusion, astrocytes are a critical cell type that participate in various physiological and pathological conditions, and their role in the history of tumor progression is beginning to be appreciated.

Acknowledgements

We thank lab members of the Developmental Vascular Biology Program for their input during numerous presentations of this subject. EG is supported by Department of Pediatrics, and Children's Research Institute. LW is partly supported by Department of Obstetrics and Gynecology funds, and Department of Defense grant # BC161839 and HL033833. DH is supported by funds from VA hospital and NIH grant HL033833. RR is partly supported by NIH grant HL123338, HL112639, HL033833, endowment funds from OBGYN and start-up funds from Department of Pediatrics and Children's Research Institute.

Author details

Emily Gronseth[1], Ling Wang[2], David R. Harder[3] and Ramani Ramchandran[1,2]*

*Address all correspondence to: rramchan@mcw.edu

1 Department of Pediatrics, Children's Research Institute, Clinical and Translational Science Institute, Medical College of Wisconsin, Milwaukee, WI, USA

2 Obstetrics and Gynecology, Children's Research Institute, Clinical and Translational Science Institute, Medical College of Wisconsin, Milwaukee, WI, USA

3 Physiology, Children's Research Institute, Clinical and Translational Science Institute, Medical College of Wisconsin, Milwaukee, WI, USA

References

[1] Sun D, Jakobs TC. Structural remodeling of astrocytes in the injured CNS. The Neuroscientist. 2012;**18**(6):567-588

[2] Liu C, Zong H. Developmental origins of brain tumors. Current Opinion in Neurobiology. 2012;**22**(5):844-849

[3] Lee JC, Mayer-Proschel M, Rao MS. Gliogenesis in the central nervous system. Glia. 2000;**30**(2):105-121

[4] Wiese S, Karus M, Faissner A. Astrocytes as a source for extracellular matrix molecules and cytokines. Frontiers in Pharmacology. 2012;**3**:120

[5] Lillien L. Changes in retinal cell fate induced by overexpression of EGF receptor. Nature. 1995;**377**(6545):158-162

[6] Kornblum HI, Hussain R, Wiesen J, Miettinen P, Zurcher SD, Chow K, Derynck R, Werb Z. Abnormal astrocyte development and neuronal death in mice lacking the epidermal growth factor receptor. Journal of Neuroscience Research. 1998;**53**(6):697-717

[7] Sibilia M, Steinbach JP, Stingl L, Aguzzi A, Wagner EF. A strain-independent postnatal neurodegeneration in mice lacking the EGF receptor. The EMBO Journal. 1998;**17**(3):719-731

[8] Collins VP. Gliomas. Cancer Surveys. 1998;**32**:37-51

[9] Rasheed BK, Wiltshire RN, Bigner SH, Bigner DD. Molecular pathogenesis of malignant gliomas. Current Opinion in Oncology. 1999;**11**(3):162-167

[10] Warren KE. Diffuse intrinsic pontine glioma: poised for progress. Frontiers in Oncology. 2012;**2**:205

[11] Yang C, Rahimpour S, AC Y, Lonser RR, Zhuang Z. Regulation and dysregulation of astrocyte activation and implications in tumor formation. Cellular and Molecular Life Sciences. 2013;**70**(22):4201-4211

[12] Tezel G, Hernandez MR, Wax MB. Vitro evaluation of reactive astrocyte migration, a component of tissue remodeling in glaucomatous optic nerve head. Glia. 2001;**34**(3):178-189

[13] Yang H, Cheng XP, Li JW, Yao Q, Ju G. De-differentiation response of cultured astrocytes to injury induced by scratch or conditioned culture medium of scratch-insulted astrocytes. Cellular and Molecular Neurobiology. 2009;**29**(4):455-473

[14] Wechsler-Reya R, Scott MP. The developmental biology of brain tumors. Annual Review of Neuroscience. 2001;**24**:385-428

[15] Altieri R, Agnoletti A, Quattrucci F, Garbossa D, Calamo Specchia FM, Bozzaro M, Fornaro R, Mencarani C, Lanotte M, Spaziante R, et al. Molecular biology of gliomas: Present and future challenges. Translational medicine @ UniSa. 2014;**10**:29-37

[16] Libermann TA, Nusbaum HR, Razon N, Kris R, Lax I, Soreq H, Whittle N, Waterfield MD, Ullrich A, Schlessinger J. Amplification and overexpression of the EGF receptor gene in primary human glioblastomas. Journal of Cell Science. Supplement. 1985;**3**:161-172

[17] Wong AJ, Bigner SH, Bigner DD, Kinzler KW, Hamilton SR, Vogelstein B. Increased expression of the epidermal growth factor receptor gene in malignant gliomas is invariably associated with gene amplification. Proceedings of the National Academy of Sciences of the United States of America. 1987;**84**(19):6899-6903

[18] Prigent SA, Lemoine NR. The type 1 (EGFR-related) family of growth factor receptors and their ligands. Progress in Growth Factor Research. 1992;**4**(1):1-24

[19] Garrett TP, McKern NM, Lou M, Elleman TC, Adams TE, Lovrecz GO, Zhu HJ, Walker F, Frenkel MJ, Hoyne PA, et al. Crystal structure of a truncated epidermal growth factor receptor extracellular domain bound to transforming growth factor alpha. Cell. 2002;**110**(6): 763-773

[20] Biernat W, Debiec-Rychter M, Liberski PP. Mutations of TP53, amplification of EGFR, MDM2 and CDK4, and deletions of CDKN2A in malignant astrocytomas. Polish Journal of Pathology: Official Journal of the Polish Society of Pathologists. 1998;**49**(4):267-271

[21] Henson JW, Schnitker BL, Correa KM, von Deimling A, Fassbender F, HJ X, Benedict WF, Yandell DW, Louis DN. The retinoblastoma gene is involved in malignant progression of astrocytomas. Annals of Neurology. 1994;**36**(5):714-721

[22] Ichimura K, Schmidt EE, Goike HM, Collins VP. Human glioblastomas with no alterations of the CDKN2A (p16INK4A, MTS1) and CDK4 genes have frequent mutations of the retinoblastoma gene. Oncogene. 1996;**13**(5):1065-1072

[23] Simon M, Koster G, Menon AG, Schramm J. Functional evidence for a role of combined CDKN2A (p16-p14(ARF))/CDKN2B (p15) gene inactivation in malignant gliomas. Acta Neuropathologica. 1999;**98**(5):444-452

[24] Yan H, Parsons DW, Jin G, McLendon R, Rasheed BA, Yuan W, Kos I, Batinic-Haberle I, Jones S, Riggins GJ, et al. IDH1 and IDH2 mutations in gliomas. The New England Journal of Medicine. 2009;**360**(8):765-773

[25] Landis SH, Murray T, Bolden S, Wingo PA. Cancer statistics, 1999. CA: a Cancer Journal for Clinicians. 1999;**49**(1):8-31 31

[26] Langley RR, Fidler IJ. The seed and soil hypothesis revisited–the role of tumor-stroma interactions in metastasis to different organs. International Journal of Cancer. 2011;**128**(11): 2527-2535

[27] Daneman R, Prat A. The blood-brain barrier. Cold Spring Harbor Perspectives in Biology. 2015;**7**(1):a020412

[28] Coomber BL, Stewart PA. Morphometric analysis of CNS microvascular endothelium. Microvascular Research. 1985;**30**(1):99-115

[29] Mittapalli RK, Manda VK, Adkins CE, Geldenhuys WJ, Lockman PR. Exploiting nutrient transporters at the blood-brain barrier to improve brain distribution of small molecules. Therapeutic Delivery. 2010;**1**(6):775-784

[30] Moody DM. The blood-brain barrier and blood-cerebral spinal fluid barrier. Seminars in Cardiothoracic and Vascular Anesthesia. 2006;**10**(2):128-131

[31] Louveau A, Smirnov I, Keyes TJ, Eccles JD, Rouhani SJ, Peske JD, Derecki NC, Castle D, Mandell JW, Lee KS, et al. Structural and functional features of central nervous system lymphatic vessels. Nature. 2015;**523**(7560):337-341

[32] Nayak L, Lee EQ, Wen PY. Epidemiology of brain metastases. Current Oncology Reports. 2012;**14**(1):48-54

[33] Wilhelm I, Fazakas C, Molnar K, Vegh AG, Hasko J, Krizbai IA. Foe or friend? Janus-faces of the neurovascular unit in the formation of brain metastases. Journal of Cerebral Blood Flow and Metabolism. 2017. 271678X17732025

[34] Cheng X, Hung MC. Breast cancer brain metastases. Cancer Metastasis Reviews. 2007;**26** (3–4):635-643

[35] Bravo Marques JM. Treatment of brain metastases in patients with HER2+ breast cancer. Advances in Therapy. 2009;**26**(Suppl 1):S18-S26

[36] Paget S. The distribution of secondary growths in cancer of the breast. Cancer Metastasis Reviews 1989. 1889;**8**(2):98-101

[37] Bos PD, Zhang XH, Nadal C, Shu W, Gomis RR, Nguyen DX, Minn AJ, van de Vijver MJ, Gerald WL, Foekens JA, et al. Genes that mediate breast cancer metastasis to the brain. Nature. 2009;**459**(7249):1005-1009

[38] Kikuchi T, Daigo Y, Ishikawa N, Katagiri T, Tsunoda T, Yoshida S, Nakamura Y. Expression profiles of metastatic brain tumor from lung adenocarcinomas on cDNA microarray. International Journal of Oncology. 2006;**28**(4):799-805

[39] Grinberg-Rashi H, Ofek E, Perelman M, Skarda J, Yaron P, Hajduch M, Jacob-Hirsch J, Amariglio N, Krupsky M, Simansky DA, et al. The expression of three genes in primary non-small cell lung cancer is associated with metastatic spread to the brain. Clinical Cancer Research: An Official Journal of the American Association for Cancer Research. 2009;**15**(5):1755-1761

[40] Hamilton R, Krauze M, Romkes M, Omolo B, Konstantinopoulos P, Reinhart T, Harasymczuk M, Wang Y, Lin Y, Ferrone S, et al. Pathologic and gene expression features of metastatic melanomas to the brain. Cancer. 2013;**119**(15):2737-2746

[41] Morita K, Furuse M, Fujimoto K, Tsukita S. Claudin multigene family encoding four-transmembrane domain protein components of tight junction strands. Proceedings of the National Academy of Sciences of the United States of America. 1999;**96**(2): 511-516

[42] McCarthy KM, Skare IB, Stankewich MC, Furuse M, Tsukita S, Rogers RA, Lynch RD, Schneeberger EE. Occludin is a functional component of the tight junction. Journal of Cell Science. 1996;**109**(Pt 9):2287-2298

[43] Taddei A, Giampietro C, Conti A, Orsenigo F, Breviario F, Pirazzoli V, Potente M, Daly C, Dimmeler S, Dejana E. Endothelial adherens junctions control tight junctions by VE-cadherin-mediated upregulation of claudin-5. Nature Cell Biology. 2008;**10**(8):923-934

[44] Stevenson BR, Siliciano JD, Mooseker MS, Goodenough DA. Identification of ZO-1: A high molecular weight polypeptide associated with the tight junction (zonula occludens) in a variety of epithelia. The Journal of Cell Biology. 1986;**103**(3):755-766

[45] Gumbiner B, Lowenkopf T, Apatira D. Identification of a 160-kDa polypeptide that binds to the tight junction protein ZO-1. Proceedings of the National Academy of Sciences of the United States of America. 1991;**88**(8):3460-3464

[46] Neuhaus J, Risau W, Wolburg H. Induction of blood-brain barrier characteristics in bovine brain endothelial cells by rat astroglial cells in transfilter coculture. Annals of the New York Academy of Sciences. 1991;**633**:578-580

[47] Prat A, Biernacki K, Wosik K, Antel JP. Glial cell influence on the human blood-brain barrier. Glia. 2001;**36**(2):145-155

[48] Tao-Cheng JH, Nagy Z, Brightman MW. Tight junctions of brain endothelium in vitro are enhanced by astroglia. The Journal of Neuroscience: The Official Journal of the Society for Neuroscience. 1987;**7**(10):3293-3299

[49] Alvarez JI, Dodelet-Devillers A, Kebir H, Ifergan I, Fabre PJ, Terouz S, Sabbagh M, Wosik K, Bourbonniere L, Bernard M, et al. The hedgehog pathway promotes blood-brain barrier integrity and CNS immune quiescence. Science. 2011;**334**(6063):1727-1731

[50] Runkle EA, Rice SJ, Qi J, Masser D, Antonetti DA, Winslow MM, Mu D. Occludin is a direct target of thyroid transcription factor-1 (TTF-1/NKX2-)1. The Journal of Biological Chemistry. 2012;**287**(34):28790-28801

[51] Lavoie JL, Sigmund CD. Minireview: Overview of the renin-angiotensin system–an endocrine and paracrine system. Endocrinology. 2003;**144**(6):2179-2183

[52] Reuss B, Dono R, Unsicker K. Functions of fibroblast growth factor (FGF)-2 and FGF-5 in astroglial differentiation and blood-brain barrier permeability: Evidence from mouse mutants. The Journal of Neuroscience: The Official Journal of the Society for Neuroscience. 2003;**23**(16):6404-6412

[53] Igarashi Y, Utsumi H, Chiba H, Yamada-Sasamori Y, Tobioka H, Kamimura Y, Furuuchi K, Kokai Y, Nakagawa T, Mori M, et al. Glial cell line-derived neurotrophic factor induces barrier function of endothelial cells forming the blood-brain barrier. Biochemical and Biophysical Research Communications. 1999;**261**(1):108-112

[54] Dohgu S, Yamauchi A, Takata F, Naito M, Tsuruo T, Higuchi S, Sawada Y, Kataoka Y. Transforming growth factor-beta1 upregulates the tight junction and P-glycoprotein of

brain microvascular endothelial cells. Cellular and Molecular Neurobiology. 2004;**24**(3):491-497

[55] Mizee MR, Wooldrik D, Lakeman KA, van het Hof B, Drexhage JA, Geerts D, Bugiani M, Aronica E, Mebius RE, Prat A, et al. Retinoic acid induces blood-brain barrier development. The Journal of Neuroscience: The Official Journal of the Society for Neuroscience. 2013;**33**(4):1660-1671

[56] Lorger M, Felding-Habermann B. Capturing changes in the brain microenvironment during initial steps of breast cancer brain metastasis. The American Journal of Pathology. 2010;**176**(6):2958-2971

[57] Kienast Y, von Baumgarten L, Fuhrmann M, Klinkert WE, Goldbrunner R, Herms J, Winkler F. Real-time imaging reveals the single steps of brain metastasis formation. Nature Medicine. 2010;**16**(1):116-122

[58] Garcia-Segura LM, Chowen JA, Duenas M, Torres-Aleman I, Naftolin F. Gonadal steroids as promoters of neuro-glial plasticity. Psychoneuroendocrinology. 1994;**19**(5–7):445-453

[59] Blutstein T, Baab PJ, Zielke HR, Mong JA. Hormonal modulation of amino acid neurotransmitter metabolism in the arcuate nucleus of the adult female rat: A novel action of estradiol. Endocrinology. 2009;**150**(7):3237-3244

[60] Haydon PG, Blendy J, Moss SJ, Rob Jackson F. Astrocytic control of synaptic transmission and plasticity: A target for drugs of abuse? Neuropharmacology. 2009;**56**(Suppl 1):83-90

[61] Bushong EA, Martone ME, Jones YZ, Ellisman MH. Protoplasmic astrocytes in CA1 stratum radiatum occupy separate anatomical domains. The Journal of Neuroscience: The Official Journal of the Society for Neuroscience. 2002;**22**(1):183-192

[62] Tabernero A, Medina JM, Giaume C. Glucose metabolism and proliferation in glia: Role of astrocytic gap junctions. Journal of Neurochemistry. 2006;**99**(4):1049-1061

[63] Sin WC, Aftab Q, Bechberger JF, Leung JH, Chen H, Naus CC. Astrocytes promote glioma invasion via the gap junction protein connexin43. Oncogene. 2016;**35**(12):1504-1516

[64] Lin Q, Balasubramanian K, Fan D, Kim SJ, Guo L, Wang H, Bar-Eli M, Aldape KD, Fidler IJ. Reactive astrocytes protect melanoma cells from chemotherapy by sequestering intracellular calcium through gap junction communication channels. Neoplasia. 2010;**12**(9):748-754

[65] Kim SJ, Kim JS, Park ES, Lee JS, Lin Q, Langley RR, Maya M, He J, Kim SW, Weihua Z, et al. Astrocytes upregulate survival genes in tumor cells and induce protection from chemotherapy. Neoplasia. 2011;**13**(3):286-298

[66] Giaume C, McCarthy KD. Control of gap-junctional communication in astrocytic networks. Trends in Neurosciences. 1996;**19**(8):319-325

[67] Rozental R, Giaume C, Spray DC. Gap junctions in the nervous system. Brain Research. Brain Research Reviews. 2000;**32**(1):11-15

[68] Theodoric N, Bechberger JF, Naus CC, Sin WC. Role of gap junction protein connexin43 in astrogliosis induced by brain injury. PLoS One. 2012;**7**(10):e47311

[69] Hossain MZ, Peeling J, Sutherland GR, Hertzberg EL, Nagy JI. Ischemia-induced cellular redistribution of the astrocytic gap junctional protein connexin43 in rat brain. Brain Research. 1994;**652**(2):311-322

[70] Goldberg GS, Lampe PD, Nicholson BJ. Selective transfer of endogenous metabolites through gap junctions composed of different connexins. Nature Cell Biology. 1999;**1**(7): 457-459

[71] De Bock M, Decrock E, Wang N, Bol M, Vinken M, Bultynck G, Leybaert L. The dual face of connexin-based astroglial Ca(2+) communication: A key player in brain physiology and a prime target in pathology. Biochimica et Biophysica Acta. 2014;**1843**(10):2211-2232

[72] Scemes E, Suadicani SO, Spray DC. Intercellular communication in spinal cord astrocytes: Fine tuning between gap junctions and P2 nucleotide receptors in calcium wave propagation. The Journal of Neuroscience: The Official Journal of the Society for Neuroscience. 2000;**20**(4):1435-1445

[73] Toyofuku T, Yabuki M, Otsu K, Kuzuya T, Hori M, Tada M. Intercellular calcium signaling via gap junction in connexin-43-transfected cells. The Journal of Biological Chemistry. 1998;**273**(3):1519-1528

[74] Chen Q, Boire A, Jin X, Valiente M, Er EE, Lopez-Soto A, Jacob L, Patwa R, Shah H, Xu K, et al. Carcinoma-astrocyte gap junctions promote brain metastasis by cGAMP transfer. Nature. 2016;**533**(7604):493-498

[75] Edsall LC, Spiegel S. Enzymatic measurement of sphingosine 1-phosphate. Analytical Biochemistry. 1999;**272**(1):80-86

[76] Van Brocklyn JR, Jackson CA, Pearl DK, Kotur MS, Snyder PJ, Prior TW. Sphingosine kinase-1 expression correlates with poor survival of patients with glioblastoma multiforme: Roles of sphingosine kinase isoforms in growth of glioblastoma cell lines. Journal of Neuropathology and Experimental Neurology. 2005;**64**(8):695-705

[77] Kaur B, Khwaja FW, Severson EA, Matheny SL, Brat DJ, Van Meir EG. Hypoxia and the hypoxia-inducible-factor pathway in glioma growth and angiogenesis. Neuro-Oncology. 2005;**7**(2):134-153

[78] Banisadr G, Skrzydelski D, Kitabgi P, Rostene W, Parsadaniantz SM. Highly regionalized distribution of stromal cell-derived factor-1/CXCL12 in adult rat brain: Constitutive expression in cholinergic, dopaminergic and vasopressinergic neurons. The European Journal of Neuroscience. 2003;**18**(6):1593-1606

[79] Sierra A, Price JE, Garcia-Ramirez M, Mendez O, Lopez L, Fabra A. Astrocyte-derived cytokines contribute to the metastatic brain specificity of breast cancer cells. Laboratory Investigation; A Journal of Technical Methods and Pathology. 1997;**77**(4):357-368

[80] Gril B, Palmieri D, Qian Y, Anwar T, Liewehr DJ, Steinberg SM, Andreu Z, Masana D, Fernandez P, Steeg PS, et al. Pazopanib inhibits the activation of PDGFRbeta-expressing

astrocytes in the brain metastatic microenvironment of breast cancer cells. The American Journal of Pathology. 2013;**182**(6):2368-2379

[81] Huang H, Colella S, Kurrer M, Yonekawa Y, Kleihues P, Ohgaki H. Gene expression profiling of low-grade diffuse astrocytomas by cDNA arrays. Cancer Research. 2000;**60**(24): 6868-6874

[82] Schwab JM, Postler E, Nguyen TD, Mittelbronn M, Meyermann R, Schluesener HJ. Connective tissue growth factor is expressed by a subset of reactive astrocytes in human cerebral infarction. Neuropathology and Applied Neurobiology. 2000;**26**(5): 434-440

[83] Halliday JJ, Holland EC. Connective tissue growth factor and the parallels between brain injury and brain tumors. Journal of the National Cancer Institute. 2011;**103**(15): 1141-1143

[84] Schultz C, Lemke N, Ge S, Golembieski WA, Rempel SA. Secreted protein acidic and rich in cysteine promotes glioma invasion and delays tumor growth in vivo. Cancer Research. 2002;**62**(21):6270-6277

[85] Chetty C, Dontula R, Ganji PN, Gujrati M, Lakka SS. SPARC expression induces cell cycle arrest via STAT3 signaling pathway in medulloblastoma cells. Biochemical and Biophysical Research Communications. 2012;**417**(2):874-879

[86] Bhoopathi P, Chetty C, Dontula R, Gujrati M, Dinh DH, Rao JS, Lakka SS. SPARC stimulates neuronal differentiation of medulloblastoma cells via the Notch1/STAT3 pathway. Cancer Research. 2011;**71**(14):4908-4919

[87] Chetty C, Dontula R, Gujrati M, Dinh DH, Lakka SS. Blockade of SOX4 mediated DNA repair by SPARC enhances radioresponse in medulloblastoma. Cancer Letters. 2012;**323**(2): 188-198

[88] Marchetti D, Li J, Shen R. Astrocytes contribute to the brain-metastatic specificity of melanoma cells by producing heparanase. Cancer Research. 2000;**60**(17):4767-4770

[89] Iozzo RV, Murdoch AD. Proteoglycans of the extracellular environment: Clues from the gene and protein side offer novel perspectives in molecular diversity and function. FASEB Journal: Official Publication of the Federation of American Societies for Experimental Biology. 1996;**10**(5):598-614

[90] Irimura T, Nakajima M, Nicolson GL. Chemically modified heparins as inhibitors of heparan sulfate specific endo-beta-glucuronidase (heparanase) of metastatic melanoma cells. Biochemistry. 1986;**25**(18):5322-5328

[91] Condorelli DF, Dell'Albani P, Mudo G, Timmusk T, Belluardo N. Expression of neurotrophins and their receptors in primary astroglial cultures: Induction by cyclic AMP-elevating agents. Journal of Neurochemistry. 1994;**63**(2):509-516

[92] Sbai O, Ould-Yahoui A, Ferhat L, Gueye Y, Bernard A, Charrat E, Mehanna A, Risso JJ, Chauvin JP, Fenouillet E, et al. Differential vesicular distribution and trafficking of MMP-2, MMP-9, and their inhibitors in astrocytes. Glia. 2010;**58**(3):344-366

[93] Gottschall PE, Yu X, Bing B. Increased production of gelatinase B (matrix metalloproteinase-9) and interleukin-6 by activated rat microglia in culture. Journal of Neuroscience Research. 1995;**42**(3):335-342

[94] Wu H, Du J, Zheng Q. Expression of MMP-1 in cartilage and synovium of experimentally induced rabbit ACLT traumatic osteoarthritis: Immunohistochemical study. Rheumatology International. 2008;**29**(1):31-36

[95] Wang L, Cossette SM, Rarick KR, Gershan J, Dwinell MB, Harder DR, Ramchandran R. Astrocytes directly influence tumor cell invasion and metastasis in vivo. PLoS One. 2013;**8**(12):e80933

[96] Mendes O, Kim HT, Lungu G, Stoica G. MMP2 role in breast cancer brain metastasis development and its regulation by TIMP2 and ERK1/2. Clinical & Experimental Metastasis. 2007;**24**(5):341-351

[97] Colombo M, Raposo G, Thery C. Biogenesis, secretion, and intercellular interactions of exosomes and other extracellular vesicles. Annual Review of Cell and Developmental Biology. 2014;**30**:255-289

[98] Simons M, Raposo G. Exosomes–Vesicular carriers for intercellular communication. Current Opinion in Cell Biology. 2009;**21**(4):575-581

[99] Camussi G, Deregibus MC, Bruno S, Cantaluppi V, Biancone L. Exosomes/microvesicles as a mechanism of cell-to-cell communication. Kidney International. 2010;**78**(9):838-848

[100] Smirnova L, Grafe A, Seiler A, Schumacher S, Nitsch R, Wulczyn FG. Regulation of miRNA expression during neural cell specification. The European Journal of Neuroscience. 2005;**21**(6):1469-1477

[101] Lafourcade C, Ramirez JP, Luarte A, Fernandez A, Wyneken U. MiRNAs in astrocyte-derived exosomes as possible mediators of neuronal plasticity. Journal of Experimental Neuroscience. 2016;**10**(Suppl 1):1-9

[102] Beveridge NJ, Gardiner E, Carroll AP, Tooney PA, Cairns MJ. Schizophrenia is associated with an increase in cortical microRNA biogenesis. Molecular Psychiatry. 2010;**15**(12): 1176-1189

[103] Perkins DO, Jeffries CD, Jarskog LF, Thomson JM, Woods K, Newman MA, Parker JS, Jin J, Hammond SM. microRNA expression in the prefrontal cortex of individuals with schizophrenia and schizoaffective disorder. Genome Biology. 2007;**8**(2):R27

[104] Cogswell JP, Ward J, Taylor IA, Waters M, Shi Y, Cannon B, Kelnar K, Kemppainen J, Brown D, Chen C, et al. Identification of miRNA changes in Alzheimer's disease brain and CSF yields putative biomarkers and insights into disease pathways. Journal of Alzheimer's Disease. 2008;**14**(1):27-41

[105] Li Y, Zhang L, Liu F, Xiang G, Jiang D, Pu X. Identification of endogenous controls for analyzing serum exosomal miRNA in patients with hepatitis B or hepatocellular carcinoma. Disease Markers. 2015;**2015**:893594

[106] Lin X, He Y, Hou X, Zhang Z, Wang R, Wu Q. Endothelial cells can regulate smooth muscle cells in contractile phenotype through the miR-206/ARF6&NCX1/exosome axis. PLoS One. 2016;**11**(3):e0152959

[107] Wu SC, Yang JC, Rau CS, Chen YC, Lu TH, Lin MW, Tzeng SL, Wu YC, Wu CJ, Hsieh CH. Profiling circulating microRNA expression in experimental sepsis using cecal ligation and puncture. PLoS One. 2013;**8**(10):e77936

[108] Ichii O, Otsuka-Kanazawa S, Horino T, Kimura J, Nakamura T, Matsumoto M, Toi M, Kon Y. Decreased miR-26a expression correlates with the progression of podocyte injury in autoimmune glomerulonephritis. PLoS One. 2014;**9**(10):e110383

[109] Cheng L, Sharples RA, Scicluna BJ, Hill AF. Exosomes provide a protective and enriched source of miRNA for biomarker profiling compared to intracellular and cell-free blood. Journal of Extracellular Vesicles. 2014;**3**:23743

[110] Huse JT, Brennan C, Hambardzumyan D, Wee B, Pena J, Rouhanifard SH, Sohn-Lee C, le Sage C, Agami R, Tuschl T, et al. The PTEN-regulating microRNA miR-26a is amplified in high-grade glioma and facilitates gliomagenesis in vivo. Genes & Development. 2009;**23**(11):1327-1337

[111] Guo P, Lan J, Ge J, Nie Q, Guo L, Qiu Y, Mao Q. MiR-26a enhances the radiosensitivity of glioblastoma multiforme cells through targeting of ataxia-telangiectasia mutated. Experimental Cell Research. 2014;**320**(2):200-208

[112] Zhang L, Zhang S, Yao J, Lowery FJ, Zhang Q, Huang WC, Li P, Li M, Wang X, Zhang C, et al. Microenvironment-induced PTEN loss by exosomal microRNA primes brain metastasis outgrowth. Nature. 2015;**527**(7576):100-104

[113] Alvarez-Buylla A, Garcia-Verdugo JM. Neurogenesis in adult subventricular zone. The Journal of Neuroscience: The Official Journal of the Society for Neuroscience. 2002;**22**(3): 629-634

[114] Kempermann G. Why new neurons? Possible functions for adult hippocampal neurogenesis. The Journal of Neuroscience: The Official Journal of the Society for Neuroscience. 2002;**22**(3):635-638

[115] Uchida N, Buck DW, He D, Reitsma MJ, Masek M, Phan TV, Tsukamoto AS, Gage FH, Weissman IL. Direct isolation of human central nervous system stem cells. Proceedings of the National Academy of Sciences of the United States of America. 2000;**97**(26): 14720-14725

[116] Lendahl U, Zimmerman LB, McKay RD. CNS stem cells express a new class of intermediate filament protein. Cell. 1990;**60**(4):585-595

[117] Wegner M. SOX after SOX: SOXession regulates neurogenesis. Genes & Development. 2011;**25**(23):2423-2428

[118] Singh SK, Clarke ID, Terasaki M, Bonn VE, Hawkins C, Squire J, Dirks PB. Identification of a cancer stem cell in human brain tumors. Cancer Research. 2003;**63**(18):5821-5828

[119] Read TA, Fogarty MP, Markant SL, McLendon RE, Wei Z, Ellison DW, Febbo PG, Wechsler-Reya RJ. Identification of CD15 as a marker for tumor-propagating cells in a mouse model of medulloblastoma. Cancer Cell. 2009;**15**(2):135-147

[120] Mao XG, Zhang X, Xue XY, Guo G, Wang P, Zhang W, Fei Z, Zhen HN, You SW, Yang H. Brain tumor stem-like cells identified by neural stem cell marker CD15. Translational Oncology. 2009;**2**(4):247-257

[121] Reynolds BA, Weiss S. Generation of neurons and astrocytes from isolated cells of the adult mammalian central nervous system. Science. 1992;**255**(5052):1707-1710

[122] Yi Y, Hsieh IY, Huang X, Li J, Zhao W. Glioblastoma stem-like cells: Characteristics, microenvironment, and therapy. Frontiers in Pharmacology. 2016;**7**:477

[123] Zeppernick F, Ahmadi R, Campos B, Dictus C, Helmke BM, Becker N, Lichter P, Unterberg A, Radlwimmer B, Herold-Mende CC. Stem cell marker CD133 affects clinical outcome in glioma patients. Clinical Cancer Research: An Official Journal of the American Association for Cancer Research. 2008;**14**(1):123-129

[124] Tamura K, Aoyagi M, Ando N, Ogishima T, Wakimoto H, Yamamoto M, Ohno K. Expansion of CD133-positive glioma cells in recurrent de novo glioblastomas after radiotherapy and chemotherapy. Journal of Neurosurgery. 2013;**119**(5):1145-1155

[125] Wilhelmsson U, Faiz M, de Pablo Y, Sjoqvist M, Andersson D, Widestrand A, Potokar M, Stenovec M, Smith PL, Shinjyo N, et al. Astrocytes negatively regulate neurogenesis through the Jagged1-mediated notch pathway. Stem Cells. 2012;**30**(10):2320-2329

[126] Seri B, Garcia-Verdugo JM, McEwen BS, Alvarez-Buylla A. Astrocytes give rise to new neurons in the adult mammalian hippocampus. The Journal of Neuroscience: The Official Journal of the Society for Neuroscience. 2001;**21**(18):7153-7160

[127] Rath BH, Fair JM, Jamal M, Camphausen K, Tofilon PJ. Astrocytes enhance the invasion potential of glioblastoma stem-like cells. PLoS One. 2013;**8**(1):e54752

[128] Rath BH, Wahba A, Camphausen K, Tofilon PJ. Coculture with astrocytes reduces the radiosensitivity of glioblastoma stem-like cells and identifies additional targets for radiosensitization. Cancer Medicine. 2015;**4**(11):1705-1716

[129] Biasoli D, Sobrinho MF, da Fonseca AC, de Matos DG, Romao L, de Moraes MR, Rehen SK, Moura-Neto V, Borges HL, Lima FR. Glioblastoma cells inhibit astrocytic p53-expression favoring cancer malignancy. Oncogene. 2014;**3**:e123

[130] Muller PA, Vousden KH. p53 mutations in cancer. Nature Cell Biology. 2013;**15**(1):2-8

[131] Kiaris H, Chatzistamou I, Trimis G, Frangou-Plemmenou M, Pafiti-Kondi A, Kalofoutis A. Evidence for nonautonomous effect of p53 tumor suppressor in carcinogenesis. Cancer Research. 2005;**65**(5):1627-1630

[132] Alexandrova A, Ivanov A, Chumakov P, Kopnin B, Vasiliev J. Changes in p53 expression in mouse fibroblasts can modify motility and extracellular matrix organization. Oncogene. 2000;**19**(50):5826-5830

[133] Wu K, Fukuda K, Xing F, Zhang Y, Sharma S, Liu Y, Chan MD, Zhou X, Qasem SA, Pochampally R, et al. Roles of the cyclooxygenase 2 matrix metalloproteinase 1 pathway in brain metastasis of breast cancer. The Journal of Biological Chemistry. 2015;**290**(15):9842-9854

[134] Boyer LA, Lee TI, Cole MF, Johnstone SE, Levine SS, Zucker JP, Guenther MG, Kumar RM, Murray HL, Jenner RG, et al. Core transcriptional regulatory circuitry in human embryonic stem cells. Cell. 2005;**122**(6):947-956

[135] Tavazoie M, Van der Veken L, Silva-Vargas V, Louissaint M, Colonna L, Zaidi B, Garcia-Verdugo JM, Doetsch F. A specialized vascular niche for adult neural stem cells. Cell Stem Cell. 2008;**3**(3):279-288

[136] Goldman SA, Chen Z. Perivascular instruction of cell genesis and fate in the adult brain. Nature Neuroscience. 2011;**14**(11):1382-1389

[137] Dawson DW, Volpert OV, Gillis P, Crawford SE, Xu H, Benedict W, Bouck NP. Pigment epithelium-derived factor: A potent inhibitor of angiogenesis. Science. 1999;**285**(5425):245-248

[138] Cao L, Jiao X, Zuzga DS, Liu Y, Fong DM, Young D, During MJ. VEGF links hippocampal activity with neurogenesis, learning and memory. Nature Genetics. 2004;**36**(8):827-835

[139] Leventhal C, Rafii S, Rafii D, Shahar A, Goldman SA. Endothelial trophic support of neuronal production and recruitment from the adult mammalian subependyma. Molecular and Cellular Neurosciences. 1999;**13**(6):450-464

[140] Folkins C, Man S, Xu P, Shaked Y, Hicklin DJ, Kerbel RS. Anticancer therapies combining antiangiogenic and tumor cell cytotoxic effects reduce the tumor stem-like cell fraction in glioma xenograft tumors. Cancer Research. 2007;**67**(8):3560-3564

[141] Lyon JG, Mokarram N, Saxena T, Carroll SL, Bellamkonda RV. Engineering challenges for brain tumor immunotherapy. Advanced Drug Delivery Reviews. 2017

[142] Abbott NJ. Dynamics of CNS barriers: Evolution, differentiation, and modulation. Cellular and Molecular Neurobiology. 2005;**25**(1):5-23

[143] Gieryng A, Pszczolkowska D, Walentynowicz KA, Rajan WD, Kaminska B. Immune microenvironment of gliomas. Laboratory Investigation; A Journal of Technical Methods and Pathology. 2017;**97**(5):498-518

[144] Sofroniew MV. Multiple roles for astrocytes as effectors of cytokines and inflammatory mediators. The Neuroscientist. 2014;**20**(2):160-172

[145] Hamby ME, Coppola G, Ao Y, Geschwind DH, Khakh BS, Sofroniew MV. Inflammatory mediators alter the astrocyte transcriptome and calcium signaling elicited by multiple G-protein-coupled receptors. The Journal of Neuroscience: The Official Journal of the Society for Neuroscience. 2012;**32**(42):14489-14510

[146] Zamanian JL, Xu L, Foo LC, Nouri N, Zhou L, Giffard RG, Barres BA. Genomic analysis of reactive astrogliosis. The Journal of Neuroscience: The Official Journal of the Society for Neuroscience. 2012;**32**(18):6391-6410

[147] Sofroniew MV. Molecular dissection of reactive astrogliosis and glial scar formation. Trends in Neurosciences. 2009;**32**(12):638-647

[148] Sobel RA, Mitchell ME, Fondren G. Intercellular adhesion molecule-1 (ICAM-1) in cellular immune reactions in the human central nervous system. The American Journal of Pathology. 1990;**136**(6):1309-1316

[149] Massa PT, Ozato K, McFarlin DE. Cell type-specific regulation of major histocompatibility complex (MHC) class I gene expression in astrocytes, oligodendrocytes, and neurons. Glia. 1993;**8**(3):201-207

[150] Aloisi F, Ria F, Columba-Cabezas S, Hess H, Penna G, Adorini L. Relative efficiency of microglia, astrocytes, dendritic cells and B cells in naive CD4+ T cell priming and Th1/ Th2 cell restimulation. European Journal of Immunology. 1999;**29**(9):2705-2714

[151] Valiente M, Obenauf AC, Jin X, Chen Q, Zhang XH, Lee DJ, Chaft JE, Kris MG, Huse JT, Brogi E, et al. Serpins promote cancer cell survival and vascular co-option in brain metastasis. Cell. 2014;**156**(5):1002-1016

[152] Lorger M. Tumor microenvironment in the brain. Cancers (Basel). 2012;**4**(1):218-243

[153] Kostianovsky AM, Maier LM, Anderson RC, Bruce JN, Anderson DE. Astrocytic regulation of human monocytic/microglial activation. Journal of Immunology. 2008;**181**(8): 5425-5432

[154] Bechmann I, Steiner B, Gimsa U, Mor G, Wolf S, Beyer M, Nitsch R, Zipp F, Astrocyte-induced T. Cell elimination is CD95 ligand dependent. Journal of Neuroimmunology. 2002;**132**(1–2):60-65

[155] Sofroniew MV, Vinters HV. Astrocytes: Biology and pathology. Acta Neuropathologica. 2010;**119**(1):7-35

[156] Voskuhl RR, Peterson RS, Song B, Ao Y, Morales LB, Tiwari-Woodruff S, Sofroniew MV. Reactive astrocytes form scar-like perivascular barriers to leukocytes during adaptive immune inflammation of the CNS. The Journal of Neuroscience: The Official Journal of the Society for Neuroscience. 2009;**29**(37):11511-11522

[157] Ekstrand AJ, James CD, Cavenee WK, Seliger B, Pettersson RF, Collins VP. Genes for epidermal growth factor receptor, transforming growth factor alpha, and epidermal growth factor and their expression in human gliomas in vivo. Cancer Research. 1991;**51**(8): 2164-2172

[158] Meco D, Servidei T, Riccardi A, Ferlini C, Cusano G, Zannoni GF, Giangaspero F, Riccardi R. Antitumor effect in medulloblastoma cells by gefitinib: Ectopic HER2 overexpression enhances gefitinib effects in vivo. Neuro-Oncology. 2009;**11**(3):250-259

[159] Kim JK, Jin X, Sohn YW, Jin X, Jeon HY, Kim EJ, Ham SW, Jeon HM, Chang SY, SY O, et al. Tumoral RANKL activates astrocytes that promote glioma cell invasion through cytokine signaling. Cancer Letters. 2014;**353**(2):194-200

[160] Seike T, Fujita K, Yamakawa Y, Kido MA, Takiguchi S, Teramoto N, Iguchi H, Noda M. Interaction between lung cancer cells and astrocytes via specific inflammatory cytokines in

the microenvironment of brain metastasis. Clinical & Experimental Metastasis. 2011;**28**(1): 13-25

[161] Huttenlocher A, Lakonishok M, Kinder M, Wu S, Truong T, Knudsen KA, Horwitz AF. Integrin and cadherin synergy regulates contact inhibition of migration and motile activity. The Journal of Cell Biology. 1998;**141**(2):515-526

[162] Yang C, Iyer RR, AC Y, Yong RL, Park DM, Weil RJ, Ikejiri B, Brady RO, Lonser RR, Zhuang Z. Beta-catenin signaling initiates the activation of astrocytes and its dysregulation contributes to the pathogenesis of astrocytomas. Proceedings of the National Academy of Sciences of the United States of America. 2012;**109**(18):6963-6968

[163] Behrens J, Jerchow BA, Wurtele M, Grimm J, Asbrand C, Wirtz R, Kuhl M, Wedlich D, Birchmeier W. Functional interaction of an axin homolog, conductin, with beta-catenin, APC, and GSK3beta. Science. 1998;**280**(5363):596-599

[164] Weidle UH, Birzele F, Kollmorgen G, Ruger R. Dissection of the process of brain metastasis reveals targets and mechanisms for molecular-based intervention. Cancer Genomics Proteomics. 2016;**13**(4):245-258

[165] Shumakovich MA, Mencio CP, Siglin JS, Moriarty RA, Geller HM, Stroka KM. Astrocytes from the brain microenvironment alter migration and morphology of metastatic breast cancer cells. FASEB Journal: Official Publication of the Federation of American Societies for Experimental Biology. 2017

[166] Cathcart J, Pulkoski-Gross A, Cao J. Targeting matrix metalloproteinases in cancer: Bringing new life to old ideas. Genes and Diseases. 2015;**2**(1):26-34

[167] Radisky ES, Raeeszadeh-Sarmazdeh M, Radisky DC. Therapeutic potential of matrix metalloproteinase inhibition in breast cancer. Journal of Cellular Biochemistry. 2017;**118**(11): 3531-3548

[168] Stark AM, Anuszkiewicz B, Mentlein R, Yoneda T, Mehdorn HM, Held-Feindt J. Differential expression of matrix metalloproteinases in brain- and bone-seeking clones of metastatic MDA-MB-231 breast cancer cells. Journal of Neuro-Oncology. 2007;**81**(1):39-48

[169] Zucker S, Cao J, Chen WT. Critical appraisal of the use of matrix metalloproteinase inhibitors in cancer treatment. Oncogene. 2000;**19**(56):6642-6650

[170] Stoletov K, Strnadel J, Zardouzian E, Momiyama M, Park FD, Kelber JA, Pizzo DP, Hoffman R, VandenBerg SR, Klemke RL. Role of connexins in metastatic breast cancer and melanoma brain colonization. Journal of Cell Science. 2013;**126**(Pt 4):904-913

[171] Hohensee I, Lamszus K, Riethdorf S, Meyer-Staeckling S, Glatzel M, Matschke J, Witzel I, Westphal M, Brandt B, Muller V, et al. Frequent genetic alterations in EGFR- and HER2-driven pathways in breast cancer brain metastases. The American Journal of Pathology. 2013;**183**(1):83-95

[172] Li J, Yen C, Liaw D, Podsypanina K, Bose S, Wang SI, Puc J, Miliaresis C, Rodgers L, McCombie R, et al. PTEN, a putative protein tyrosine phosphatase gene mutated in human brain, breast, and prostate cancer. Science. 1997;**275**(5308):1943-1947

[173] Hohensee I, Chuang HN, Grottke A, Werner S, Schulte A, Horn S, Lamszus K, Bartkowiak K, Witzel I, Westphal M, et al. PTEN mediates the cross talk between breast and glial cells in brain metastases leading to rapid disease progression. Oncotarget. 2017;**8**(4):6155-6168

[174] Shipman L. Microenvironment: Astrocytes silence PTEN to promote brain metastasis. Nature Reviews Cancer. 2015;**15**(12):695

[175] Le MT, Hamar P, Guo C, Basar E, Perdigao-Henriques R, Balaj L, Lieberman J. miR-200-containing extracellular vesicles promote breast cancer cell metastasis. The Journal of Clinical Investigation. 2014;**124**(12):5109-5128

[176] Neman J, Choy C, Kowolik CM, Anderson A, Duenas VJ, Waliany S, Chen BT, Chen MY, Jandial R. Co-evolution of breast-to-brain metastasis and neural progenitor cells. Clinical & Experimental Metastasis. 2013;**30**(6):753-768

[177] Neman J, Termini J, Wilczynski S, Vaidehi N, Choy C, Kowolik CM, Li H, Hambrecht AC, Roberts E, Jandial R. Human breast cancer metastases to the brain display GABAergic properties in the neural niche. Proceedings of the National Academy of Sciences of the United States of America. 2014;**111**(3):984-989

[178] Attwell D, Laughlin SB. An energy budget for signaling in the grey matter of the brain. Journal of Cerebral Blood Flow and Metabolism. 2001;**21**(10):1133-1145

[179] Belanger M, Allaman I, Magistretti PJ. Brain energy metabolism: Focus on astrocyte-neuron metabolic cooperation. Cell Metabolism. 2011;**14**(6):724-738

[180] Menon S, Shin S, Dy G. Advances in cancer immunotherapy in solid Tumors. Cancers (Basel). 2016;**8**(12)

[181] Papaioannou NE, Beniata OV, Vitsos P, Tsitsilonis O, Samara P. Harnessing the immune system to improve cancer therapy. Annals of Translational Medicine. 2016;**4**(14):261

[182] Khong H, Overwijk WW. Adjuvants for peptide-based cancer vaccines. Journal for ImmunoTherapy of Cancer. 2016;**4**:56

[183] Mitchell DA, Batich KA, Gunn MD, Huang MN, Sanchez-Perez L, Nair SK, Congdon KL, Reap EA, Archer GE, Desjardins A, et al. Tetanus toxoid and CCL3 improve dendritic cell vaccines in mice and glioblastoma patients. Nature. 2015;**519**(7543):366-369

[184] Ishida Y, Agata Y, Shibahara K, Honjo T. Induced expression of PD-1, a novel member of the immunoglobulin gene superfamily, upon programmed cell death. The EMBO Journal. 1992;**11**(11):3887-3895

[185] Topalian SL, Hodi FS, Brahmer JR, Gettinger SN, Smith DC, McDermott DF, Powderly JD, Carvajal RD, Sosman JA, Atkins MB, et al. Safety, activity, and immune correlates of anti-PD-1 antibody in cancer. The New England Journal of Medicine. 2012;**366**(26):2443-2454

[186] Iwai Y, Hamanishi J, Chamoto K, Honjo T. Cancer immunotherapies targeting the PD-1 signaling pathway. Journal of Biomedical Science. 2017;**24**(1):26

[187] Berghoff AS, Kiesel B, Widhalm G, Rajky O, Ricken G, Wohrer A, Dieckmann K, Filipits M, Brandstetter A, Weller M, et al. Programmed death ligand 1 expression and tumor-infiltrating lymphocytes in glioblastoma. Neuro-Oncology. 2015;**17**(8):1064-1075

[188] Bloch O, Crane CA, Kaur R, Safaee M, Rutkowski MJ, Parsa AT. Gliomas promote immunosuppression through induction of B7-H1 expression in tumor-associated macrophages. Clinical Cancer Research: An Official Journal of the American Association for Cancer Research. 2013;**19**(12):3165-3175

[189] Mishra V, Schuetz H, Haorah J. Differential induction of PD-1/PD-L1 in Neuroimmune cells by drug of abuse. International Journal of Physiology, Pathophysiology and Pharmacology. 2015;**7**(2):87-97

[190] Duchnowska R, Peksa R, Radecka B, Mandat T, Trojanowski T, Jarosz B, Czartoryska-Arlukowicz B, Olszewski WP, Och W, Kalinka-Warzocha E, et al. Immune response in breast cancer brain metastases and their microenvironment: The role of the PD-1/PD-L axis. Breast Cancer Research : BCR. 2016;**18**(1):43

[191] Berghoff AS, Ricken G, Widhalm G, Rajky O, Dieckmann K, Birner P, Bartsch R, Holler C, Preusser M. Tumour-infiltrating lymphocytes and expression of programmed death ligand 1 (PD-L1) in melanoma brain metastases. Histopathology. 2015;**66**(2):289-299

[192] Harter PN, Bernatz S, Scholz A, Zeiner PS, Zinke J, Kiyose M, Blasel S, Beschorner R, Senft C, Bender B, et al. Distribution and prognostic relevance of tumor-infiltrating lymphocytes (TILs) and PD-1/PD-L1 immune checkpoints in human brain metastases. Oncotarget. 2015;**6**(38):40836-40849

[193] Langley RR, Fidler IJ. Tumor cell-organ microenvironment interactions in the pathogenesis of cancer metastasis. Endocrine Reviews. 2007;**28**(3):297-321

[194] Gupta GP, Massague J. Cancer Metastasis: Building a framework. Cell. 2006;**127**(4):679-695

[195] Walker AE, Robins M, Weinfeld FD. Epidemiology of brain tumors: the national survey of intracranial neoplasms. Neurology. 1985;**35**(2):219-226

[196] Percy AK, Elveback LR, Okazaki H, Kurland LT. Neoplasms of the central nervous system. Epidemiologic considerations. Neurology. 1972;**22**(1):40-48

[197] Counsell CE, Collie DA, Grant R. Incidence of intracranial tumours in the Lothian region of Scotland, 1989-90. Journal of Neurology, Neurosurgery, and Psychiatry. 1996;**61**(2):143-150

[198] Ostrom QT, Gittleman H, Xu J, Kromer C, Wolinsky Y, Kruchko C, Barnholtz-Sloan JS. CBTRUS statistical report: Primary brain and other central nervous system tumors diagnosed in the United States in 2009–2013. Neuro-Oncology. 2016;**18**(suppl_5):v1-v75

Chapter 9

Astrocytes in Aceruloplasminemia

Hiroaki Miyajima

Additional information is available at the end of the chapter

http://dx.doi.org/10.5772/intechopen.71831

Abstract

In neurons, iron plays an important role in the signal transduction related to synaptic plasticity. The neuronal iron supply is tightly controlled and depends not only on transferrin-bound iron but also on non-transferrin-bound iron (NTBI). Ceruloplasmin is bound to the cell membranes of astrocytes, where it plays a role in iron efflux from astrocytes due to the activity of ferroxidase, which oxidizes ferrous iron after its transfer to the cell surface via ferroportin, and which delivers ferric iron to extracellular transferrin, which is transported to neurons. Aceruloplasminemia is an autosomal recessive neurodegenerative disorder in which iron accumulates in the brain due to the complete lack of ceruloplasmin ferroxidase activity. Redox-active iron accumulation was found to be more prominent in astrocytes than in neurons. Neurons take up iron from alternative sources of NTBI because astrocytes without ceruloplasmin cannot transport iron to transferrin. Neuronal cell loss may result from iron starvation in the early stage of aceruloplasminemia and may result from iron-mediated oxidation in the late stage of the condition. The excess iron in astrocytes can result in oxidative damage to these cells, thereby disrupting the neuronal cell protection offered by astrocytes in patients with aceruloplasminemia.

Keywords: ceruloplasmin, iron, ferroxidase, non-transferrin-bound iron (NTBI), neurodegeneration

1. The role of iron in brain

Iron is a bioactive metal that is essential for a normal brain function. It participates in a variety of cellular functions, including the biosynthesis of many neurotransmitters, myelin formation and electron transport, which sustains the brain's energy metabolism. On the other hand, excessive iron in the brain causes neuronal injury, because redox-active ferrous iron (Fe^{2+}) enhances oxidative stress due to the generation of the highly cytotoxic hydroxyl radical [1, 2]. A deficiency or excess of iron can cause impaired cellular functions and eventually cell death.

However, the precise mechanisms underlying the metabolism of iron and its regulation in the brain remain unknown. Iron deficiency in the developing human has been clearly established as a causative factor of long-term developmental and cognitive impairment. Late fetal and early postnatal iron deficiency is a condition that causes learning and memory impairments in humans, which persist after iron repletion [3–6]. Two other factors that are important in determining the degree of cognitive deficit are the magnitude and the duration of iron deficiency [7]. In contrast, while several prominent neurodegenerative disorders, including Alzheimer's disease and Parkinson's disease, have been reported to be associated with the excessive accumulation of iron in specific brain regions, the relationship of this accumulation to the pathogenesis of these diseases is far from clear. The iron control in the brain is virtually independent of the rest of the body. Indeed, it has been reported that neither systemic iron-overload nor systemic iron deficiency has a significant effect on the brain in adulthood [1, 8].

Despite the critical and diverse role of iron in the brain function, the molecular and cellular details of neuronal iron metabolism remain poorly understood; however, current studies have started to uncover the participation of iron in signal transduction mechanisms related to synaptic plasticity and that iron is needed for long-term potentiation (LTP), and have provided a potential model to account for the learning and memory deficits exhibited by humans with iron deficiency. Iron-generated reactive oxygen species (ROS) could be a new class of molecules that act as second messengers in the signaling cascades related to synaptic plasticity, the putative cellular substrate of memory [9]. These ROS are involved in the calcium signaling initiated by the stimulation of NMDA receptors. On the other hand, an excess of iron, with the ensuing uncontrolled production of ROS, is detrimental to neuronal survival. In the presence of elevated iron, increased synaptic activity can cause iron overload and contribute to the development of cytotoxic effects [10], as was suggested to occur in Alzheimer's disease [11]. A direct coupling between synaptic activity and iron entry can properly address these requirements. This is a double-edged sword in that iron entry—if not properly controlled—represents a harmful condition, because Fe^{2+} is capable of catalyzing the Fenton reaction, which occurs primarily at the mitochondrial level with the production of the highly toxic hydroxyl radical [12]. Astrocytes that can uptake iron, and which thereby buffer its concentration in the synaptic environment, may play a protective role. Astrocytes are endowed with a strong detoxifying defense system that makes them more resistant to oxidative insults than neurons [13].

2. Ceruloplasmin

Ceruloplasmin consists of a single chain of 1046 amino acids and is a member of the multicopper oxidase family. This protein is a glycoprotein of the $\alpha 2$ globulin fraction of the serum, and contains 95% of the copper in the plasma [14]. There were precisely six copper ions present in the molecule, and that there was an important three-copper catalytic center—the so-called 'trinuclear cluster'—which plays an important role in the oxidase reaction [15]. Despite the need for copper for the functions of ceruloplasmin, this protein plays no essential role in the transport or metabolism of copper. Copper depletion resulted in a marked decrease in the circulating serum ceruloplasmin in association with iron deficiency anemia that could only be corrected by the administration of copper and by the accumulation of iron in parenchymal tissues, while the administration of exogenous ceruloplasmin resulted in the prompt release of iron from tissue with subsequent incorporation into circulating transferrin. The essential function of ceruloplasmin is as a ferroxidase, which utilizes the electron chemistry of bound copper ions to couple the oxidation of ferrous iron (Fe^{2+}) to the reduction of oxygen bound to the trinuclear cluster [16, 17].

Two isoforms of this protein are generated by alternative splicing: a secretory form (serum ceruloplasmin) and a glycosylphosphatidylinositol (GPI)-linked form [18]. The secretory form is mostly expressed in hepatocytes, while the GPI-linked form is expressed in the brain, liver, and several other organs [19]. Although the GPI-linked form is strongly expressed within the brain, several other tissues are known to express it at relatively low levels (i.e., the spleen, kidney, heart, and liver). In the brain, most ceruloplasmin is derived from astrocytes and is located on the surface of astrocytes in the GPI-linked form [20].

Serum transferrin-bound iron is endocytosed by brain endothelial cells, which are dependent on transferrin receptor 1, and iron is released to the brain interstitial fluid through the basolateral iron exporter, ferroportin. Extracellular iron is oxidized due to GPI-linked ceruloplasmin, which is found in the foot processes of astrocytes, and then iron binds to the transferrin and is transported to neurons [21]. The GPI-linked ceruloplasmin likely plays an important role in the mobilization of iron and the antioxidant effects in the central nervous system [20, 22]. GPI-linked ceruloplasmin may be associated with iron homeostasis and the antioxidant defense by protecting the central nervous system from iron-mediated free radical injury. The ferroxidase activity of GPI-linked ceruloplasmin is also essential for the stability of cell surface ferroportin [23, 24]. The importance of ceruloplasmin in human biology is underscored by aceruloplasminemia, which is an inherited disease of iron homeostasis. This disease reveals an essential role of ceruloplasmin in brain iron homeostasis. It is known that (1) ceruloplasmin regulates the efficiency of iron efflux, (2) ceruloplasmin functions as a ferroxidase and regulates the oxidation of ferrous iron (Fe^{2+}) to ferric iron (Fe^{3+}), (3) ceruloplasmin does not bind to transferrin directly, (4) ceruloplasmin stabilizes the cell surface iron transporter, ferroportin, and (5) GPI-linked ceruloplasmin is the predominant form expressed in the brain [19].

3. Aceruloplasminemia

In 1987, we described the first case of aceruloplasminemia in a 52-year-old Japanese woman suffering from blepharospasm, retinal degeneration, and diabetes mellitus (DM) [25]. Subsequent evaluations revealed the presence of anemia and low serum iron concentrations, despite the fact that the patient had high levels of serum ferritin and marked iron accumulation in the brain and liver on T2-weighted magnetic resonance imaging (MRI, **Figure 1**), as well as the complete absence of serum ceruloplasmin. The lack of serum ceruloplasmin was

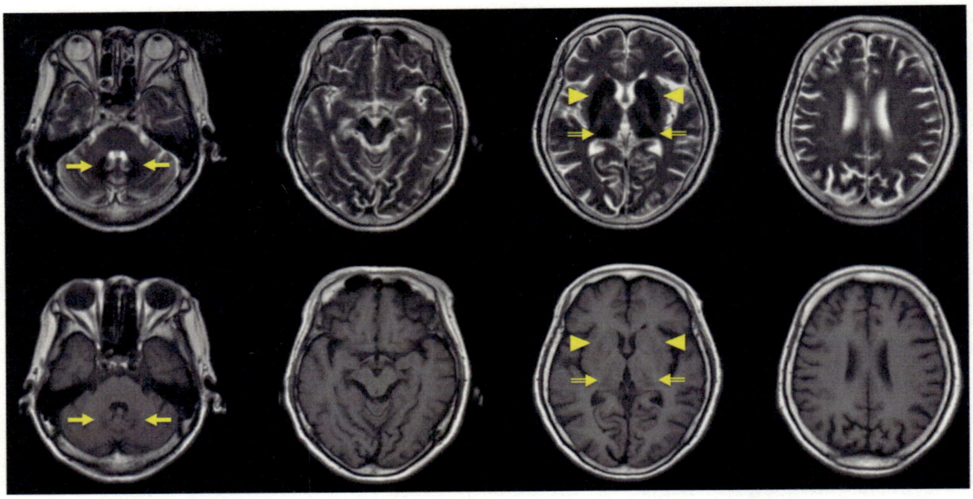

Figure 1. The brain MRI findings in a patient with aceruloplasminemia. T1-weighted (lower row) and T2-weighted (upper row) axial images of the brain showed signal attenuation of the dentate nucleus of the cerebellum (arrows), basal ganglia (arrowheads), and thalami (double arrows).

inherited in an autosomal recessive fashion. A direct connection between iron accumulation in both the brain and liver and the complete absence of serum ceruloplasmin was hypothesized. A genetic analysis of the ceruloplasmin gene revealed that this patient was homozygous, with a 5-base insertion in exon 7 (c.1286_90insTACAC), which resulted in a frame shift mutation and a truncated open reading frame [26]. The clinical findings and the identification of a mutation in the ceruloplasmin gene confirmed that the disorder was a novel disorder of iron metabolism, which resulted from a lack of ceruloplasmin in the serum. The disorder was termed aceruloplasminemia (MIM 604290). The patient died from pancreatic cancer at 66 years of age. We examined the pathological studies that were performed in this case [27]. Brown pigmentation of the basal ganglia was observed in a coronal section of the brain (**Figure 2**). Severe iron deposition was observed in the basal ganglia, thalamus, and cerebellum, and neuronal loss was observed in the regions with the highest iron accumulation. The iron deposition in astrocytes was more severe than that in neurons (**Figure 2**). The globular structures (inclusions) were identified in the cerebral cortices as well as the basal ganglia. These structures included many oxidatively damaged proteins that were derived from astrocytes. Intense redox-active iron deposition was mainly demonstrated in the inclusions in the astrocytes (**Figure 2**).

Aceruloplasminemia is classified as an inherited neurodegenerative disorder with systemic iron-overload syndrome. The clinical manifestations of aceruloplasminemia are the triad of retinal degeneration, DM, and neurological signs/symptoms [27]. The neurological manifestations (in order of frequency) include ataxia, involuntary movement, cognitive dysfunction and parkinsonism; these correspond to the specific regions of brain iron accumulation. These symptoms generally appear in the fourth or fifth decade of life. More than 40% of involuntary movement is dystonia, and approximately 25% of cases exhibit chorea and choreoathetosis.

http://dx.doi.org/10.5772/intechopen.71831

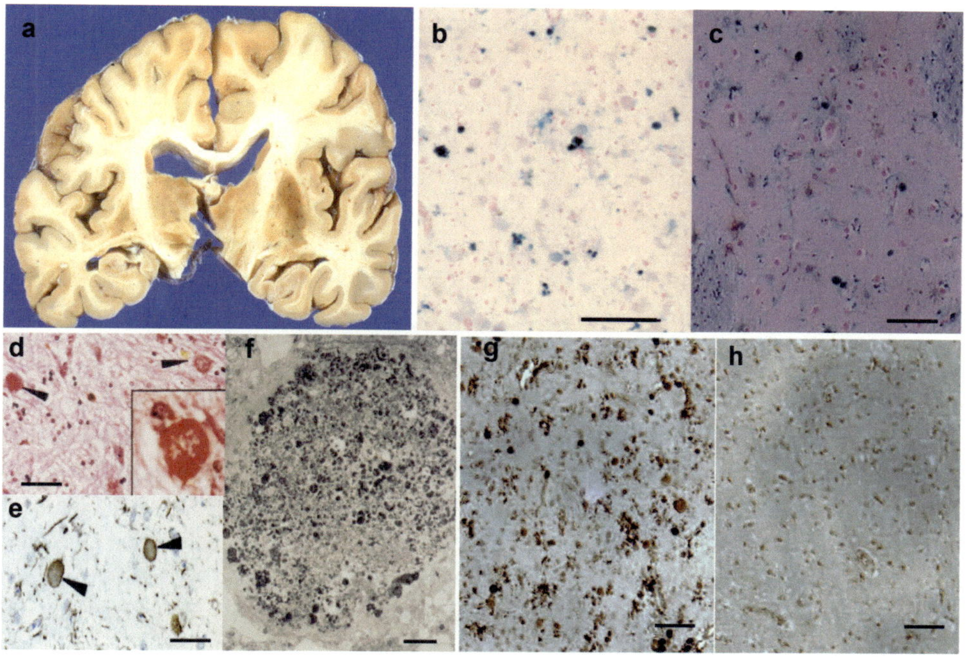

Figure 2. The histopathological findings in a patient with aceruloplasminemia. A coronal section of the brain shows brown pigmentation of the basal ganglia (a). Severe ferric iron deposition is noted in the putamen (b: Berlin blue stain). Iron deposition is mainly observed in the astrocytes, and a small amount of ferric iron is seen in the neurons (c: Berlin blue staining + H&E staining). Globular structures, indicated by arrowheads, are seen in the astrocytes (d: H&E staining) and were positive for anti-HNE antibody (e). The electron microscopic findings of the globular structures indicate that they contain many electron-dense bodies (f). The marked accumulation of redox-active iron is shown in the globus pallidus of an aceruloplasminemic brain (g) in comparison to the brain of a control subject (h) (redox-active iron staining: A modified Perl's technique). Scale bars: b-e, g, h =100 μm; f = 5 μm.

The cognitive dysfunction includes forgetfulness, mental slowing, and apathy. The neuroimaging studies of aceruloplasminemia patients are strongly supported by the characteristic abnormally low intensity on MRI, reflecting the accumulation of iron in the liver and brain. In Japan, the prevalence of aceruloplasminemia was estimated to be approximately one per 2,000,000 in individuals with non-consanguineous parents [28]. Genetic testing can confirm the diagnosis. Worldwide, genetic analyses of patients with aceruloplasminemia have identified more than 50 distinct mutations in the ceruloplasmin gene [29]. The majority of mutations are truncated mutations, which lead to the formation of a premature stop codon. The human ceruloplasmin gene contains 20 exons. The ferroxidase activity of ceruloplasmin is dependent upon the trinuclear copper cluster, the ligands for which are encoded by exon 18 [30]. The truncated mutations identified are predicted to result in the formation of a protein lacking the copper cluster sites that are presumed to be critical for the enzymatic function. The clinical phenotype in most patients shows little variation, regardless of the specific mutation [31]. The precise pathogenesis of iron deposition in the brain has been unclear, but evidence from several studies suggests that the enhanced oxidative stress induced by excess iron causes neuronal cell death [32, 33].

4. The role of astrocytes in aceruloplasminemia

In the brain of aceruloplasminemia patients, abnormal astrocytes were more frequently observed in the basal ganglia, where the accumulation of iron was marked than that in the frontal cortex. Intense ferrous iron deposition was demonstrated in the inclusions, many of which were positive for glia fibrillary acidic protein (GFAP) and which were stained by anti-4-hydroxynoneal (HNE) antibody. GFAP is most severely modified by oxidative stress in the brains of patients with aceruloplasminemia [34]. Intense ferrous iron deposition was demonstrated in the inclusions. The morphological changes in the astrocytes may be related to iron-induced tissue damage.

GPI-linked ceruloplasmin is bound to the cell membranes of astrocytes, where it plays an important role in the mobilization of iron from the blood to the extracellular space in the brain through astrocytes due to the ferroxidase activity. Ferroportin is a cell membrane-bound protein that is expressed in the brain as well as several organs and which transports intracellular ferrous iron to transferrin via the oxidization of ferrous iron to ferric iron via the ferroxidase of ceruloplasmin. GPI-linked ceruloplasmin likely plays an important role in the mobilization of iron from astrocytes to neurons. A ceruloplasmin homolog, hephaestin, is also expressed on neurons and functions as a ferroxidase to interact with neuronal ferroportin. Ceruloplasmin and ceruloplasmin/hephaestin knockout mice exhibited a neurodegenerative phenotype and retinal degeneration, consistent with that seen in aceruloplasminemia patients [35, 36]. The brain requires iron at concentrations that are several times higher than that obtained from the blood in order to maintain its normal function [2]. Taken together, the known functions of iron metabolic molecules suggest the presence of a cycle of iron storage and reutilization within the brain [37]. The neuronal iron supply is tightly controlled and mainly neurons take up iron from transferrin and alternative sources of non-transferrin-bound iron (NTBI). The pathological findings in the brain of patients with aceruloplasminemia included severe iron deposition in both the astrocytes and neurons, and neuronal loss. The iron accumulation observed in the neurons indicates that the neurons take up significant amounts of iron due to alternative sources of NTBI, because astrocytes without any expression of ceruloplasmin cannot transport iron to the transferrin that binds to transferrin receptor 1 on neurons. A ceruloplasmin-deficient model showed that neuronal cell loss may result from iron starvation in regions where the iron in astrocytes is not effectively mobilized for the uptake into neurons, and the accumulation of excess iron in astrocytes may also result in oxidative damage to these cells, with the subsequent loss of the glial-derived growth factors that are critical for neurons [36]. Neuronal cell injury may therefore result from iron deficiency in the early stage as well as iron-mediated oxidation in the late stage (**Figure 3**). NTBI is mainly composed of Fe^{3+} that is loosely bound to buffering molecules (mainly citrate and ascorbate). The high concentrations of ascorbate in the cerebrospinal fluid, which are up to 100 times higher than the concentrations in plasma, result in a reducing environment that increases the ratio Fe^{2+}/Fe^{3+} ratio in NTBI [38]. Thus, in addition to its physiological role in the brain, NTBI can acquire a pathological relevance, as NTBI levels increase during aging. NTBI has been thought to be an important contributor to the pathogenesis of cancer, cardiovascular diseases, and neurodegenerative disorders. The high propensity of NTBI to induce the generation of ROS makes it a potentially toxic form of iron; it is responsible for cellular damage not only at the plasma membrane level but also toward different intracellular organelles [39]. High levels of NTBI

http://dx.doi.org/10.5772/intechopen.71831

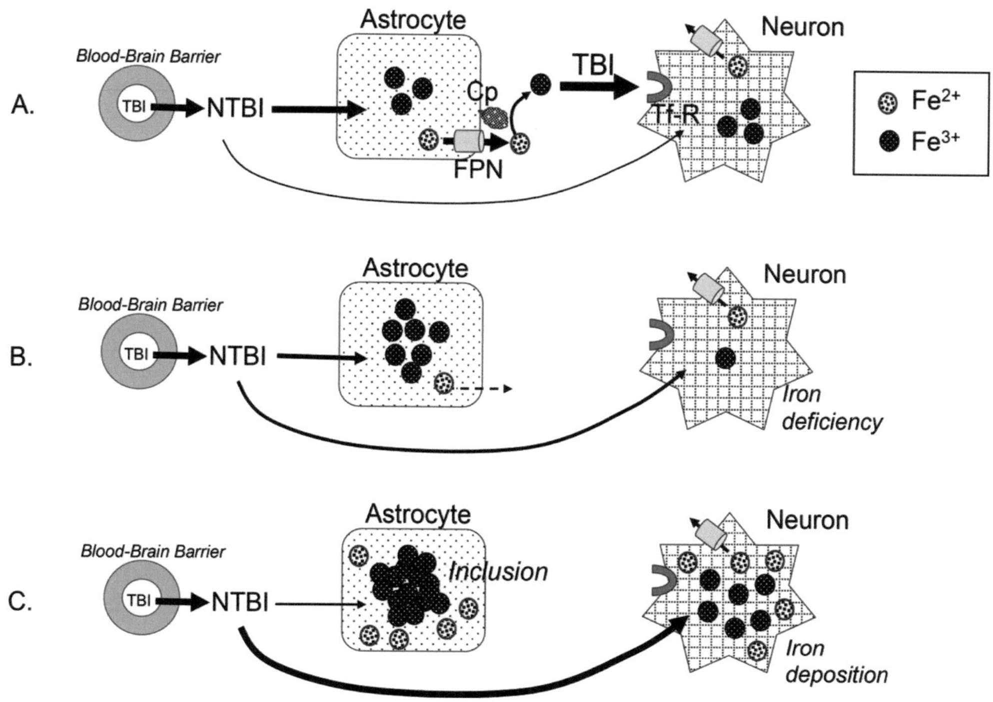

Figure 3. A model of the iron metabolic cycle in the brain. In the normal brain (a), iron may be recycled between astrocytes and neurons. Transferrin acts as a shuttle to deliver iron from astrocytes to neurons. The GPI-linked ceruloplasmin on astrocytes is a ferroxidase that mediates the oxidation of ferrous iron and its subsequent transfer to transferrin. Neurons take up the transferrin-bound iron and also take up iron from alternative sources (non-transferrin-bound iron; NTBI). Hephaestin also plays a role as a ferroxidase and interacts with neuronal ferroportin. In the brain of a patient with aceruloplasminemia, neuronal cell loss may result from iron deficiency in regions where the iron in astrocytes cannot be mobilized for the uptake into neurons in the early stage of the disease (b). Iron accumulation is subsequently observed in neurons as well as astrocytes, since neurons take up iron from NTBI, not from transferrin, in the late stage of the disease (c), because astrocytes without GPI-linked ceruloplasmin cannot transport iron to transferrin. TBI, transferrin-bound iron; NTBI, non-transferrin-bound iron; FPN, iron transporter of ferroportin; Cp, ceruloplasmin; Tf-R, transferrin receptor 1.

accumulate in the brains of patients with neurodegenerative disorders, including patients with Parkinson's disease and Alzheimer's disease [40]. Oxidative stress, which is closely related to the increased iron levels in the brain, and which may also occur due to defects in the antioxidant defense mechanism, is widely believed to be associated with neuronal cell death in patients with these diseases [41]. Astrocyte dysfunction may contribute to neuronal cell loss, in addition to the direct effects of free radicals on neurons. GPI-linked ceruloplasmin may be associated with astrocyte homeostasis and neuronal survival in the brain.

5. Conclusion

Astrocytes play an important role in iron homeostasis in the brain. They participate in the synaptic plasticity through the supply of iron to neurons and by buffering iron. The excess iron in astrocytes can result in oxidative damage to these cells, thereby disrupting the neuronal cell protection offered by astrocytes in patients with aceruloplasminemia.

Author details

Hiroaki Miyajima

Address all correspondence to: miyajima@hama-med.ac.jp

First Department of Medicine, Hamamatsu University School of Medicine, Hamamatsu, Japan

References

[1] Sipe JC, Beutler E. Brain iron metabolism and neurodegenerative disorders. Developmental Neuroscience. 2002;**24**:188-196. DOI: 10.1159/000065701

[2] Moos T, Rosengren Nielsen T, Skjørringe T, Morgan EH. Iron trafficking inside the brain. Journal of Neurochemistry. 2007;**103**:1730-1740. DOI: 10.1111/j.1471-4159.2007.04976.x

[3] Palti H, Meijer A, Adler B. Learning achievement and behavior at school of anemic and non-anemic infants. Early Hum. 1985;**10**:217-223. DOI: 10.1016/0378-3782(85)90052-0

[4] Lozoff B, Wol AW, Jimenez E. Iron-deficiency anemia and infant development: Effects of extended oral iron therapy. The Journal of Pediatrics. 1996;**129**:382-389. DOI: 10.1016/S0022-3476(96)70070-7

[5] Grantham-McGregor S, Ani C. A review of studies on the effect of iron deficiency on cognitive development in children. The Journal of Nutrition. 2001;**131**:649S-668S. DOI: 10.3945/jn.131/2/649S

[6] Beard JL, Connor JR. Iron status and neural functioning. Annual Review of Nutrition. 2003;**23**:41-58. DOI: 10.1146/annurev.nutr.23.020102.075739

[7] Pollitt E. Timing and vulnerability in research on malnutrition and cognition. Nutrition Reviews. 1996;**54**:S49-S55. DOI: 10.1111/j.1753-4887.1996.tb03870.x

[8] Russo N, Edwards M, Andrews T, O'Brien M, Bhatia KP. Hereditary haemochromatosis is unlikely to cause movement disorders—a critical review. Journal of Neurology. 2004;**251**:849-852. DOI: 10.1007/s00415-004-0445-9

[9] Muñoz P, Humeres A, Elgueta C, Kirkwood A, Hidalgo C, Núñez MT. Iron mediates N-methyl-Daspartate receptor-dependent stimulation of calciuminduced pathways and hippocampal synaptic plasticity. The Journal of Biological Chemistry. 2011;**286**:13382-13392. DOI: 10.1074/jbc.M110.213785

[10] Pelizzoni I, Macco R, Zacchetti D, Grohovaz F, Codazzi F. Iron and calcium in the central nervous system: A close relationship in health and sickness. Biochemical Society Transactions. 2008;**36**:1309-1312. DOI: 10.1042/BST0361309

[11] Altamura S, Muckenthaler MU. Iron toxicity in diseases of aging: Alzheimer's disease, Parkinson's disease and atherosclerosis. Journal of Alzheimer's Disease. 2009;**16**:879-895. DOI: 10.3233/JAD-2009-1010

[12] Halliwell B. Oxidative stress and neurodegeneration: Where are we now? Journal of Neurochemistry. 2006;**97**:1634-1658. DOI: 10.1111/j.1471-4159.2006.03907.x

[13] Pelizzoni I, Macco R, Morini MF, Zacchetti D, Grohovaz F, Codazzi F. Iron handling in hippocampal neurons: Activity-dependent iron entry and mitochondria-mediated neurotoxicity. Aging Cell. 2011;**10**:172-183. DOI: 10.1111/j.1474-9726.2010.00652.x

[14] Hellman NE, Gitlin JD. Ceruloplasmin metabolism and function. Annual Review of Nutrition. 2002;**22**:439-458. DOI: 10.1146/annurev.nutr.22.012502.114457

[15] Zaitsev VN, Zaitseva I, Papiz M, Lindley PF. An X-ray crystallographic study of the binding sites of the azide inhibitor and organic substrates to ceruloplasmin, a multicopper oxidase in the plasma. Journal of Biological Inorganic Chemistry. 1999;**4**:579-587. DOI: 10.1007/s007750050380

[16] Ragan HA, Nacht S, Lee GR, Bishop CR, Cartwright GE. The role of ceruloplasmin in iron metabolism. The Journal of Clinical Investigation. 1970;**49**:2408-2417. DOI: 10.1172/JCI106460

[17] Osaki S, Johnson DA, Frieden E. The possible significance of the ferrous oxidase activity of ceruloplasmin in normal human serum. The Journal of Biological Chemistry. 1966;**241**:2746-2751. DOI: 10.1172/JCI106460

[18] Patel BN, Dunn RJ, David S. Alternative RNA splicing generates a glycosylphosphatidylinositol-anchored form of ceruloplasmin in mammalian brain. The Journal of Biological Chemistry. 2000;**275**:4305-4310. DOI: 10.1074/jbc.275.6.4305

[19] Kono S. Aceruloplasminemia. Current Drug Targets. 2012;**13**:1190-1199. DOI: 10.2174/138945012802002320

[20] Jeong SY, David S. Glycosylphosphatidylinositol-anchored ceruloplasmin is required for iron efflux from cells in the central nervous system. The Journal of Biological Chemistry. 2003;**278**:27144-27148. DOI: 10.1074/jbc.M301988200

[21] Rouault TA, Cooperman S. Brain iron metabolism. Seminars in Pediatric Neurology. 2006;**13**:142-148. DOI: 10.1016/j.spen.2006.08.002

[22] Patel BN, Dunn RJ, Jeong SY, Zhu Q, Julien JP, David S. Ceruloplasmin regulates iron levels in the CNS and prevents free radical injury. The Journal of Neuroscience. 2002;**22**:6578-6586 DOI: 20026652

[23] Kono S, Yoshida K, Tomosugi N, Terada T, Hamaya Y, Kanaoka S, Miyajima H. Biological effects of mutant ceruloplasmin on hepcidin-mediated internalization of ferroportin. Biochimica et Biophysica Acta. 2010;**1802**:968-975. DOI: 10.1016/j.bbadis.2010.07.011

[24] De Domenico I, Ward DM, di Patti MC, Jeong SY, David S, Musci G, Kaplan J. Ferroxidase activity is required for the stability of cell surface ferroportin in cells expressing GPI-ceruloplasmin. The EMBO Journal. 2007;**26**:2823-2831. DOI: 10.1038/sj.emboj.7601735

[25] Miyajima H, Nishimura Y, Mizoguchi K, Sakamoto M, Shimizu T, Honda N. Familial apoceruloplasmin deficiency associated with blepharospasm and retinal degeneration. Neurology. 1987;**37**:761-767. DOI: 10.1212/WNL.37.5.761

[26] Harris ZL, Takahashi Y, Miyajima H, Serizawa M, MacGillivray RT, Gitlin JD. Aceruloplasminemia: Molecular characterization of this disorder of iron metabolism. Proceedings of the National Academy of Sciences of the United States of America. 1995;**92**:2539-2543. DOI: 10.1073/pnas.92.7.2539

[27] Miyajima H. Aceruloplasminemia, an iron metabolic disorder. Neuropathology. 2003;**23**:345-350. DOI: 10.1046/j.1440-1789.2003.00521.x

[28] Miyajima H, Kohno S, Takahashi Y, Yonekawa O, Kanno T. Estimation of the gene frequency of aceruloplasminemia in Japan. Neurology. 1999;**53**:617-619. DOI: 10.1212/WNL.53.3.617

[29] Kono S, Miyajima H. Aceruloplasminemia. In: Rosenberg RN, Pascual JM, editors. Rosenberg's Molecular and Genetic Basis of Neurological and Psychiatric Disease. 5th ed. London: Elsevier, Academic Press; 2015. pp. 495-506. DOI: 10.1016/B978-0-12-410529-4.00045-0

[30] Vachette P, Dainese E, Vasyliev VB, Di Muro P, Beltramini M, Svergun DI, De Filippis V, Salvato B. A key structural role for active site type 3 copper ions in human ceruloplasmin. The Journal of Biological Chemistry. 2002;**277**:40823-40831. DOI: 10.1074/jbc.M207188200

[31] McNeill A, Pandolfo M, Kuhn J, Shang H, Miyajima H. The neurological presentation of ceruloplasmin gene mutations. European Neurology. 2008;**60**:200-205. DOI: 10.1159/000148691

[32] Yoshida K, Kaneko K, Miyajima H, Tokuda T, Nakamura A, Kato M, Ikeda S. Increased lipid peroxidation in the brains of aceruloplasminemia patients. Journal of the Neurological Sciences. 2000;**175**:91-95. DOI: 10.1016/S0022-510X(00)00295-1

[33] Miyajima H, Adachi J, Kohno S, Takahashi Y, Ueno Y, Naito T. Increased oxysterols associated with iron accumulation in the brains and visceral organs of acaeruloplasminaemia patients. QJM. 2001;**94**:417-422. DOI: 10.1093/qjmed/94.8.417

[34] Kaneko K, Nakamura A, Yoshida K, Kametani F, Higuchi K, Ikeda S. Glial fibrillary acidic protein is greatly modified by oxidative stress in aceruloplasminemia brain. Free Radical Research. 2002;**36**:303-306. DOI: 10.1080/10715760290019327

[35] Hahn P, Qian Y, Dentchev T, Chen L, Beard J, Harris ZL, Dunaief JL. Disruption of ceruloplasmin and hephaestin in mice causes retinal iron overload and retinal degeneration with features of age-related macular degeneration. Proceedings of the National Academy of Sciences of the United States of America. 2004;**101**:13850-13855. DOI: 10.1073/pnas.0405146101

[36] Jeong SY, David S. Age-related changes in iron homeostasis and cell death in the cerebellum of ceruloplasmin-deficient mice. The Journal of Neuroscience. 2006;**26**:9810-9819. DOI: 10.1523/JNEUROSCI.2922-06.2006

[37] Miyajima H. Aceruloplasminemia. Neuropathology. 2015;**35**:83-90. DOI: 10.1111/neup.12149

[38] Tulpule K, Robinson SR, Bishop GM, Dringen R. Uptake of ferrous iron by cultured rat astrocytes. Journal of Neuroscience Research. 2010;**88**:563-571. DOI: 10.1002/jnr.22217

[39] Brissot P, Ropert M, Le Lan C, Loreal O. Non-transferrin bound iron: A key role in iron overload and iron toxicity. Biochimica et Biophysica Acta. 2012;**1820**:403-410. DOI: 10.1016/j.bbagen.2011.07.014

[40] Zecca L, Youdim MB, Riederer P, Connor JR, Crichton RR. Iron, brain ageing and neurodegenerative disorders. Nature Reviews. Neuroscience. 2004;**5**:863-873. DOI: 10.1038/nrn1537

[41] Gaeta A, Hider RC. The crucial role of metal ions in neurodegeneration: The basis for a promising therapeutic strategy. British Journal of Pharmacology. 2005;**146**:1041-1059. DOI: 10.1038/sj.bjp.0706416

Chapter 10

Astrocyte Pathophysiology in Liver Disease

Carlos Pérez-Monter and Aldo Torre-Delgadillo

Additional information is available at the end of the chapter

http://dx.doi.org/10.5772/intechopen.72506

Abstract

Liver disease is one of the major chronic disabilities around the world. It is known that global casualties are increasing because of virus C infection, alcohol consumption, or non-alcoholic circumstances. One of the main derived comorbidities of liver disease is the hepatic encephalopathy (HE), a severe neuropsychological syndrome derived from the acute or chronic liver disease. A key feature accounting for HE symptoms in cirrhotic patients is brain edema, which is triggered by hyperammonemia. In basal conditions, ammonia can be metabolized in the central nervous system (CNS) by astrocytes, which synthetize glutamine using ammonia and glutamate as substrates. In hyperammonemic conditions, astrocytes synthetize large amounts of glutamine generating a hyperosmotic condition, inducing these cells to become swollen in shape, invoking the characteristic symptom clinically manifested in patients with HE, as brain edema; this condition is regulated by water channels called aquaporins (AQPs) and by other molecules such as myoinositol. Experimental evidence suggests that some small non-coding RNAs may regulate AQPs expression both *in vivo* an *in vitro* and that some pharmacological interventions improve cognitive impairment in cirrhotic patients. It is undeniable that astrocytes and the different signaling pathways beneath its plasma membrane play a crucial role in liver disease-derived HE and represent some of the novel pharmacological targets to treat comorbidities of the liver disease.

Keywords: liver, hyperammonemia, encephalopathy, astrocytes, astrogliosis

1. Introduction

1.1. General aspects of liver disease and hepatic encephalopathy

Liver disease is one of the leading non-infectious pathologies affecting people around the world. In its report from 2015, WHO indicates that the advanced form of liver disease, meaning cirrhosis, is among the 20 most frequent (2%) causes of death (~1.62×10^6) around the globe (http://www.who.int/). Hepatic encephalopathy (HE) is a pathological condition that represents the neuropsychiatric disorder derived from liver disease. It is known that about 80% of patients with liver disease (depending on severity), may develop HE, which represents one of the major complications leading to death in about 90% of patients with acute liver failure (ALV) [1]. HE has been classified by the Hepatic Encephalopathy consensus Group, at the World Congress of Gastroenterology in 1998, in type A, associated with ALV; type B related to porto-systemic bypass; and type C related with chronic liver disease, mainly cirrhosis [2]. Further classification includes the severity of symptoms that includes the subcategory called covert (CHE, also known as minimal), persistent (PHE), and overt (OHE). The former is mild in manifestations and is hard to diagnose without specific neurophysiological and neuropsychological tests, such as the visual-based flicker test, the psychometric hepatic encephalopathy score (PHES), the repeatable battery for assessment of neuropsychological status (RBANS), the inhibitory control test (ICT), the cognitive drug research (CDR), and the most recent STROOP App test (*EncephalApp_Stroop*), a practical smartphone App tool for HE screening to be used by the own patients [3, 4]. The PHE and OHE involve more specific clinical symptoms, including seizures, hyperreflexia, rigidity, myoclonus (sudden involuntary jerking of a muscle or a group of muscles), asterixis (hand tremor when wrist is extended), and stupor, which can be detected or reported by the clinician or patient as well [5]. In all of these cases, the main gross causative is the liver failure and the metabolic pathways affected thereafter. In general terms, HE is a debilitating condition in which patients gradually became less psychologically independent and more psychiatrically dependent. The majority of the symptoms in HE are triggered by molecular events within the central nervous system (CNS), and several hypotheses have been proposed in order to understand the pathophysiology. Some of them suggest that metabolites such as ammonia, myoinositol, glutamine, manganese, inflammatory mediators (IL-1, IL-6, and TNFα), and amino acids (Tyr, Phe, Val, Ile, and Leu) [6], regarding its effects over astrocytes and neuronal cells, are responsible of the clinical manifestations of the disease [6–8].

2. Astrocytes as mediators of the pathophysiology of HE

In this and further sections, we will try to introduce to the reader into a review about recent findings that illustrates how the physiological functions of the liver, or to a better extent, a lack of them, may harm at different levels, the metabolic and physiological homeostasis over brain cells and function.

2.1. Ammonium metabolism

The liver is responsible to detoxify the majority of endogenous or exogenous toxic compounds produced by the metabolic or catabolic activity within the organism, including pharmacological metabolites, ammonium, bilirubin, bile salts, etc. Several factors may affect liver functions, such as increased consumption of a fat diet, another one is the chronic alcohol abuse; while the infection by hepatitis C virus (HCV), pharmacological intoxication (mainly paracetamol), complete the pathological scenario. The fatty liver, also known as steatosis (non-alcoholic fatty liver disease or NAFLD), has been called the first hit in liver damage, which when not properly attended, could result in a chronic inflammation or steatohepatitis (NASH). NASH could evolve to fibrosis and eventually to a more critical stage, cirrhosis. Cirrhotic patients suffer a wide spectrum of comorbidities [9]. Among them is hepatic encephalopathy (HE), a debilitating psychological condition where the patients present a variety of symptoms including loss of memory, mild or manifested tremors, and most importantly, increased plasma levels of ammonia. In basal conditions, ureotelic organisms like humans, should contend with the ammonia derived from the gastrointestinal bacterial activity and muscle metabolism, by converting it to carbamoyl-phosphate (CP), a substrate of the urea cycle, CP is then converted to citrulline, the precursor of arginosuccinate; arginosuccinate is then transformed to arginine and by the action of arginase, arginine is converted to urea and ornithine; all of these reactions takes place within the mitochondria and cytosol of the hepatocytes, resulting in the release of urea into the bloodstream and then in urine [10]. However, in pathological conditions like cirrhosis, hepatocytes are unable to produce urea; therefore, ammonium in its form of gas (NH_3) easily diffuses to the blood brain barrier (BBB). Once within CNS, ammonium is metabolized primarily by the astrocytes, a group of specialized glial cells capable of modulate inhibitory and excitatory neurotransmission. In its form of ion (NH_4^+), ammonia reaches the astrocytes where a different transporter mediates its translocation throughout the plasma membrane. Among this transporters are the Na^+/K^+-ATPase pump, the Na^+/H^+-ATPase antiporter and $Na^+/K^+/2Cl^-$, K^+/Cl^- symporters [5]. Astrocytes metabolize the ammonium by the so-called glutamate-glutamine cycle (GGC). The GGC produces glutamine (Gln) through the action of glutamine synthetase (GS), delivering it to neighboring glutamatergic neurons (**Figure 1**). In neurons, glutamine is subject to the opposite reaction, mediated by the enzyme glutaminase, whose products are glutamate and ammonium. Glutamate is packaged into synaptic vesicles and released to the synaptic cleft in response to electrochemical stimulus, while ammonium is released to the extracellular space [11]. Once released, glutamate binds to ionotropic (N-methyl-D-aspartate (NMDA) or AMPA) receptors, or metabotropic (mGluR1 and mGluR2) receptors in the postsynaptic neuron and astrocytes [11]. Unbound released glutamate can be

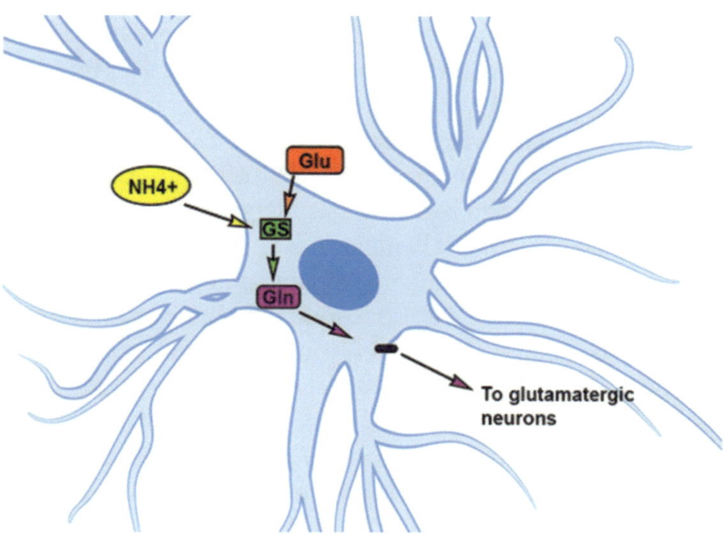

Figure 1. The glutamine (Gln)-glutamate (Glu) cycle within astrocytes. Glutamine synthase (GS) mediates the reaction of ammonia ($NH4^+$) and Glu to produce Gln. Gln is then exported by a specific transporter (illustrated here as a small black cylinder) to the glutamatergic neurons near the astrocyte. The cycle completes when Glu is released to the synaptic cleft and then binds to NMDA receptors or is recaptured by astrocytes to began the cycle. See text for details.

recycled when captured by the excitatory amino acid transporters (EAAT) located in the astrocytes membrane. These events represent the final step in the GGC.

On the other hand, besides GGC, astrocytes may use other systems to titrate ammonium from bloodstream. Those based in the use of the branched chain amino acids (BCAA) on one side, or the use of L-ornithine and L-aspartate in the other. In the first case, BCAA are metabolized by the enzyme branched-chain amino acid transaminase (BCAT) particularly enriched in the cytoplasm and axons of glutamatergic and GABAergic neurons [12]; cytoplasmic BCAT enzymatically mediates the synthesis of branched-chain ketoacids (BCKA), which in turn generates both, a precursor for the tri-carboxylic acid cycle (TCA) in the form of Acetyl-CoA and the excitatory amino acid glutamate; glutamate in turn, can be metabolized by means of the GS to produce glutamine; glutamine is deaminated by the phosphate-activated glutaminase (PAG) which is also present in the cytoplasm of neuronal and glial cells [13]. The second one, the L-Ornithine and L-Aspartate system, operates to generate glutamate by means of the ornithine- or aspartate-aminotransferase (OAT, AAT); both enzymes are enriched in the skeletal muscle, thus contributing to stimulate the glutamine production in this tissue by the GS, diminishing the ammonia derived from circulation [5]. L-ornithine and L-aspartate represent one of the most frequent therapeutic approaches to improve ammonia levels in cirrhotic patients, as we shall see later.

2.2. Astrocytes and the effect of hyperammonemic conditions within CNS

It is known that NH_4^+ and K^+ have comparable physical and chemical properties, so that any change or increase in NH_4^+ concentrations may activate the Na^+ transport by the Na^+/K^+-ATPase pump, leading to abnormal neurotransmission in neurons or even astrocytes [14]. NH_4^+ enters to the astrocytes and induces the increase in the activity of the GS; this event results in the accumulation of glutamine. As intracellular glutamine concentrations rise, the osmotic pressure does it in parallel, provoking the astrocytes to become swelling and to activate two main mechanisms to counteract this morphological change [15]. The first one consists of the release of an osmotic regulator, myoinositol; myoinositol leaves the astrocyte to redress the osmotic balance within the cell to prevent astrocyte and cerebral edema; while the other one is to increase the activity of the water channels called aquaporins (AQPs). One of the main water channel transporters related with regulation of the osmotic response in astrocytes, is the aquaporin 4 (AQP4) [16]. It has been reported that AQP4 increases its activity under hyperammonemic conditions, allowing the H_2O molecules to enter into the cell, thus relieving the osmotic pressure induced by the accumulation of glutamine [17]. Until then, it was not clear whether the increased activity of AQP4 was the result of a higher transcriptional activity or an increased rate of mRNA translation [18]. Evidence in favor of both options had been reported. In two separate reports, Jalan et al. and Norenberg et al. demonstrated independently the increased expression of AQP4 protein, in a chronic or acute *in vivo* models of liver failure based on the bile duct ligation (BLD) or the use of thioacetamide (TAA) or acetaminophen (AAP), respectively [19, 20]. Accordingly, *in vitro* evidence indicates that ammonia-treated astrocytes also increase AQP4 protein levels [21]. On the other hand and in favor of transcription, additional evidence indicates that ammonium or mannitol, both osmotic stressors, increase the expression of AQP4 mRNA *in vitro* and *in vivo*, probably mediated by the p38-MAPK signaling pathway, which stimulates the tonicity-enhancer binding protein (TonEBP) to interact with the responsive enhancer element (TonE) over the AQP4 gene promoter region

[17, 19, 22]. Further evidence indicates that other AQPs are direct targets of the hypothalamic arginine-vasopressin peptide (AVP) and the angiotensin II (ANGII) hormone; for instance, AVP controls the expression of AQP2 in the renal collecting duct cells under basal conditions, increasing the intracellular levels of cAMP that in turns modifies the activity of one of its targets, PKA; PKA phosphorylates the CREB protein allowing its translocation to the nucleus and its transcriptional activity [23]. It remains to be elucidated if AQP4 gene expression in hepatic encephalopathy conditions is also regulated by similar mechanisms.

As we have seen, hepatic failure is closely related to astrocyte low grade and brain edema mediated by water movement throughout the AQP4 channel. Among the pathogenic factors contributing to aggravate this condition are the free radical production, the MAP-kinase activity, and the induction of the mitochondrial permeability transition (MPT) process. MPT is well known to occur in response to the sudden intra-cytoplasmic increase of molecules around 1.5 kDa in size that enters the mitochondria mediated by the so-called permeability transition pore (PTP), which is located at the inner membrane [24]. These phenomena critically compromises mitochondria homeostasis and the metabolic function of many crucial processes like the TCA and ATP synthesis, promoting the generation of reactive oxygen species (ROS). It seems that HE promotes the generation of ROS, therefore inducing the MPT due to the oxidative stress, because indirect evidence demonstrates that antioxidants are able to reduce MPT. Norenberg et al. demonstrated that MPT is involved in the ammonium-induced astrocyte swelling after their *in vitro* experiments based on the use of cyclosporine A (CsA), a well-known inhibitor of MPT [25]; in this study, the expression of the AQP4 protein was also inhibited by CsA, indicating a plausible crosstalk between different signaling pathways, such as the MAP-kinases or that conformed by the protein kinase A (PKA)/CREB, both of which might be related to the control of cell swelling in hyperammonemic conditions.

2.3. Systemic and local inflammatory pathway effects on astrocyte disturbances

Another important mechanism of regulation of astrocyte physiology in response to hepatic failure is the activation of the pro-inflammatory response. In recent years, an increasing role of the inflammatory-related pathways in response to ammonia-induced brain dysfunction has been reported. The cytokines promoting brain damage are TNFα, interlukin-6 (IL-6), interlukin1-beta (IL-1β), IL-18, and many others. However, there is controversy about the role between these pro-inflammatory cytokines in both acute and chronic hepatic failure. Several groups have provided evidence of a positive correlation in this interaction in human subjects or animal models. In 2007, Wright and colleagues determined the TNFα, IL-6, and IL-1β artery blood levels and found a positive correlation of these cytokines with intracranial pressure in ALF-affected humans [26]. Further evidence indicates that the same cytokines are elevated, at least at the transcriptional level, in the brains of a rat ALF model [27]. A recent interesting proposal about the role of these circulating inflammatory interleukins indicates that they might interact with certain blood-brain barrier (BBB) endothelial cells to reach the CNS, acting synergistically with ammonia. This synergistic model has been expanded through the identification of additional factors such as GABA produced by certain bacterial families within the gut, contributing to modify the GABAergic tone that reach the CNS via the vagal afferent pathway [28]. In view of these facts, systemic inflammation is in part responsible for the astrocyte and neuronal network alterations in both acute and chronic liver disease. A major player in the systemic inflammation effects over CNS in these pathologies is a member of the danger-associated molecular patterns (DAMPS) called high mobility group box protein 1 (HMGB1), which in basal conditions regulates transcriptional activity [29]; however, in pathological conditions, it can be released passively from damaged cells into the extracellular space in response to pro-inflammatory stimuli, such as LPS; HMGB1 can also be actively released by a JAK/STAT acetylation-mediated process, from immunocompetent cells [30]. In a recent study, Ohnishi et al. showed that HMGB1 significantly decrease the expression of AQP4 mRNA and protein in cultured astrocytes; conversely, the intra-cerebroventricular injection of HMGB1 in adult rats, slightly increase AQP4 protein expression and as expected, the brain edema; further, exposure of microglia to a HMGB had a significant effect over IL-1β mRNA expression and protein release, which apparently regulates AQP4 increased expression; the authors suggest that the pathway IL-1β-NF-κB-AQP4 in microglia might regulate the brain edema in response to HMGB1-mediated systemic inflammation [31]. Whether this pathway might occur with other pro-inflammatory cytokines such as TNFα, IL-6, or IFNγ, remains to be investigated.

The unusual extracellular histone proteins represent another piece in the puzzle of the systemic inflammation response. It has been showed that in ALF or HBV infected patients, increased concentrations of circulating histones correlates with an immunostimulatory effect, leading to multiple organ injuries [32–34]. *In vitro* experiments with hepatic or monocyte cell lines stimulated with sera obtained from ALF patients, elicit cell death or release of inflammatory cytokines, respectively; interestingly, these effects were abolished with heparin—a histone-binding anticoagulant—suggesting that histone proteins are key players in the cellular injury and systemic inflammation observed in ALF-affected patients [32]. In addition to previously described consequences of the liver disease, including hyponatremia, sepsis, variceal bleeding, and renal failure; is the activation of microglial cells, the resident macrophages of the brain. Microglia increase the synthesis and release of inflammatory cytokines in a process called microgliosis [35]. Microgliosis is part of the most general response gliosis, which involves the astrocytes, the microglia, and oligodendrocyte cells; microgliosis is the local response to brain insults and typically represents the scar-promoting mechanism within the CNS.

Along with systemic and local brain inflammation, the increased ammonia and manganese levels in the brain also alter the TCA cycle, promoting lactate accumulation and the promotion of dopaminergic cell death, as well as the generation of reactive oxygen species (ROS) in basal ganglia, and contributing in this way to the parkinsonism-like behavior and cognitive impairment observed in cirrhotic patients [36]. In this line of evidence, oxidative stress is thought to be of relevance for ammonia toxicity in HE. Molecular studies indicate that acute ammonia loading, mechanical or drugs stressors like hypo-osmolarity, diazepam, and TNFα, *in vitro* and *in vivo*, increases ribonucleic acid (RNA) oxidation. Among the oxidized RNA species, the 18 s rRNA and the glutamate/aspartate transporter (GLAST/SLC1A3) mRNA have been described; strikingly, the cerebral RNA oxidation in liver-injured rats predominates in the transport RNA granules located in close vicinity with postsynaptic spines, where learning and memory-associated protein synthesis occurs [37]. These data strongly suggest that ammonia-induced inflammation and RNA oxidation might impair both cognitive events in cirrhotic patients. In addition, it has been demonstrated that ammonia inhibits astrocyte proliferation promoting senescence both *in vitro* and *in vivo*, by means of the multidrug resistance-associated protein (Mrp) 4 and by a p38/MAPK-dependent activation of the cell cycle inhibitor genes GADD45α and p21 [38, 39].

2.4. The role of the intestinal microbiota in the gut-liver-brain axis

The intestinal microbiota has evolved as a new and relevant player in the pathogenesis of several intestinal and non-intestinal diseases. As the liver is the organ in closest contact with the intestinal tract, it is potentially exposed to bacterial components and metabolites. In physiological conditions, nutrients and bacterial compounds translocate to the liver via the portal circulation and contribute to the host homeostasis. As the epithelial wall and mucus layer act as physical barrier to impede that the most of the bacterial components or even bacteria reach the blood flow, it is usually accepted that a small quantity of these compounds enter the portal venous flow, and a tight balance on the immune response is achieved in order to fight against potential exogenous insults. However, in pathological conditions, such a physical barrier can become more permeable to bacterial components, specially lipopolysaccharide (LPS), flagellin, peptidoglycan, and microbial nucleic acids [40]. Evidence about the effect of gut microbiota over hepatic physiology has been demonstrated. In 2010, Gupta and co-workers found that small intestine bacterial overgrowth (SIBO) was a hallmark in cirrhotic patients suffering of HE [41]; in the same year, Jun et al. published evidence about the direct association of SIBO with the peripheral founding of bacterial DNA in cirrhotic patients [42]; later on, in 2012, Henao-Mejia et al. demonstrated that genetic deficiency of inflammasome, a protein complex considered the sensor of endogenous and exogenous pathogen-associated molecular patterns (PAMPS), induced the accumulation of bacterial components in the portal circulation, with the consequent liver damage effect [43]. One important fact about the bacterial overgrowth in cirrhotic patients is that the translocation of bacteria or any of its components promotes and aggravates the liver illness. There are several reports indicating the differences in the fecal microbiota of various populations around the globe, specifically in patients with liver cirrhosis in comparison with healthy subjects. In general, these studies coincides in founding that the *phyla Proteobacteria* and *Fusobacteria*, significantly increases in cirrhotic patients, compared with its healthy counterparts [44–46]; while at the genus level, the pathogenic *Enterobacteriaceae*, *Alcaligenaceae*, *Porphyromonadaceae*, *Veillonellaceae*, and *Streptococcaceae* families prevail and the beneficial taxa such as *Lachnospiraceae* and *Bifidobacteriaceae*, diminished in cirrhotic samples [45, 47]. In our laboratory, we conducted a pilot study in order to explore the changes in the microbiota of cirrhotic patients. Preliminary results indicate that some of these taxa previously reported are also present in the cirrhotic group of VHC-infected patients based in Mexico city; but we have also found that some other taxa have not been reported in other population (unpublished data); our findings are in concordance with the idea that additional variables, such as ethnicity or geographical location and even food ingestion habits, should be taken into account in order to interpret microbiome-derived studies, which eventually can be used in future clinical trials.

Another significant consequence of SIBO is the higher tendency of the microbial community to increase the synthesis and release of organic compounds with a metabolic effect over a wide number of host cells. For example, it has been demonstrated that ingestion of *L. rhamnosus*, diminishes the expression of gamma-amino-butyric acid (GABA) receptor ($GABA_B$) in the cingulate and prelimbic cortical regions of mice brain; this $GABA_B$ regulation implies a direct effect over neuronal physiology, which reflects in less anxiety and more antidepressant-like behavior in mice; moreover, vagotomised mice were unable to respond to *L. rhamnosus*, indicating that vagus nerve acts as an interface between gut bacteria and the brain [28]. Whether these bacteria produce a GABA-like neurotransmitter or directly modify the fire-threshold from vagus nerve remains a matter of study. Nowadays, molecular studies contributing to explain partially the mechanics behind the role of GABA and the intestinal microbiota have been published. Butterworth and colleagues in 1990 and 2008, found that brain samples from cirrhotic patients who died from HE, had unusual elevated levels of the peripheral-type benzodiazepine receptors (PTBZR) and of neurosteroids such as allopregnanolone (ALLO) or tetrahydrodeoxycorticosterone (THDOC) [48, 49]; interestingly, these neurosteroids are synthesized in the brain following activation of the translocator protein (TSPO), whose main activity is the cholesterol transport through the mitochondria, where stimulates the steroid biosynthesis [50]. Further evidence from Noremberg and co-workers indeed, indicates that astrocyte exposure to ammonia and manganese, significantly increase the TSPO activity, at least *in vitro* [51], indicating that neurosteroids are one of the main metabolites synthetized in response to hyperammonemic conditions as a result of dysbiosis and a lack of a functional urea cycle. However, there is some evidence indicating that some other metabolites produced by gut microbiota, such as the bile acids, tryptophan precursors, serotonin and catecholamine, might be able to signal through membrane receptors located in local cells of the gut epithelium or by a neurocrine or endocrine pathways; among these metabolites are the carbohydrate derivatives butyrate, acetate and propionate, which might be converted to short chain fatty acids (SCFAs); these SCFA in turn can reduce food intake and modulate the immune system response in the host [52, 53]. Different reports indicate that SCFAs are present in the enteroendocrine cells and on neurons of the submucosal and myenteric ganglia [54, 55]. Besides the SCFAs, it cannot be ruled out the possibility that some Gram-positive cell wall components are also capable of inducing neuronal or glial cell damage within the CNS of cirrhotic patients. In 2005, a report indicated that lipoteichoic acid (LTA) and muramyl dipeptide from *Staphylococcus aureus* induce a strong inflammatory response that ultimately lead to neuronal death by increasing nitric oxide (NO), superoxide (O_2-), peroxynitrite (ONOO-), TNFα, IL-1β and IL-6, within astrocytes and microglia [56].

Here, we can say that the net result of the so-called "*dysbiosis*" in cirrhotic patients is that a plethora of metabolic compounds like urea, methanol, short-chain fatty acids (SCFAs), and other volatile compounds are delivered or restricted to the host via the gastrointestinal tract. Altogether, these data indicate that intestinal bacteria play key roles in development and pathophysiology of hepatic liver over the CNS.

2.5. Genetic and epigenetic effects induced by HE in astrocytes

Epigenetic modifications are heritable and reversible stable marks that do not modify gene sequences *per se*, but have tremendous impact over the gene expression process. These marks allow the genome to adapt its transcriptional repertoire to different cellular and molecular conditions in response to environmental cues for fine-tuning of gene expression, and encompass a myriad of processes including histone, DNA and RNA modifications. One of the best-studied DNA modifications is the methylation (5-mC) and 5-hidroxy-methylation (5-hmC) of cytosine bases at the CpG dinucleotide sequence, mediated by the DNA methyltransferase (DNMT) or by the translocated in liposarcoma, Ewing's sarcoma and TATA-binding protein-associated factor 15 (TET)-family of proteins, respectively [57]. It is widely accepted that the first mark, 5-mC, is a negative signal for gene expression to occur, while the 5-hydroxy-mC indicates the opposite. The role of DNA methylation dynamics within astrocytes is not yet known, at least in the context of HE derived from liver disease; however, specific data indicate that the NMDA receptor NR2B gene is negatively regulated by the neuron restrictive silencer factor (NRSF) in ethanol-exposed cortical neurons *in vitro* [58]; although specific analysis in this study indicates that NRSF directly interacts with the NR2B gene promoter region, there is no evidence of how ethanol regulates NRSF gene expression. Further evidence about the role of methylation or acetylation of glutamatergic or gabaergic-mediated signaling pathways affected by hyperammonemia remains to be elucidated.

On the other hand, we know that non-coding RNAs (ncRNA) are important players in epigenetic mechanisms regulating cell fate and metabolism. Among the ncRNAs with relevant physiological roles are small RNAs and the long non-coding-RNAs (lncRNAs). A variant of small RNAs includes the microRNAS (miRNAs), which are beginning to acquire significant roles in coordinating astrocyte gene expression. miRNAs are small RNAs (~22 nt in length) that controls gene expression through their binding to the 3′-untranslated region (UTR) in mRNAs, leading transcripts to degradation or translational repression [59]. Long noncoding RNAs (lncRNA) on the other side are sequences of about 200 nt in length, which regulate the expression of neighbor protein-coding-genes in a phenomenon called "transvection" (for a systematic review see [60]). In the last decade, there has been an increase in the number of reports demonstrating the role of both miRNAs and lncRNAs in the physiopathology of HE. Two of the first reports regarding the role of two specific miRNA in the regulation of astrocyte cell swelling came from Singapore; in 2010 and 2012, Jeyaseelan and colleagues published in separate papers that miR-130a and miR-320a directly affect the AQP4 expression in the CNS. In the first case, the role of miR-130a is a non-canonical regulation, because the repression mechanism occurs at the transcriptional level over the AQP4 M1 gene promoter [61], while the mir320a was described as a modulator of AQP1 and AQP4 in a model of cerebral ischemia [62]. In a more wide recent study, Häussinger and co-workers explored the global miRNA profile using NH4Cl stimulated rat brain astrocytes *in vitro*. They were interested in the ammonia-dependent senescence observed in astrocytes and its relationship with miRNAs. By means of miRNA array experiments, they found that 43 of 336 miRNAs were significantly downregulated in hyperammonemic conditions, six of which (miR-31a-5p, miR-221-3p miR-221-5p, miR-222-3p, miR-326-3p, and miR-365-3p) seem to bind and regulate the mRNA encoding the heme oxygenase 1 (HO-1) protein; four of these miRNAs (miR-31a-5p, miR-221-3p, miR-222-3p, and miR-326-3p) were prevented to be downregulated by NH4Cl treatment, when astrocytes were exposed to the glutamine synthase inhibitor, methionine sulfoximine (MSO); moreover, the NADPH oxidase inhibitor, apocynin, fully prevented NH4Cl-mediated downregulation of the four miRNAs predicted to target HO-1, indicating that senescence is regulated by miRNA expression in cultured astrocytes and partly regulated by glutamine synthesis and NADPH-oxidase activity [63]. Data recently obtained in our laboratory indicate that three miRNAs (miR-29a-5p, miR-29b-3p, and miR-148b-3p) are repressed in brain tissue of a mouse model of liver cirrhosis. Interestingly, we found that the same miRNAs were downregulated in *in vitro* experiments using primary astrocytes incubated in the presence of NH4Cl (**Figure 2**); thus indicating that these miRNAs are strongly correlated with the physiological regulation of AQP4, both in basal and pathological conditions. Future experiments will allow us to demonstrate whether overexpression of these miRNAs by means of systemic or direct injection in hyperammonemic conditions counteracts the astrocyte cytotoxic edema.

The lncRNAs, on the other hand, had been more less studied in the context of liver-associated CNS pathologies; however, in a recent study in which 35,923 lncRNAs were screened using

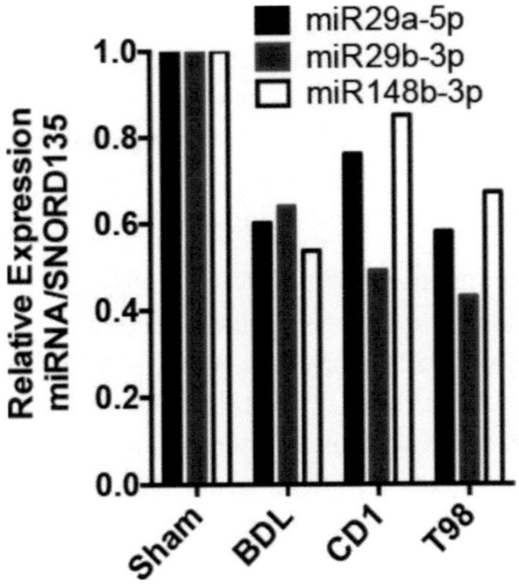

Figure 2. The expression of miR-29 and miR-148 diminished in response to hyperammonemia in vivo and in vitro. Total RNA extracted from the whole brain of bile duct ligated (BDL) mice or control mice (Sham), as well as primary astrocytes (CD1) or the astrocytoma cell line T-98 in the presence or absence of NH_4Cl, was used to evaluate the expression by means of qPCR. The data represent the mean expression of at least three replicates in each case (unpublished data).

microarrays, Silva and colleagues found that 380 and 486 transcripts were upregulated or downregulated in a mouse model of acute liver failure. The authors found that some of these lncRNAs might be related to the cytokine-receptor interaction, MAPK, insulin, NFκB, and TNFα signaling pathways, all of them related to the inflammatory response; the authors also found that the lncRNA uc007pjf.1 associated with a guanine nucleotide exchange factor (NET1), which regulates RhoA, is involved in the cytoskeleton dynamics, suggesting a relationship of this factor with the astrocyte cell swelling observed in HE [64]; these data are of relevance because contributes to corroborate the role of some genetic pathways already related with ALF and certainly established the roots to new discoveries; however, these findings are the result of a combination of cellular phenotypes within CNS and are hardly extrapolated solely to astrocytes, neurons, microglia or even to non-differentiated precursor cells residing in the frontal cortex; complementary *in vitro* or FACS-sorted cells experiments, should be carried out in order to acutely assign the contribution of each of these cell phenotypes to the physiopathology of liver disease.

2.6. Clinical data in osmoregulation and systemic infections in cirrhotic patients with HE

The maintenance of a constant cell volume is a critical problem of all cells. Cell swelling or shrinkage is undesirable for normal cellular function. Changes in the cell volume mostly occur due to changes in the extra or intracellular osmolarity. As most cell membranes are freely permeable to water and do not possess water pumps in their membranes, cells will shrink or swell in response to changes in the tonicity of the extracellular fluid (ECF) [65]. Cells will shrink in a hypertonic ECF, while they swell in a hypotonic ECF. Similarly, when the tonicity of the intracellular space of the cells increases, the cells try to compensate it and increase the osmolarity by the uptake of water from the ECF—and consequently swell. Extra- and intracellular osmolarity is determined by the concentrations of several compounds, such as ions, amino acids, etc. Consistent with the adaption against the rise of intracellular osmolarity in patients affected by CLF, it has been proposed that reductions in brain concentrations of myoinositol are implicated in the pathogenesis of ammonia-induced brain edema [66].

In the same line of evidence, it is difficult to elucidate whether the release of taurine (an atypical aminoacid with osmoregulatory properties) from the astrocytes to the ECF is an osmoregulatory response to increased intracellular glutamine and/or cell swelling, since other mechanisms that increased intracellular osmolarity may lead to the cellular release of taurine and taurine may also be released from neurons. Taurine has been related with reversal of hepatic hypertension in a rat model of liver cirrhosis; in a study from 2009, Liang and colleagues found that natural taurine significantly decreased the portal venous pressure, resistance and flow, and markedly decrease the nitric oxide (NO) and cyclic guanine-monophosphate (cGMP), with a concomitant reduction in the pathological status of liver tissue damage and the expression of collagen 1 (COL-1), COL-III, and transforming growth factor-β1 (TGF-β1) [67]. Taurine also have clinical uses in the form of a hydrophilic bile acid called tauroursodeoxycholate (TUDCA) for treatment of primary biliary cirrhosis (PBC). In a randomized cross-over study with 12 female patients suffering from PBC, the use of TUDCA showed to improve the enrichment of biliary ursodeoxycholate (UDCA) and was better absorbed than ursodeoxycholate and undergoes less biotransformation than UDCA, thus suggesting that TUDCA is clinically relevant for the treatment of cholestatic liver diseases [68]. As taurine is synthetized in both liver and brain it is plausible that HE might impact on taurine metabolism and biological action. Several reports have indeed described the pathological disturbances in patients with chronic liver disease as well as in liver failure murine models. In both cases, the taurine concentrations were significantly diminished [69, 70]. Astrocytes synthetize and stored taurine, which is involved in ion movement across CNS, mainly K^+ and Ca^{2+}; therefore, is not rare to consider that neural excitability modifications in cirrhotic patients occurs. Evidence in favor of this hypothesis was reported in an experimental model of ALF, in which CSF taurine concentrations significantly increased in a positive correlation with early progression of HE [71]. As taurine has osmoregulatory actions any increase or decrease in its extracellular concentrations could have an impact in the pathogenesis of acute liver failure as has been demonstrated [72]. In contrast, taurine concentrations in chronic liver failure are not changed, but the release of taurine into the extracellular space could represent a control mechanism for volume regulation of astrocytes [73, 74].

Another important metabolite that has been related with HE is the acidic calcium binding protein S100β, produced by astrocytes in the CNS and apparently secreted in response to oxidative stress, exerting its paracrine or autocrine effects on glia, neurons, and microglia [75–77]. S100β is a multifunctional protein that can be measured in basal conditions in CSF and is barely detected in circulating blood flow; however, in pathological conditions, its serum levels might increase, indicating neuronal or astrocytic damage. Our group and others have begun to investigate the diagnostic efficacy of S100β as a biomarker to detect low grade HE in cirrhotic patients. Recent findings from our laboratory indicate that cirrhotic subjects with OHE have higher serum levels of S100β when compared with non-HE cirrhotic or cirrhotic patients with MHE or control subjects, and that 0.13 ng/mL of S100β is the best cut-off for the diagnosis of HE (83 and 64% of sensitivity and specificity, respectively) [78]. These results are in accordance with previous data in which S100β and neuron-specific enolase (NSE) were evaluated in a small Egyptian cohort of 52 subjects, where 62 and 38% of 29 cirrhotic patients had HE grade 1 or 2, respectively; these groups were compared with non-HE cirrhotic or healthy subjects. Here, NSE showed non-significant differences among the groups, but S100β was increased in serum samples from grade 1 and 2 HE, compared with cirrhotic or healthy subjects; in addition, a significant positive correlation was found between S100β levels and plasma ammonia, in all patients; the main conclusion in this report was that S100β serum levels could be a useful surrogate marker with more than 90 and 50% of specificity and sensitivity, respectively, for detection of mild cognitive impairment in cirrhotic patients, before they progress to more advanced stages of HE [79]. In a similar study, Wiltfang et al. reported that a cut-off value of 112 pg./mL or 0.11 ng/mL of serum S100β, practically the same value found in our group of patients, is able to predict subclinical porto-systemic encephalopathy with a 100 and 57% of specificity and sensitivity, respectively [80].

Osmotic abnormalities account for the cognitive impairment in cirrhotic patients and some clinicians are using the magnetic resonance (MR) in order to clearly demonstrate a relationship among water, manganese, glutamate, glutamine, and myoinositol levels and the degree of brain damage in patients with liver disease. MR might be useful to diagnose brain abnormalities elicited by hyperammonemia, especially in specific regions like the *globus pallidum* and the temporal region. It has been documented that N-acetylaspartate (NAA) is a good biomarker for neuronal loss and phosphocholine (Cho) concentrations reflects phospholipid metabolism and osmotic regulation due to its role in membrane synthesis and myelin destruction. Low levels of Cho have been associated with osmotic changes in the brain of cirrhotic patients. The majority of these metabolites have different echo times in MR spectroscopy with glutamate (Glu), glutamine (Gln), and phosphocreatine (PPC) being some of most constant correlation findings between patients with or without HE. However, in patients with OHE, the MR is difficult to perform because many confounding factors might co-exist, such as infection, renal failure, anemia, alcohol consumption, and other factors [81]. Our group recently conducted a pilot study in which non-infected compensated, infected cirrhotic, and healthy patients were evaluated to assess for cerebral changes in myoinositol and NAA by means of proton magnetic resonance spectroscopy (^{1}H–MRs). Here, we have found that 40 and 30% of the infected patients were by spontaneous bacterial peritonitis or urinary tract infection, respectively; we also registered a significant decrease of myoinositol levels in the temporal region of non-infected cirrhotic and infected cirrhotic patients when compared with the healthy control group; in addition, we found a similar pattern whit NAA, which significantly diminished in the former groups (**Figure 3**) (unpublished data). When we sought over basal ganglia, Creatine, Cho as well as myoinositol levels did also significantly diminished in infected cirrhotic patients; altogether these results strongly suggests that acute infection in cirrhotic patients contributes to regulate brain metabolites and may be a factor related with development of HE (unpublished data).

Besides those data indicating that brain metabolites are also implicated in the pathophysiology of HE, another important issue in end-stage liver disease is the local blood flow. Cirrhotic patients with portal hypertension suffering ascites, hepatorenal syndrome and HE, usually also had distorted cerebral blood flow (CBF), which severely impact their skeletal muscle, brain, and kidney irrigation as a result of vascular resistance. It has been a long way since the 1960s decade, when one of the first studies about cerebral hemodynamics in cirrhosis came into light [82]. Since then, a plenty of studies have contributed to understand the role of vascular pressure over the pathology associated with HE. In 1969, Bianchi-Porro and co-workers reported that after portacaval shunt surgery, cirrhotic patients, had a significance increase in

http://dx.doi.org/10.5772/intechopen.72506

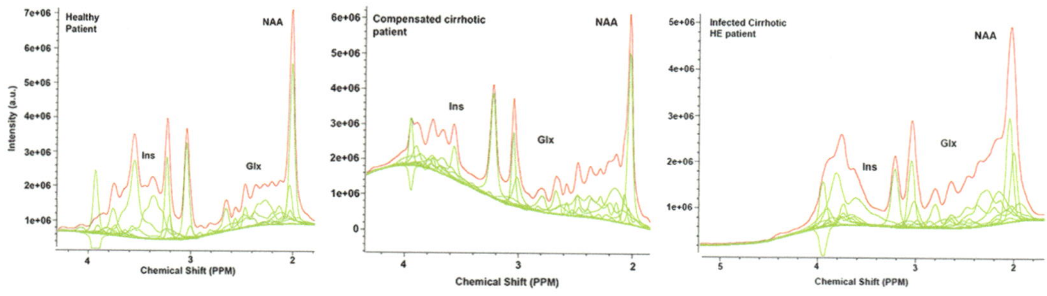

Figure 3. Cirrhotic infected patients have significant abnormalities in the glutamine/glutamate (Glx) ratio and NAA brain levels. See text for details.

CBF and a significant decrease in cerebral vascular resistance (a measure of CBF and metabolism) and the metabolic rate of glucose and the glucose:oxygen quotient did also increase in these patients; the authors suggested that the increased CBF was related to metabolic problems, and that this increase accelerates the removal of toxic substances and allows the disposal of brain metabolites capable of neutralize toxic compounds [83]. It is now well accepted that cirrhotic patients have decreased CBF, portal hypertension, and splanchnic vasodilatation, associated with a hyperdynamic circulatory state, all of which can affect CBF. In a more recent study, we described a maneuver in which we used the transcranial Doppler (TCD) technique (transmission of ultrasound beam through the skull using a pulsed Doppler sectorial probe with a 2 MHz transducer), to measure in an non-invasive and reliable way, the cerebral autoregulation, meaning the physiological mechanisms that maintain CBF at an appropriate levels in response to vasoconstrictors or vasodilators and the middle cerebral artery (MCA) velocities. From here, two functional cerebral hemodynamic indexes were evaluated, (a) the pulsatility index (PI) which assesses the arteriolar vascular integrity and (b) the breath holding index (BHI), which measures cerebrovascular reactivity (CVR). We compared the TCD measures of cirrhotic non HE ($n = 30$), cirrhotic HE ($n = 30$) and healthy subjects ($n = 30$). Here, we found that major basal vessel integrity was not compromised because there were no differences among the three groups when the left and right cerebral arteries were evaluated. However, we observed significant differences in PI and BHI between cirrhotic and control subjects and when the compensated status was taken into account, the PI and BHI was significantly increased and decreased, respectively, when decompensated (CTP > 7 and MELD score ≥ 14) patients were compared with compensated and healthy groups. Similarly and more importantly, when HE status was included in the analysis, the results were the same as before, which means that disturbances in CBF is a novel pathophysiological pathway in HE, and opens an new way for treatment and prevention. Patients with decompensated cirrhosis or HE have a higher risk of cerebral hypoperfusion related with microvascular damage and the ability for autoregulation, which is and important feature for systemic blood pressure sudden changes, particularly hypotension, which can promotes HE [84]. These findings were similar to those reported by two separated groups, one located in Turkey, were 50 decompensated group of cirrhotic patients was compared with 50 healthy volunteers using the same TCD approach [85]; while other in China recruited a healthy control group ($n = 40$), a cirrhotic without HE group ($n = 52$), a cirrhotic with MHE group ($n = 21$) and a cirrhotic with OHE group ($n = 19$) [86]. Here, in the first case, the authors analyzed the spectra signal derived from the systolic velocity, diastolic velocity, mean flow velocity (MFV in cm/s), pulsatility, and the resistive indexes (PI = Peak systolic velocity (V_p) – end-diastolic velocity (V_d)/MVF; and RI = $V_p - V_d/V_d$) of intracranial arteries. Patients with cirrhosis had a lower MFV compared to control healthy group, while cirrhotic patients had a higher PI and RI values and a positive correlation exists with the model for end-stage liver disease (MELD) score and the RI values of patients with ascites, which were higher than those without ascites [85]. In the second case, authors found that mean velocity (V_m), V_d, PI, and RI, as well as the serum ammonia levels, were decreased in the group of cirrhotic patients with MHE subject to lactulose treatment, when compared with the placebo group, while a positive correlation was found between ammonia and PI, RI, cognitive test results and V_d; authors propose that cerebral hemodynamics is related with the severity of HE and that lactulose treatment is able to significantly improve this parameter in cirrhotic patients [86].

3. Novel pharmacological findings over HE treatment

Despite being one of the most frequent and best studied associated pathologies of liver dysfunction, HE still represents a bigger challenge to clinicians due to its devastating effects over cognitive functions. Still, there is no clear consensus about its appropriate treatment because of its complex physiology involving inflammatory responses, neurosteroid-like compounds, reactive oxygen species, etc. In addition, there is another layer of complexity represented by the co-infections and organ failure that many patients develop in the course of the pathology. Nowadays, there had been a lot of attempts to circumvent the signs and symptoms of HE, both experimentally and clinically. One example of this is the use of one of the most popular anti-inflammatory drugs used to treat cirrhotic patients, infliximab, which reduces peripheral inflammation, directly impacts over neuroinflammation, and restores the altered neurotransmission and cognitive impairment, as well as the reversal of activation of microglia and astrocyte GABA transporters (GAT1, GAT3). Infliximab also reduces the synthesis and release of pro-inflammatory cytokines, such as TNFα, IL-1β, etc., as demonstrated by Dadsetan et al. in a murine model of HE [87, 88]. These data are still scarce in human subjects, although some advance have been reported. In an initial trial, Sharma and co-workers reported that patients with severe alcohol-associated hepatitis, who received a single dose of infliximab (5 mg/kg IV), have an improvement of the Maddrey's discriminant factor (DF)—useful in the prediction of short-term prognosis—serum TNFα, C reactive protein (CRP), MELD score and total neutrophil count compared with the before-treatment parameters; interestingly, among the patients who survived only 8% had HE at admission, while among those who died, 67% suffer from HE; the authors concluded that HE at admission of the trial, Lille score and delta bilirubin, predicted 2-month mortality and that infliximab should be carefully used to treat alcoholic hepatitis [89]. Besides the use of infliximab, other therapies aimed to reduce the production of ammonia by the intestinal microbiota, especially the coliforms, have been widely reported. Treatment with lactulose (a non-absorbable disaccharide) or non-absorbable antibiotic rifaximin, are two of the most frequent therapies for cirrhotic patients suffering from HE. The metabolic activity of colonic bacteria which produce short-chain organic acids when metabolize lactulose lowering the pH of the gastrointestinal tract, is the main effect of the disaccharide for the removal of nitrogen; the acidic environment also results in the change of ammonia to ammonium (NH_4^+) a non-absorbable form of nitrogen which diminishes the circulating ammonia. Further mechanisms include the laxative effect for removal of nitrogen-containing compounds from the gut. In a concise Cochrane review from last year, 38 clinical trials were evaluated and their findings indicate that non-absorbable disaccharides have beneficial effects when compared with placebo/no intervention on mortality, HE, liver failure, hepatorenal syndrome and variceal bleeding; secondary outcomes such as quality of life, also were favored when non-absorbable disaccharides were administered [90]. Additionally, experimental data indicates that lactulose promotes neuro- and astrogenesis in the hippocampus of rats with HE as well as the reduction of plasma ammonia, the locomotor activity impairment and neuronal hyperactivity in brain areas related with locomotor activity [91]. These data are in accordance with those data indicating that Lactulose do also improved cognitive function in MHE patients, as reviewed by Luo et al. [92]. The non-absorbable antibiotic, rifaximin, is the most common additive therapy along with lactulose to treat cirrhotic patients with HE. In a recent prospective observational study, 60 HE patients were divided into two groups, one receiving rifaximin alone and the other one received rifaximin plus lactulose for 7–15 days until discharge from hospital or death. In this study, the authors found that both groups were effectively improved in their mental scores, although they conclude that the combination of both substances was effective, but not superior to lactulose alone in the treatment of HE [93]. The resolution of overt HE has also been tested using rifaximin in comparison with other antibiotics. A meta-analysis of these trials indicates that rifaximin treatment was more likely to resolve an episode in patients with OHE besides an improvement in secondary prevention of HE [94]. Other treatment regimes devoted to reduce the serum ammonia levels, such as polyethylene glycol (PEG), sodium benzoate, odium phenylacetate, glycerol-phenylbutyrate (GPB), ornithine-phenylacetate (OP), phenyl-acetyl-glutamine (PAGN), and a carbon microsphere adsorbent (AST-120) among others, had been also tested for nitrogen removal (for a concise review see [95]).

On the other hand, it is more common to see the rise of many biological compounds that previously were used to treat distinct pathologies; an example of this is Artesunate, a water-soluble hemisuccinate derivative of the Chinese herb *Artemisia annua*, that has been recommended for its use as an antimalarial drug, but it seems that also have anti-inflammatory properties because its use in cancerous cells inhibits its replication and interferes with the expression of pro-inflammatory genes [96, 97]. Artesunate do also have anti-profibrotic properties as was demonstrated recently by Wang and colleagues. Here, Wang et al. investigate the role of treatment with artesunate in a lung fibrosis rodent model; the authors found that artesunate treatment successfully reverted the expression of pro-fibrotic genes such as transforming growth factor (TGFβ), Smad3, and α-smooth muscle actin (α-SMA) as well as the heat shock protein 47 (HSP47) at the protein level, when compared with control animals [98]; these results are in accordance with those of Wang et al., whose findings in the RLE-6TN cell line indicates that TGFβ and Smad3 are inhibited after artesunate exposure [99]. The effect of artesunate on the CNS of rats with HE has been tested too. Rats administered with artesunate (50 or 100 mg/kg), significantly improved its spatial learning ability in the Morris water maze test, while *in vitro*, cerebellar granule neurons treated with artesunate (100 μM) significantly reduced its glutamate release, as well as the Na^+K^+-ATPase activity, indicating that artesunate has a neuroprotective effect, although the effect over astrocytes was not evaluated in this work [100]. Additional evidence about the effect of artesunate over glial cells is lacking, but this drug has a relevant role in the field of the HE treatment choices. A synthetic drug called GR3027 has been tested *in vivo* in a rat model of HE. This new compound has antagonist properties over the $GABA_A$ receptors when subcutaneously administered and effectively reverses the motor coordination and spatial memory impairment in rats with experimental HE, offering a new way to prevent the ammonia-induced neurological GABA-related damage [101]. These findings are similar to those reported by Turkmen et al. using the UC1011 $GABA_A$ receptor antagonist, who also observed a reduced allopregnanolone effect on the learning test [102].

Although the mechanisms of astrocyte cell swelling are still controversial, some authors propose that the plasma membrane depolarization plays a crucial role, while others suggest that the ionic homeostasis is equally important [103, 104]. In addition, glutamine, manganese, pH changes, and the neurosteroids are also implicated in this process. However, both, *in vivo* and *in vitro* experimental evidence strongly suggests that astrocyte swelling is the primary response to hyperammonemia. One additional factor is the oxidative stress derived from the altered mitochondria. It has been shown that astrocytes exposed to ammonia, results in the activation of the mitochondrial permeability transition pore (MPT), a process related to generation of ROS within the cell. The permeability transition is a sudden increase in the inner mitochondrial membrane to solutes >1.5 kDa and it is known that adenine nucleotides inhibit this process. The MPT is a Ca^{2+}-dependent process that usually culminates in necrosis or apoptosis in hepatocytes; in mammals, cyclophilin D (CyPD) (a conserved cis-trans isomerase) acts as the mitochondrial receptor for cyclosporine A (CsA) (a very well-known immunosuppressive agent). The MTP is a multiprotein complex whose formation is ultimately inhibited by the CyPD/CsA complex. Pre-treatment of astrocytes with CsA completely reverts the cell swelling after treatment with ammonia [25]; in a similar manner, sodium pyruvate, minocycline, magnesium sulfate, and trifluoparazine (TFP), decreased the ammonia-induced MTP-dependent cell swelling, in a significant manner [105]. Other antioxidant compounds have been tested in order to revert the cognitive impairment in HE. For example, the multifunctional soy isoflavone, genistein, has an important activity as an oxygen-derived free radicals scavenger, and as a potent inhibitor of pro-inflammatory cytokines such as IL-4, IL-10, IL-1β, TNFα, etc., as well as the expression of $GABA_A$ and GluR2 receptors in the hippocampus of a rat model of HE, restoring the altered neurotransmission, neuroinflammation and the DNA damage observed in the rat's brain [106, 107]. Further evidence indicates that genistein may inhibit astrocyte swelling by inhibiting the protein tyrosine kinase (PTK) activity and repression of NF-κB-mediated inducible nitric oxide synthase (iNOS)-derived nitric oxide (NO) accumulation [108]. Resveratrol, lipoic acid (LA), and N-acetyl-cysteine (NAC) are important anti-oxidants that can, at least *in vitro*, modulate the expression and activity of the glutamate transporters, increase the glutamate release, reduce the activity of GS and GSH content as well as the ammonia-induced pro-inflammatory response in glial cells [109].

A most recent study, conducted *in vivo*, indicates that TNFα and its receptors, TNFR1 and TNFR2, play major roles in acute ammonia intoxication. In TNFα-deficient or double TNFR1/TNFR2 knock-out mice, ammonia challenge is unable to trigger astrocyte cell swelling, an affect that seems to be related to the expression of the Na^+, K^+, $2Cl^-$ (NKCCl) co-transporter, which is closely related to the NH_4^+ hepatic clearance [110].

L-ornithine and L-aspartate (LOLA) are urea cycle substrates that can lower ammonia levels in cirrhotic patients. The first is a substrate of the ornithine-aminotransferase (OAT) enzyme, which converts ornithine into glutamate or glutamate-semialdehyde, while L-aspartate is converted by the aspartate-aminotransferase into glutamate or oxaloacetate [5]. A complete review about the effect of LOLA in cirrhotic patients has been published and one of the main conclusions was that LOLA is effective in patients with OHE and less beneficial for those having MHE and had no effects on patients with acute liver failure [111, 112].

An intriguing method to treat liver-affected patients is based in Ayurveda. According to Wikipedia, Ayurveda is a system of medicine with roots in India, where medical knowledge is transmitted from gods to sages and then to humans. Ayurveda therapies are based on complex herbal compounds, minerals, and metal substances. In a clinical research paper, Ayurveda was put into practice to treat a case of HE in India. The report indicates that Ayurvedic therapy, consisting on a mix of four substances (*Siddha Makar Dhwaja, Brihat Vata Chintamani Rasa, Phyllanthus niruri* extract and a syrup of "*hepatoprotective herbs*"), was administered to a grade three HE male patient currently receiving "*modern therapies.*" After a 3-day period of treatment, the patient was found more oriented and awake. The hepatic aminotransferases and bilirubin significantly improved after almost 1 month of treatment [113]. This report, according to authors, is interesting enough to begin a new debate in the area of practice of Ayurvedic medicine. The debate is open.

4. Concluding remarks

Hepatic encephalopathy is a very devastating disease associated with liver failure. Besides the detrimental effects over astrocyte and neuron physiology, HE had a direct impact over the quality of life of affected patients. Recent evidence suggests that many pro-inflammatory pathways are related to these pathology and therapeutic interventions are devoted to counteract it. In this chapter, many of the molecular and pathological events related with ammonia and its effects over astrocytes cells had been addressed. Indeed, ammonia is one of the main factors contributing to the pathophysiology of HE, responsible of the astrocyte swelling along with other metabolites such as myoinositol, manganese, etc. (**Figure 4**). Ammonia is a toxic compound mainly produced by the bacteria in the gastrointestinal tract or by metabolism of ammonium-containing substances. In healthy subjects, urea is the final metabolite of ammonium metabolism in the liver, which is then excreted in urine. Hepatic failure is a one of the most common public concerns in western economies and is beginning to become a major problem in the next 10–15 years. Some of the most feasible and easy-to-implement therapies against liver disease is prevention. Public health policies must be strengthened regarding preventive information not only for liver but also to different metabolic-related illness. The stress and inappropriate feeding habits in general population has enormous impact not only in adults, but also in young or even in elementary-school grade childhood. One of the main tasks of public health should be informative and not only the medical practice. If we want to succeed in our struggle against different maladies affecting human beings, we must to begin to turn the sight to the basics of having a proper balanced diet and to make regular physical activity; this actions would improve and prevent any metabolic imbalance in the short to median term. The society has the future in their hands.

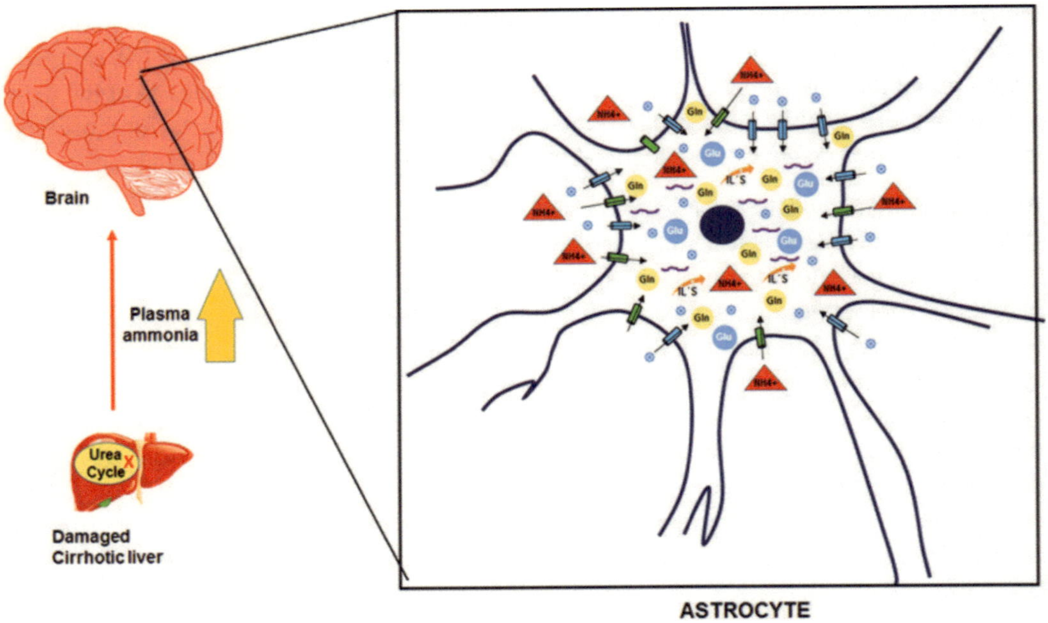

Figure 4. Proposed model of astrocyte dynamic during hyperammonemic conditions. Here, the ammonia (triangle) molecules are increased in the extracellular space and they easily diffuse through the plasma membrane or by means of the NKCC1 channels (dark gray cylinders) once inside ammonia is conjugated with glutamate (**Glu**) by the enzyme glutamine synthase (not shown) to generate glutamine (**Gln**). This is the GGC previously described (see **Figure 1**). In hyperammonemic conditions, such as that resulting from liver cirrhosis, the amount of Gln exceeds the astrocyte capacity to export it. Then, astrocyte increase the expression of the water channel AQP_4 (light gray cylinders) in order to let water (snow flake-like spots) to get inwards. These process is accompanied by the increase of different interleukines like TNFα, IL-1β, IFNγ, and other pro-inflammatory cytokines (**IL´s**), which promotes the mitochondria to become less effective in its metabolic functions, leading the astrocyte to an stressed state. This process generates reactive oxygen species (ROS) and reactive nitrosative species (RNS), as well as oxidized RNAs (**short lines**) that eventually impairs the astrocyte overall function. The whole process generates a condition of low-grade cellular edema and astrocyte cell swelling. See text for additional details: (NH_4^+), (Glu), (Gln), (dark gray cilinders), (light gray cylinders), (snow flake-like spots).

Author details

Carlos Pérez-Monter[1,2]* and Aldo Torre-Delgadillo[1,2]

*Address all correspondence to: carlos.perezm@incmnsz.mx

1 Department of Gastroenterology, National Institute of Medical Sciences, Salvador Zubiran, Tlalpan, Mexico

2 Faculty of Medicine, National University of Mexico, Ciudad de México, Mexico

References

[1] Ferenci P, Herneth A, Steindl P. Newer approaches to therapy of hepatic encephalopathy. Seminars in Liver Disease. 1996;**16**(3):329-338

[2] Mullen KD, Prakash RK. New perspectives in hepatic encephalopathy. Clinics in Liver Disease. 2012;**16**(1):1-5

[3] Nabi E, Bajaj JS. Useful tests for hepatic encephalopathy in clinical practice. Current Gastroenterology Reports. 2014;**16**(1):362

[4] Zhan T, Stremmel W. The diagnosis and treatment of minimal hepatic encephalopathy. Deutsches Arzteblatt international. 2012;**109**(10):180-187

[5] Rose CF. Ammonia-lowering strategies for the treatment of hepatic encephalopathy. Clinical Pharmacology and Therapeutics. 2012;**92**(3):321-331

[6] Wakim-Fleming J. Hepatic encephalopathy: Suspect it early in patients with cirrhosis. Cleveland Clinic Journal of Medicine. 2011;**78**(9):597-605

[7] Khungar V, Poordad F. Hepatic encephalopathy. Clinics in Liver Disease. 2012;**16**(2):301-320

[8] Zielinska M, Popek M, Albrecht J. Roles of changes in active glutamine transport in brain edema development during hepatic encephalopathy: An emerging concept. Neurochemical Research. 2014;**39**(3):599-604

[9] Younossi ZM, Koenig AB, Abdelatif D, Fazel Y, Henry L, Wymer M. Global epidemiology of nonalcoholic fatty liver disease-meta-analytic assessment of prevalence, incidence, and outcomes. Hepatology. 2016;**64**(1):73-84

[10] Morris SM Jr. Regulation of enzymes of the urea cycle and arginine metabolism. Annual Review of Nutrition. 2002;**22**:87-105

[11] Popoli M, Yan Z, McEwen BS, Sanacora G. The stressed synapse: The impact of stress and glucocorticoids on glutamate transmission. Nature Reviews. Neuroscience. 2011;**13**(1):22-37

[12] Hull J, Hindy ME, Kehoe PG, Chalmers K, Love S, Conway ME. Distribution of the branched chain aminotransferase proteins in the human brain and their role in glutamate regulation. Journal of Neurochemistry. 2012;**123**(6):997-1009

[13] Cardona C, Sanchez-Mejias E, Davila JC, Martin-Rufian M, Campos-Sandoval JA, Vitorica J, Alonso FJ, Mates JM, Segura JA, Norenberg MD, et al. Expression of Gls and Gls2 glutaminase isoforms in astrocytes. Glia. 2015;**63**(3):365-382

[14] Hertz L, Song D, Peng L, Chen Y. Multifactorial effects on different types of brain cells contribute to ammonia toxicity. Neurochemical Research. 2017;**42**(3):721-736

[15] Lachmann V, Gorg B, Bidmon HJ, Keitel V, Haussinger D. Precipitants of hepatic encephalopathy induce rapid astrocyte swelling in an oxidative stress dependent manner. Archives of Biochemistry and Biophysics. 2013;**536**(2):143-151

[16] Shawcross D, Jalan R. The pathophysiologic basis of hepatic encephalopathy: Central role for ammonia and inflammation. Cellular and Molecular Life Sciences. 2005;**62**(19-20):2295-2304

[17] Eefsen M, Jelnes P, Schmidt LE, Vainer B, Bisgaard HC, Larsen FS. Brain expression of the water channels aquaporin-1 and -4 in mice with acute liver injury, hyperammonemia and brain edema. Metabolic Brain Disease. 2010;**25**(3):315-323

[18] Blei AT. The pathophysiology of brain edema in acute liver failure. Neurochemistry International. 2005;**47**(1-2):71-77

[19] Wright G, Soper R, Brooks HF, Stadlbauer V, Vairappan B, Davies NA, Andreola F, Hodges S, Moss RF, Davies DC, et al. Role of aquaporin-4 in the development of brain oedema in liver failure. Journal of Hepatology. 2010;**53**(1):91-97

[20] Rama Rao KV, Verkman AS, Curtis KM, Norenberg MD. Aquaporin-4 deletion in mice reduces encephalopathy and brain edema in experimental acute liver failure. Neurobiology of Disease. 2014;**63**:222-228

[21] Rama Rao KV, Chen M, Simard JM, Norenberg MD. Increased aquaporin-4 expression in ammonia-treated cultured astrocytes. Neuroreport. 2003;**14**(18):2379-2382

[22] Arima H, Yamamoto N, Sobue K, Umenishi F, Tada T, Katsuya H, Asai K. Hyperosmolar mannitol simulates expression of aquaporins 4 and 9 through a p38 mitogen-activated protein kinase-dependent pathway in rat astrocytes. The Journal of Biological Chemistry. 2003;**278**(45):44525-44534

[23] Thai TL, Blount MA, Klein JD, Sands JM. Lack of protein kinase C-alpha leads to impaired urine concentrating ability and decreased aquaporin-2 in angiotensin II-induced hypertension. American journal of physiology Renal physiology. 2012;**303**(1):F37-F44

[24] Norenberg MD, Rao KV, Jayakumar AR. Mechanisms of ammonia-induced astrocyte swelling. Metabolic Brain Disease. 2005;**20**(4):303-318

[25] Rama Rao KV, Chen M, Simard JM, Norenberg MD. Suppression of ammonia-induced astrocyte swelling by cyclosporin A. Journal of Neuroscience Research. 2003;**74**(6):891-897

[26] Wright G, Shawcross D, Olde Damink SW, Jalan R. Brain cytokine flux in acute liver failure and its relationship with intracranial hypertension. Metabolic Brain Disease. 2007;**22**(3-4):375-388

[27] Jiang W, Desjardins P, Butterworth RF. Direct evidence for central proinflammatory mechanisms in rats with experimental acute liver failure: Protective effect of hypothermia. Journal of Cerebral Blood Flow and Metabolism. 2009;**29**(5):944-952

[28] Bravo JA, Forsythe P, Chew MV, Escaravage E, Savignac HM, Dinan TG, Bienenstock J, Cryan JF. Ingestion of Lactobacillus strain regulates emotional behavior and central GABA receptor expression in a mouse via the vagus nerve. Proceedings of the National Academy of Sciences of the United States of America. 2011;**108**(38):16050-16055

[29] Klune JR, Dhupar R, Cardinal J, Billiar TR, Tsung A. HMGB1: Endogenous danger signaling. Molecular Medicine. 2008;**14**(7-8):476-484

[30] Yang R, Zou X, Tenhunen J, Tonnessen TI. HMGB1 and extracellular histones significantly contribute to systemic inflammation and multiple organ failure in acute liver failure. Mediators of Inflammation. 2017;**2017**:5928078

[31] Ohnishi M, Monda A, Takemoto R, Fujimoto Y, Sugitani M, Iwamura T, Hiroyasu T, Inoue A. High-mobility group box 1 up-regulates aquaporin 4 expression via microglia-astrocyte interaction. Neurochemistry International. 2014;**75**:32-38

[32] Wen Z, Lei Z, Yao L, Jiang P, Gu T, Ren F, Liu Y, Gou C, Li X, Wen T. Circulating histones are major mediators of systemic inflammation and cellular injury in patients with acute liver failure. Cell Death & Disease. 2016;**7**(9):e2391

[33] Li X, Gou C, Yao L, Lei Z, Gu T, Ren F, Wen T. Patients with HBV-related acute-on-chronic liver failure have increased concentrations of extracellular histones aggravating cellular damage and systemic inflammation. Journal of Viral Hepatitis. 2017;**24**(1):59-67

[34] Allam R, Kumar SV, Darisipudi MN, Anders HJ. Extracellular histones in tissue injury and inflammation. Journal of Molecular Medicine. 2014;**92**(5):465-472

[35] Carson MJ, Thrash JC, Walter B. The cellular response in neuroinflammation: The role of leukocytes, microglia and astrocytes in neuronal death and survival. Clinical Neuroscience Research. 2006;**6**(5):237-245

[36] Butterworth RF. The liver-brain axis in liver failure: Neuroinflammation and encephalopathy. Nature Reviews. Gastroenterology & Hepatology. 2013;**10**(9):522-528

[37] Gorg B, Qvartskhava N, Keitel V, Bidmon HJ, Selbach O, Schliess F, Haussinger D. Ammonia induces RNA oxidation in cultured astrocytes and brain in vivo. Hepatology. 2008;**48**(2):567-579

[38] Gorg B, Karababa A, Shafigullina A, Bidmon HJ, Haussinger D. Ammonia-induced senescence in cultured rat astrocytes and in human cerebral cortex in hepatic encephalopathy. Glia. 2015;**63**(1):37-50

[39] Jordens MS, Keitel V, Karababa A, Zemtsova I, Bronger H, Haussinger D, Gorg B. Multidrug resistance-associated protein 4 expression in ammonia-treated cultured rat astrocytes and cerebral cortex of cirrhotic patients with hepatic encephalopathy. Glia. 2015

[40] Dhiman RK. Gut microbiota and hepatic encephalopathy. Metabolic Brain Disease. 2013;**28**(2):321-326

[41] Gupta A, Dhiman RK, Kumari S, Rana S, Agarwal R, Duseja A, Chawla Y. Role of small intestinal bacterial overgrowth and delayed gastrointestinal transit time in cirrhotic patients with minimal hepatic encephalopathy. Journal of Hepatology. 2010;**53**(5):849-855

[42] Jun DW, Kim KT, Lee OY, Chae JD, Son BK, Kim SH, Jo YJ, Park YS. Association between small intestinal bacterial overgrowth and peripheral bacterial DNA in cirrhotic patients. Digestive Diseases and Sciences. 2010;**55**(5):1465-1471

[43] Henao-Mejia J, Elinav E, Jin C, Hao L, Mehal WZ, Strowig T, Thaiss CA, Kau AL, Eisenbarth SC, Jurczak MJ, et al. Inflammasome-mediated dysbiosis regulates progression of NAFLD and obesity. Nature. 2012;**482**(7384):179-185

[44] Wei X, Yan X, Zou D, Yang Z, Wang X, Liu W, Wang S, Li X, Han J, Huang L, et al. Abnormal fecal microbiota community and functions in patients with hepatitis B liver cirrhosis as revealed by a metagenomic approach. BMC Gastroenterology. 2013;**13**:175

[45] Bajaj JS, Heuman DM, Hylemon PB, Sanyal AJ, White MB, Monteith P, Noble NA, Unser AB, Daita K, Fisher AR, et al. Altered profile of human gut microbiome is associated with cirrhosis and its complications. Journal of Hepatology. 2014;**60**(5):940-947

[46] Bajaj JS, Ridlon JM, Hylemon PB, Thacker LR, Heuman DM, Smith S, Sikaroodi M, Gillevet PM. Linkage of gut microbiome with cognition in hepatic encephalopathy. American Journal of Physiology Gastrointestinal and Liver Physiology. 2012;**302**(1):G168-G175

[47] Preveden T, Scarpellini E, Milic N, Luzza F, Abenavoli L. Gut microbiota changes and chronic hepatitis C virus infection. Expert Review of Gastroenterology & Hepatology. 2017;**11**(9):813-819

[48] Lavoie J, Layrargues GP, Butterworth RF. Increased densities of peripheral-type benzodiazepine receptors in brain autopsy samples from cirrhotic patients with hepatic encephalopathy. Hepatology. 1990;**11**(5):874-878

[49] Ahboucha S, Butterworth RF. The neurosteroid system: Implication in the pathophysiology of hepatic encephalopathy. Neurochemistry International. 2008;**52**(4-5):575-587

[50] Midzak A, Zirkin B, Papadopoulos V. Translocator protein: Pharmacology and steroidogenesis. Biochemical Society Transactions. 2015;**43**(4):572-578

[51] Hazell AS, Desjardins P, Butterworth RF. Chronic exposure of rat primary astrocyte cultures to manganese results in increased binding sites for the 'peripheral-type' benzodiazepine receptor ligand 3H-PK 11195. Neuroscience Letters. 1999;**271**(1):5-8

[52] Cani PD, Everard A, Duparc T. Gut microbiota, enteroendocrine functions and metabolism. Current Opinion in Pharmacology. 2013;**13**(6):935-940

[53] Cummings JH, Pomare EW, Branch WJ, Naylor CP, Macfarlane GT. Short chain fatty acids in human large intestine, portal, hepatic and venous blood. Gut. 1987;**28**(10):1221-1227

[54] Nohr MK, Pedersen MH, Gille A, Egerod KL, Engelstoft MS, Husted AS, Sichlau RM, Grunddal KV, Poulsen SS, Han S, et al. GPR41/FFAR3 and GPR43/FFAR2 as cosensors for short-chain fatty acids in enteroendocrine cells vs FFAR3 in enteric neurons and FFAR2 in enteric leukocytes. Endocrinology. 2013;**154**(10):3552-3564

[55] Foster AC, Kemp JA. Glutamate- and GABA-based CNS therapeutics. Current Opinion in Pharmacology. 2006;**6**(1):7-17

[56] Kinsner A, Pilotto V, Deininger S, Brown GC, Coecke S, Hartung T, Bal-Price A. nflammatory neurodegeneration induced by lipoteichoic acid from *Staphylococcus aureus* is mediated by glia activation, nitrosative and oxidative stress, and caspase activation. Journal of Neurochemistry. 2005;**95**(4):1132-1143

[57] Feinberg AP, Tycko B. The history of cancer epigenetics. Nature Reviews Cancer. 2004;**4**(2):143-153

[58] Qiang M, Rani CS, Ticku MK. Neuron-restrictive silencer factor regulates the N-methyl-D-aspartate receptor 2B subunit gene in basal and ethanol-induced gene expression in fetal cortical neurons. Molecular Pharmacology. 2005;**67**(6):2115-2125

[59] Winter J, Jung S, Keller S, Gregory RI, Diederichs S. Many roads to maturity: MicroRNA biogenesis pathways and their regulation. Nature Cell Biology. 2009;**11**(3):228-234

[60] Mercer TR, Dinger ME, Mattick JS. Long non-coding RNAs: Insights into functions. Nature Reviews Genetics. 2009;**10**(3):155-159

[61] Sepramaniam S, Ying LK, Armugam A, Wintour EM, Jeyaseelan K. MicroRNA-130a represses transcriptional activity of aquaporin 4 M1 promoter. The Journal of Biological Chemistry. 2012;**287**(15):12006-12015

[62] Sepramaniam S, Armugam A, Lim KY, Karolina DS, Swaminathan P, Tan JR, Jeyaseelan K. MicroRNA 320a functions as a novel endogenous modulator of aquaporins 1 and 4 as well as a potential therapeutic target in cerebral ischemia. The Journal of Biological Chemistry. 2010;**285**(38):29223-29230

[63] Oenarto J, Karababa A, Castoldi M, Bidmon HJ, Gorg B, Haussinger D. Ammonia-induced miRNA expression changes in cultured rat astrocytes. Scientific Reports. 2016;**6**:18493

[64] Silva VR, Secolin R, Vemuganti R, Lopes-Cendes I, Hazell AS. Acute liver failure is associated with altered cerebral expression profiles of long non-coding RNAs. Neuroscience Letters. 2017;**656**:58-64

[65] Strange K. Cellular volume homeostasis. Advances in Physiology Education. 2004;**28**(1-4): 155-159

[66] Cordoba J, Gottstein J, Blei AT. Glutamine, myo-inositol, and organic brain osmolytes after portocaval anastomosis in the rat: Implications for ammonia-induced brain edema. Hepatology. 1996;**24**(4):919-923

[67] Liang J, Deng X, Lin ZX, Zhao LC, Zhang XL. Attenuation of portal hypertension by natural taurine in rats with liver cirrhosis. World Journal of Gastroenterology. 2009; **15**(36):4529-4537

[68] Invernizzi P, Setchell KD, Crosignani A, Battezzati PM, Larghi A, O'Connell NC, Podda M. Differences in the metabolism and disposition of ursodeoxycholic acid and of its taurine-conjugated species in patients with primary biliary cirrhosis. Hepatology. 1999;**29**(2):320-327

[69] Swain MS, Bergeron M, Audet R, Blei AT, Butterworth RF. Monitoring of neurotransmitter amino acids by means of an indwelling cisterna magna catheter: A comparison of two rodent models of fulminant liver failure. Hepatology. 1992;**16**(4):1028-1035

[70] Bosman DK, Deutz NE, Maas MA, van Eijk HM, Smit JJ, de Haan JG, Chamuleau RA. Amino acid release from cerebral cortex in experimental acute liver failure, studied by in vivo cerebral cortex microdialysis. Journal of Neurochemistry. 1992;**59**(2):591-599

[71] Swain M, Butterworth RF, Blei AT. Ammonia and related amino acids in the pathogenesis of brain edema in acute ischemic liver failure in rats. Hepatology. 1992;**15**(3):449-453

[72] Hagberg H, Lehmann A, Sandberg M, Nystrom B, Jacobson I, Hamberger A. Ischemia-induced shift of inhibitory and excitatory amino acids from intra- to extracellular compartments. Journal of Cerebral Blood Flow and Metabolism. 1985;**5**(3):413-419

[73] Heins J, Zwingmann C. Organic osmolytes in hyponatremia and ammonia toxicity. Metabolic Brain Disease. 2010;**25**(1):81-89

[74] Pasantes Morales H, Schousboe A. Volume regulation in astrocytes: A role for taurine as an osmoeffector. Journal of Neuroscience Research. 1988;**20**(4):503-509

[75] Hamed SA, Hamed EA, Zakary MM. Oxidative stress and S-100B protein in children with bacterial meningitis. BMC Neurology. 2009;**9**:51

[76] Zenaide PV, Gusmao-Flores D. Biomarkers in septic encephalopathy: A systematic review of clinical studies. Revista Brasileira de Terapia Intensiva. 2013;**25**(1):56-62

[77] Adami C, Sorci G, Blasi E, Agneletti AL, Bistoni F, Donato R. S100B expression in and effects on microglia. Glia. 2001;**33**(2):131-142

[78] Duarte-Rojo A, Ruiz-Margain A, Macias-Rodriguez RU, Cubero FJ, Estradas-Trujillo J, Munoz-Fuentes RM, Torre A. Clinical scenarios for the use of S100beta as a marker of hepatic encephalopathy. World Journal of Gastroenterology. 2016;**22**(17):4397-4402

[79] Saleh A, Kamel L, Ghali A, Ismail A, El Khayat H. Serum levels of astroglial S100-beta and neuron-specific enolase in hepatic encephalopathy patients. Eastern Mediterranean Health Journal = La revue de sante de la Mediterranee orientale = al-Majallah al-sihhiyah li-sharq al-mutawassit. 2007;**13**(5):1114-1123

[80] Wiltfang J, Nolte W, Otto M, Wildberg J, Bahn E, Figulla HR, Pralle L, Hartmann H, Ruther E, Ramadori G. Elevated serum levels of astroglial S100beta in patients with liver cirrhosis indicate early and subclinical portal-systemic encephalopathy. Metabolic Brain Disease. 1999;**14**(4):239-251

[81] Cordoba J, Sanpedro F, Alonso J, Rovira A. 1H magnetic resonance in the study of hepatic encephalopathy in humans. Metabolic Brain Disease. 2002;**17**(4):415-429

[82] Feruglio FS, Migheli B, Campus S, Pandol Fo G, Bert G, Pupita F. Hemodynamic and metabolic aspects of the cerebral circulation in hepatic cirrhosis. Minerva Cardioangiologica. 1961;**9**:429-431

[83] Bianchi Porro G, Maiolo AT, Della Porta P. Cerebral blood flow and metabolism in hepatic cirrhosis before and after portacaval shunt operation. Gut. 1969;**10**(11):894-897

[84] Macias-Rodriguez RU, Duarte-Rojo A, Cantu-Brito C, Sauerbruch T, Ruiz-Margain A, Trebicka J, Green-Gomez M, Diaz Ramirez JB, Sierra Beltran M, Uribe-Esquivel M, et al. Cerebral haemodynamics in cirrhotic patients with hepatic encephalopathy. Liver International. 2015;**35**(2):344-352

[85] Oncel C, Yilmaz M. Cerebral hemodynamics in patients with cirrhosis. The Turkish Journal of Gastroenterology: The Official Journal of Turkish Society of Gastroenterology. 2016;**27**(3):264-267

[86] Zhou Y, Dong Q, Zhang R, Zhou S, Li L, Cheng K, Kong R, Yu Q, Xu S, Li J, et al. Cerebral hemodynamics and cognitive function in cirrhotic patients with hepatic encephalopathy. Gastroenterology Research and Practice. 2016;**2016**:8485032

[87] Dadsetan S, Balzano T, Forteza J, Agusti A, Cabrera-Pastor A, Taoro-Gonzalez L, Hernandez-Rabaza V, Gomez-Gimenez B, ElMlili N, Llansola M, et al. Infliximab reduces peripheral inflammation, neuroinflammation, and extracellular GABA in the cerebellum and improves learning and motor coordination in rats with hepatic encephalopathy. Journal of Neuroinflammation. 2016;**13**(1):245

[88] Dadsetan S, Balzano T, Forteza J, Cabrera-Pastor A, Taoro-Gonzalez L, Hernandez-Rabaza V, Gil-Perotin S, Cubas-Nunez L, Garcia-Verdugo JM, Agusti A, et al. Reducing peripheral inflammation with infliximab reduces neuroinflammation and improves cognition in rats with hepatic encephalopathy. Frontiers in Molecular Neuroscience. 2016;**9**:106

[89] Sharma P, Kumar A, Sharma BC, Sarin SK. Infliximab monotherapy for severe alcoholic hepatitis and predictors of survival: An open label trial. Journal of Hepatology. 2009;**50**(3):584-591

[90] Gluud LL, Vilstrup H, Morgan MY. Non-absorbable disaccharides versus placebo/no intervention and lactulose versus lactitol for the prevention and treatment of hepatic encephalopathy in people with cirrhosis. The Cochrane Database of Systematic Reviews. 2016;**4**:CD003044

[91] Yang N, Liu H, Jiang Y, Zheng J, Li DM, Ji C, Liu YY, Zuo PP. Lactulose enhances neuroplasticity to improve cognitive function in early hepatic encephalopathy. Neural Regeneration Research. 2015;**10**(9):1457-1462

[92] Luo M, Li L, Lu CZ, Cao WK. Clinical efficacy and safety of lactulose for minimal hepatic encephalopathy: A meta-analysis. European Journal of Gastroenterology & Hepatology. 2011;**23**(12):1250-1257

[93] Ahire K, Sonawale A. Comparison of Rifaximin plus lactulose with the lactulose alone for the treatment of hepatic encephalopathy. The Journal of the Association of Physicians of India. 2017;**65**(8):42-46

[94] Kimer N, Krag A, Moller S, Bendtsen F, Gluud LL. Systematic review with meta-analysis: The effects of rifaximin in hepatic encephalopathy. Alimentary Pharmacology & Therapeutics. 2014;**40**(2):123-132

[95] Rahimi RS, Rockey DC. Novel ammonia-lowering agents for hepatic encephalopathy. Clinics in Liver Disease. 2015;**19**(3):539-549

[96] Karpel-Massler G, Westhoff MA, Kast RE, Dwucet A, Nonnenmacher L, Wirtz CR, Debatin KM, Halatsch ME. Artesunate enhances the antiproliferative effect of temozolomide on U87MG and A172 glioblastoma cell lines. Anti-Cancer Agents in Medicinal Chemistry. 2014;**14**(2):313-318

[97] Xu H, He Y, Yang X, Liang L, Zhan Z, Ye Y, Yang X, Lian F, Sun L. Anti-malarial agent artesunate inhibits TNF-alpha-induced production of proinflammatory cytokines via inhibition of NF-kappaB and PI3 kinase/Akt signal pathway in human rheumatoid arthritis fibroblast-like synoviocytes. Rheumatology. 2007;**46**(6):920-926

[98] Wang C, Xuan X, Yao W, Huang G, Jin J. Anti-profibrotic effects of artesunate on bleomycin-induced pulmonary fibrosis in Sprague Dawley rats. Molecular Medicine Reports. 2015;**12**(1):1291-1297

[99] Wang CM, Chen J, Jiang M, Xuan XP, Li HX. Relationship between artesunate influence on the process of TGF-beta1 induced alveolar epithelial cells transform into mesenchymal cells and on idiopathic pulmonary fibrosis. Yao xue xue bao = Acta pharmaceutica Sinica. 2014;**49**(1):142-147

[100] Wu YB, Zhang L, Li WT, Yang Y, Zhao JM. Artesunate restores spatial learning of rats with hepatic encephalopathy by inhibiting ammonia-induced oxidative damage in neurons and dysfunction of glutamate signaling in astroglial cells. Biomedicine & Pharmacotherapy = Biomedecine & Pharmacotherapie. 2016;**84**:972-978

[101] Johansson M, Agusti A, Llansola M, Montoliu C, Stromberg J, Malinina E, Ragagnin G, Doverskog M, Backstrom T, Felipo V. GR3027 antagonizes GABAA receptor-potentiating neurosteroids and restores spatial learning and motor coordination in rats with chronic

hyperammonemia and hepatic encephalopathy. American Journal of Physiology Gastrointestinal and Liver Physiology. 2015;**309**(5):G400-G409

[102] Turkmen S, Lundgren P, Birzniece V, Zingmark E, Backstrom T, Johansson IM. 3beta-20beta-dihydroxy-5alpha-pregnane (UC1011) antagonism of the GABA potentiation and the learning impairment induced in rats by allopregnanolone. The European Journal of Neuroscience. 2004;**20**(6):1604-1612

[103] Allert N, Koller H, Siebler M. Ammonia-induced depolarization of cultured rat cortical astrocytes. Brain Research. 1998;**782**(1-2):261-270

[104] Norenberg MD. Astrocytes and ammonia in hepatic encephalopathy. In: Vellis JD, editor. Neuroglia in the Aging Brain. 1st ed. Vol. XIII. New York: Springer Science + Business Media, Humana Press; 2002. p. 513

[105] Reddy PV, Rama Rao KV, Norenberg MD. Inhibitors of the mitochondrial permeability transition reduce ammonia-induced cell swelling in cultured astrocytes. Journal of Neuroscience Research. 2009;**87**(12):2677-2685

[106] Ganai AA, Husain M. Genistein alleviates neuroinflammation and restores cognitive function in rat model of hepatic encephalopathy: Underlying mechanisms. Molecular Neurobiology. 2017

[107] Ganai AA, Husain M. Genistein attenuates D-GalN induced liver fibrosis/chronic liver damage in rats by blocking the TGF-beta/Smad signaling pathways. Chemico-Biological Interactions. 2017;**261**:80-85

[108] Dai H, Jia G, Wang W, Liang C, Han S, Chu M, Mei X. Genistein inhibited ammonia induced astrocyte swelling by inhibiting NF-kappaB activation-mediated nitric oxide formation. Metabolic Brain Disease. 2017;**32**(3):841-848

[109] Bobermin LD, Hansel G, Scherer EB, Wyse AT, Souza DO, Quincozes-Santos A, Goncalves CA. Ammonia impairs glutamatergic communication in astroglial cells: Protective role of resveratrol. Toxicology In Vitro: An International Journal Published in Association with BIBRA. 2015;**29**(8):2022-2029

[110] Pozdeev VI, Lang E, Gorg B, Bidmon HJ, Shinde PV, Kircheis G, Herebian D, Pfeffer K, Lang F, Haussinger D, et al. TNFalpha induced up-regulation of Na^+, K^+, $2Cl^-$ cotransporter NKCC1 in hepatic ammonia clearance and cerebral ammonia toxicity. Scientific Reports. 2017;**7**(1):7938

[111] Acharya SK, Bhatia V, Sreenivas V, Khanal S, Panda SK. Efficacy of L-ornithine L-aspartate in acute liver failure: A double-blind, randomized, placebo-controlled study. Gastroenterology. 2009;**136**(7):2159-2168

[112] Jiang Q, Jiang XH, Zheng MH, Chen YP. L-ornithine-l-aspartate in the management of hepatic encephalopathy: A meta-analysis. Journal of Gastroenterology and Hepatology. 2009;**24**(1):9-14

[113] Rastogi S, Srivastav PS. Ayurveda in critical care: Illustrating Ayurvedic intervention in a case of hepatic encephalopathy. Ayu. 2011;**32**(3):345-348